Living Longer and Stronger with CBD

—∽—

James H. Collins, PhD

Copyright © 2021 James H. Collins, PhD

All rights reserved. This book or any portion thereof may not be reproduced or used in any manner whatsoever without the express written permission of the publisher except for the use of brief quotations in a book review.

ISBN: 978-0-578-91067-3 (paperback)

Library of Congress Control Number: 2021907737

Contents

Medical Disclaimer		vii
Foreword		ix
1	Cannabidiol (CBD)—An Introduction	1
2	The Very Long and Fascinating History of Cannabis as Medicine	15
3	The Endocannabinoid System and Phytocannabinoids Explained	39
4	The Connection Between CBD and the Aging Process	51
5	CBD and Arthritis, Cancer, Cardiovascular Disease, Diabetes, Endocrine Disorders, Fibromyalgia, and Gastrointestinal Disorders	59
6	CBD and Headaches and Migraines, Lupus, Menopause, Pain, Respiratory Disorders, Seizures and Epilepsy, and Skin Conditions	101
7	CBD and Addiction, Anxiety, Depression, and Eating Disorders	139
8	CBD and Obsessive-Compulsive Disorder, Post-Traumatic Stress Disorder, Schizophrenia, and Late-Onset Schizophrenia	181
9	CBD and Sleep Disorders	209
10	CBD and Neurodegenerative Disorders	219
11	CBD and End-of-Life Care	263
12	CBD for Your Pets	271
13	How to Buy and Use CBD	279
14	The Future of CBD and Other Cannabinoids	289
Acknowledgments		301
About the Author		303
References		305

Medical Disclaimer

The information in this book is not medical advice, and the author in no way prescribes the use of cannabidiol for any physical, emotional, or medical condition. Use of this book is for information and education only and in no way should be substituted for medical care or advice from your physician or other health care professional. No information in this book is meant to serve as a treatment method for any disease, disorder, or ailment. It is intended to provide information and choices concerning nutritional supplements. The author's intent is to provide a source of general information to assist you in maximizing your quality of physical, mental, and emotional well-being by providing science-based and practical information. The author assumes no responsibility for action taken based on information in this book. Always consult your physician or other health care provider before taking new supplements, particularly in you are pregnant, nursing, or elderly, or if you have chronic health conditions. Using any information in this book is completely at the reader's discretion and risk. The author assumes no responsibility in using any information from this book. There are no guarantees of well-being made by the author.

Foreword

You are about to read a book that brings clarity to a newly recognized system of the body, which has obviously been in existence for thousands of years. As will be explained below, the discovery came about while exploring how the components of the marijuana plant function within us. One of those components, CBD, has become popularized due to its healing potential. Dr. Collins explains in a factual and clear manner the potential of CBD as both a general support for our health, as well as a treatment adjunct for several clinical disorders.

How is it possible that CBD could have properties that are anti-inflammatory, antioxidant, anti-anxiety, antipsychotic, antispasmodic, and analgesic? These properties combat the major mechanisms that contribute to both the aging process and the development of a variety of disorders and diseases, which are discussed thoroughly in this book. In order to explain this mystery, I wish to share an intriguing story with you.

In the year 2002, while researching the first edition of my textbook, we interviewed Dr. Raphael Mechoulam, a professor at Hebrew University in Jerusalem. In the 1970s, he elucidated the structure of the major chemical that possesses psychoactive properties (tetrahydrocannabinol, or THC) in the marijuana plant. Dr. William Devane discovered and characterized the cellular receptor for THC (the discovery was published in 1988). A curious scientist will reason that if there is a receptor in the body for a plant or drug, shouldn't there be a chemical or hormone that the body produces that will also fit into the receptor? During Dr. Devane's contemplation and meditation, he predicted that the molecule would have the structure of an amide and named the neuropeptide "anandamide (the amide of bliss)." He then contacted Dr. Mechoulam and traveled from his lab at St. Louis University Medical School to Israel. The research team in Israel, working along with Dr. Devane, discovered the existence of anandamide in pig brain tissue, and their findings were published in the journal *Science* in 1992—hence the birth of the discovery of the endocannabinoid system. Anandamide and an additional neuropeptide have been found to be present in the human brain as well.

As an endocrinologist, I have spent my career feeling comfortable with a "system" that interacts with all other systems in order to promote health and well-being. The THC receptor is now referred to as the cannabinoid receptor, of which there are two, with a potential new one on the horizon. CBD interacts with these receptors, as does our own anandamide. It is my contention that the endocannabinoid system is a signaling system that enhances the function of the endocrine system in order to "fine tune" healthy function in all body systems. In disease states, in the presence of emotional or physical stress, or due to the aging process, the production of our own cannabinoids (endocannabinoids) becomes deficient. CBD therefore comes to the rescue and makes up for the deficiency, thus having a major positive impact on virtually all body systems.

The discovery of the endocannabinoid system is a remarkable advance in medical science that, although newly discovered, has been with us since we began to stand erect as Homo sapiens. It is exciting to speculate the rich information regarding this system that is yet to be discovered. University research centers have been formed to study this system and the use of cannabis and its derivatives at the University of California, University of Colorado, and Thomas Jefferson University in Philadelphia, as well as other institutions.

Please allow me to render a bit of personal advice. If you take medications or have a specific medical condition, please inform your physician that you plan to take CBD. As you improve, your medications may need to be altered by your doctor (never by yourself). I also suggest that you inform your physician of this excellent book, as it contains multiple scientific references to substantiate the information provided by Dr. Collins.

Enjoy, learn, and feel well!

—Len Wisneski, MD, FACP
Author, *The Scientific Basis of Integrative Health*
Georgetown University, George Washington University, University of Colorado
Member, the International Cannabinoid Research Society
Member, the Society of Cannabis Clinicians

1

Cannabidiol (CBD)— An Introduction

I don't know where I'm going from here, but I promise it won't be boring.
—David Bowie

Introduction

You are the reason I wrote this book—a book solely focused on a new and very exiting molecule from the hemp plant. It is popularly referred to as CBD, which is short for *cannabidiol*, and it's the second most abundant component of the cannabis plant after THC. You've probably heard about CBD or know someone who is using it, and that's the reason you're reading this book. Perhaps you've read about the many health benefits of this miraculous molecule and want to learn more about how it can positively impact your health and emotional well-being. While there is a lot of information out there, particularly on the internet, some of it can be misleading, unverifiable, and downright wrong. It's important to understand that, regardless of what you may learn from other sources, all CBD products are not created equal. With so much information and so many products to choose from, it can be challenging to find the truth, not to mention to determine the best products to use for your own personal health and wellness. Since we are all aging, it would be nice to pick up a book written by a gerontologist who has researched this topic, scanned through hundreds of medical articles, and read stacks of books, one who presents accurate, scientifically derived, and no-nonsense information about CBD, aging, and quality of life. Well, that's exactly what you're holding in your hands right now! And as I began this paragraph, your physical and mental health are the reasons I wrote this book.

Just like David Bowie said, I'm not sure where we're going with CBD and health, but I'm pretty sure it's going to be interesting and exciting. I'd like to introduce a few key concepts that will help you navigate the rest of the book so that reading it makes sense to you. Since CBD is in the title of the book, I'd like to spend a little time describing what it is and how it works. I'd also like to address what THC is and differentiate it from CBD, because there still lies some confusion about the two, but they are completely different substances. Concepts including cannabinoids, phytocannabinoids, and the endocannabinoid system will also be introduced.

Cannabidiol (CBD)

CBD, or cannabidiol, has received a tidal wave of attention over the past few years—and for some very good reasons. Although we will get more specific later about what CBD is, it's good to know that CBD is a cannabinoid or more precisely, a *phytocannabinoid*, which naturally occurs in both marijuana and hemp plants.

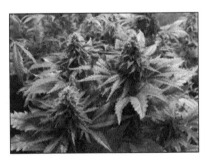 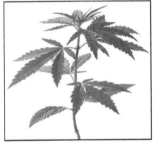

*Marijuana or cannabis plants pictured on the left and
a single hemp plant on the right*

As you can quickly see, the marijuana plants on the left show broader leaves and tight bud nuggets with tiny hairs and shiny crystals. They are also shorter and fatter than the hemp plant shown on the right, which is taller and has skinnier and fewer leaves or branches below the top of the plant.

CBD is the most important cannabinoid from these plants due to its potential physical and emotional health benefits. CBD is only one of over one hundred currently identified cannabinoids, and researchers are consistently on the hunt for more of them. Below is a graphic illustration of the chemical structure of CBD and that of THC.

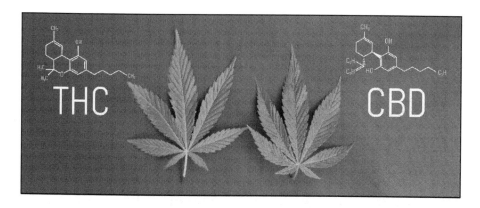

Molecular structures of THC and CBD molecules

You may be more familiar with the most abundant molecule from cannabis plants known as THC, or *tetrahydrocannabinol*. This is the potent active ingredient in marijuana that produces either a mental or a bodily "high." It is important to know the difference between CBD and THC. They are not the same. THC generally is found in marijuana, which is grown specifically because of its higher THC content, whereas CBD comes mainly from hemp, which contains trace amounts or less of THC, roughly around 0.3% or less. Most of the research on cannabis and health has historically focused on THC, and it is only recently that CBD has gained attention for its potential to reduce the symptoms of numerous illnesses without any high. CBD has become a supplement that is safe, has few to no unpleasant side effects, and according to a number of scientific studies, has anti-inflammatory, antioxidant, anti-anxiety, antipsychotic, antispasmodic, and analgesic effects. There are a number of dietary nutrients in CBD oil, including protein; fiber; essential fatty acids; vitamins A, C, D, E, B1, B2, B3, and B6; iron; beta carotene; zinc; potassium; calcium; selenium; phosphorus; manganese; magnesium; omega-3 and omega-6; flavonoids; and terpenes. It almost seems too good to be true, but there is a lot of science behind these claims. This is where the *endocannabinoid system* comes in, and although I will cover this in greater detail later in the book, it is good to know what it is and how it works.

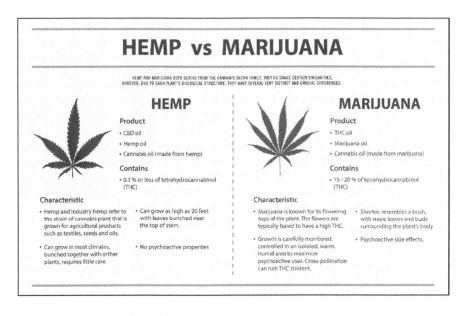

Some differences between hemp and marijuana

Cannabidiol (CBD) is a naturally occurring cannabinoid or chemical compound found in certain strains of the cannabis plant. CBD comes from hemp oil and is further extracted and refined to produce higher quantities of it, while minimizing or removing other cannabinoids like THC and various other terpenes (substances that provide color and aroma). It is one of numerous compounds and happens to be the second most abundant, right after THC, or tetrahydrocannabinol. CBD is also known as a phytocannabinoid, which simply means a plant-based cannabinoid. THC is also a phytocannabinoid, and while many people may associate the two, they are completely different.

> *Marijuana has a long and stigmatized history in the United States. Fortunately, more and more people are now associating it with health and wellness benefits. CBD does not carry the same stigma and is generally viewed as a safer alternative for everyday physical and emotional health issues.*

While THC can make the user "high," CBD does not and is therefore considered very valuable for research and practical everyday use. Cannabidiol actually reduces the psychoactive or euphoric effects of THC. Experts agree that CBD has a far greater impact on health than THC. Once such expert is Dr. Gregory L. Smith,[1] who reports that over 80% of the health benefits from cannabis actually come from CBD; we'll examine some of them later in this chapter.

CBD is the most prevalent on the flowers or buds of the plant but is also found to a lesser degree in the stalk and stems. Although the exact number of cannabinoids found in the cannabis plant are not fully known, experts believe that CBD is only one of over one hundred cannabinoids. Others, including CBG (cannabigerol), CBC (cannabichromene), and CBN (cannabinol), are also gaining more attention in research as having potential health benefits. THC, CBD, and CBG are the three main cannabinoids found in the greatest quantity in the plant.

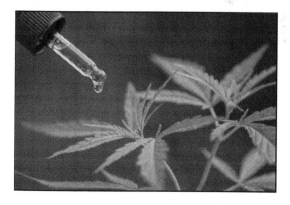

Typical CBD oil dropper

CBD has certainly grown in popularity and, after the signing of the 2018 Farm Bill, is legal in every state, as long as it is derived from plants containing

0.3% THC or less. There are medicinal hemp plants that contain zero percent THC, and most people would find this an attractive feature. The 2018 Farm Bill changed the classification of hemp and related compounds from Schedule I substances to nutritional supplements. This, too, eases the consumer's mind while building confidence in trying CBD for the first time. You're not doing anything illegal! It is simply a new food supplement that is safe and legal and has many promising health and research applications. Now you just need to learn about them.

> *The Ancient Egyptians used cannabis to treat inflammation, sore eyes, cataacts, and glaucoma. Even Cleopatra used hemp seed oil as a health and beauty product.*

Scientists used to believe that CBD was a precursor to the formation of THC in the cannabis plant. Since THC was a controlled substance, they treated CBD the same way. However, they were wrong. As a result, CBD was ignored as a viable molecule to be researched for its medical benefits, while THC became the main star because it was assumed to be the key active ingredient in cannabis. CBD is completely unrelated to the chemical chain that results in THC, and while they do share some characteristics, they also show differences at the molecular level.

After many years of minimal to no research, there are now thousands of studies on the physical and emotional health benefits of CBD, THC, and other cannabinoids. This is a very interesting time because these cannabinoids have become a major part of medicine for some medical and health care practitioners (i.e., chiropractors) and will likely become more mainstream in the health and wellness industry in the near future. It makes sense that something natural like cannabis could have so many benefits for the body. And as we will see, people have used it throughout history to treat a number of illnesses and diseases.

The Differences between Hemp and Marijuana

This is probably a good time to fully distinguish the two substances even more, because many people remain confused about the differences between hemp and marijuana, especially when you throw the word "cannabis" into the discussion. Hemp and marijuana are actually two distinct varieties of the cannabis plant. There are only three types of cannabis plants: cannabis sativa, cannabis indica, and cannabis ruderalis. These grow on every continent except Antarctica.

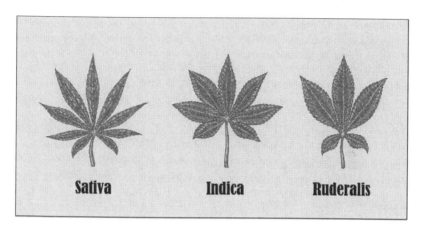

Illustration of various types of leaves per cannabis plant

Cannabis sativa is a plant that grows tall and thin with long, thin leaves. If it contains 0.3% THC by weight or less, it is considered hemp, and if it contains more THC, it is marijuana. Hemp has been used for nutritional and health benefits and industrial materials, while marijuana has been used for both medical and recreational purposes. Cannabis indica, on the other hand, is a short and rounder plant producing short wide leaves. Cannabis ruderalis isn't a medically significant plant.

Generally speaking, sativa plants have less THC and more CBD, while indica has the opposite. After years of research, farming, and cross-breeding, there are now hundreds of hybrid strains of cannabis that contain characteristics of both sativa and indica. It is important to note that CBD and THC have no odor, so the only real way to know how much of either substance is in the plant is through laboratory testing. The aroma of the plants actually come from their terpenes. When you purchase a CBD product, make sure it has been independently lab tested. Look up the "certificate of analysis" on the company's website. It is also good to know that CBD has a far broader impact on health and wellness than THC.

Who Is Using CBD, and Why?

A very recent and interesting article by Corroon and Phillips provides a cross-sectional snapshot of cannabidiol (CBD) users.[2] They report that almost 62% of participants in their study use CBD for very specific medical conditions, including pain (chronic pain, arthritis, and joint pain), anxiety, depression, and sleep disorders. Around 36% of respondents said that CBD treats their conditions "very well by itself." Only 4.3% reported that CBD did not treat their symptoms effectively. Women used CBD to treat specific conditions more than men. The participants also used CBD for other health conditions, including headaches, PTSD, nausea, cancer, allergies, asthma, epilepsy or seizure disorders, multiple sclerosis, COPD and other lung conditions, Parkinson's disease, Alzheimer's disease, and others.

Respondents reported various ways of using CBD. The majority used CBD oils and applied them sublingually, or under the tongue. This is an effective way to get CBD into your bloodstream, as the sublingual vein under the tongue acts like a sponge and gets the supplement into your system quickly. The second most common way of using CBD was by "vaping" it or using a smokeless device that produces a steam so it is inhaled into the lungs. Other methods used include pills or capsules, liquids, smoking devices, edibles, and topical products.

The article closes by reporting that CBD seems to be taken for specific medical conditions instead of preventive reasons. The most common condition cited was pain: "In preclinical studies, CBD-based analgesia is associated with potent immune-modulatory, anti-inflammatory, and antioxidant activity." Some respondents also reported that they take CBD for both anxiety and depression. Over 74% stated they take it daily or more than daily. Around 50% report using CBD for more than a year, and a little over 10% report taking it for over five years.

Note about Vaping

Although vaping has become somewhat popular, is not recommended and is associated with many health risks.

In conclusion, the majority of respondents reported that CBD was effective in treating their condition(s), and without any serious side effects. These findings, combined with thousands of research papers, should encourage more work on the potential benefits of CBD on a number of disorders, including chronic pain, anxiety and depression, sleep disorders, Alzheimer's disease, multiple sclerosis, and many other conditions.

CBD and Health

One of the reasons I wrote this book and continue to research the potential physical and emotional health benefits of CBD is because the list of conditions and symptoms impacted by it continues to grow, and more compelling research-based evidence is published monthly. When my interest in medical marijuana and CBD began several years ago, it was clear that CBD had a number of beneficial pharmacological effects. It has anti-inflammatory, analgesic, antioxidant, anxiolytic (anti-anxiety), antiemetic (antinausea and vomiting), and neuroprotective properties. Some experts believe that CBD is such a powerful antioxidant that it is more effective than both vitamins C and E as a neuroprotective antioxidant. Some studies report that it can even help with skin problems like acne and eczema. To think that a naturally occurring substance in hemp could be so effective is quite impressive.

According to recent research findings, CBD given at higher doses can be effective in treating more serious disorders like schizophrenia, dementia, and diabetes. Numerous studies show CBD's positive impact on neurodegenerative disorders like Alzheimer's disease, Parkinson's disease, Huntington's disease, multiple sclerosis, and amyotrophic lateral sclerosis (ALS). Studies also continue to show the potential for CBD to help alleviate pain associated with conditions including arthritis, sports injuries, neuropathy, and cancer. It may also benefit people who have seizure disorders, epilepsy, fibromyalgia, glaucoma, and cardiovascular conditions.

Various psychological conditions may also be improved through the use of CBD, including more serious forms of depression, anxiety, post-traumatic stress disorder (PTSD), obsessive-compulsive disorder (OCD), addiction, as well as everyday stress and strain. It seems that CBD is almost too good to be true, and I began to fear that it was just another flash in the pan, or a fad that would prove to be modern-day snake oil. I had to ask myself, "Is it possible for thousands of research studies to be wrong?" The answer: Not a chance.

Dr. Michael Moskowitz, in his book *Medical Cannabis: A Guide for Patients, Practitioners, and Caregivers*, provides a graphic example of health benefits of CBD based on a review of the medical literature.[3] In this illustration he demonstrates that CBD can be an active agent to treat the following:

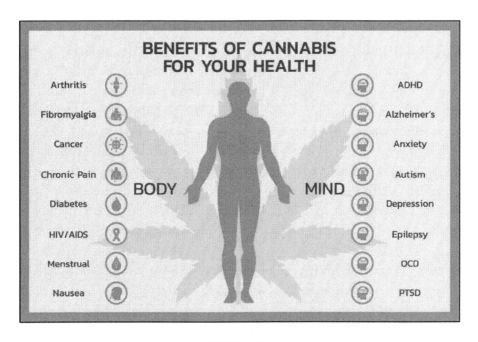

CBD benefits

You can see why I began to doubt the effects of CBD. But after doing my own research into this little-known substance, I am now a full believer and have seen positive results on the health and wellness of both family and friends. As a gerontologist, my next logical question was, "OK, CBD works. But is it safe?" Let's take a look at what I discovered.

Is CBD Safe?
Researchers have reviewed hundreds of studies and have concluded that CBD is a valid treatment option for an extraordinary range of symptoms and

conditions, and that it's both effective and safe. Physicians are now looking into CBD for its medical applications and are doing so for many reasons. CBD has almost no side effects whatsoever, there is little to no risk of addiction, and there is virtually no risk of overdosing on it. When you compare these benefits to the potentially serious and sometimes deadly side effects of many prescription drugs, including opioids, CBD seems to be the better alternative. There is also research indicating that CBD can be taken with many prescription medications. But as always, before taking any supplement or new product, ask your physician to be on the safe side. Remember, neither is medicine "one size fits all," nor is the prescribing dose.

The World Health Organization (WHO) released a report on cannabidiol in 2018 remarking on its safety.[4] It concludes that CBD has no abuse or dependency potential. It is generally well tolerated by most people and has a good safety profile. The report closes by stressing that no evidence has been found of recreational use of CBD or any public health-related issues connected to the use of CBD. In other words, people don't abuse it because it doesn't make anyone high. There would be no reason to use it "recreationally." The majority of people use it for specific health or emotional problems or as a preventive nutritional supplement for enhancing physical, emotional, mental, and even neurological health.

Summary

Although research in this area is considered to be in its infancy, researchers, physicians, and other experts are looking into the very real potential this cannabinoid has for numerous health conditions as well as general wellness. Almost every finding to date has been remarkably positive, and research has yet to find any negative or dangerous side effects. It can, for some people, induce a sense of relaxation and soothe the body without producing euphoria.

There is little to no concern about addiction, dependency, abuse, overdose, or development of problems from taking CBD. It can be considered an adjunct supplement to be taken with other medications. Perhaps one day, CBD will be considered a true preventive medicine that can delay or prevent a wide range of physiological and mental disorders.

I want this book to be enjoyable, informative, and readable. Some of the content will be a bit technical at times and based on research. Other parts of the book will be more anecdotal and casual. Either way, I will try my best to give you as much science-based information on CBD and health, emotional, mental, and neurodegenerative conditions as they pertain to aging as I can. My goal is to make the book both informative and practical, so that you walk away with a real understanding of CBD and how it might benefit you and your family, friends, and colleagues. Here is an outline of the chapters.

Chapter 1, "Cannabidiol (CBD)—An Introduction," provides an overview of cannabidiol, or CBD, and the rise of its popularity. It also examines the differences between hemp and marijuana, who is using CBD and why, and how safe CBD is reported to be. The chapter then provides a brief look at CBD and health.

Chapter 2, "The Very Long and Fascinating History of Cannabis as Medicine," dives into the history of cannabis and how it was used as medicine in ancient China, India, Egypt, and Greece. It also provides a snapshot at more recent history in the modern world. It examines Mexico's role in bringing cannabis to the United States and the laws and politics that made it illegal. The chapter ends with California's legalization of marijuana and the 2018 Farm Bill.

Chapter 3, "The Endocannabinoid System and Phytocannabinoids Explained," gets a little technical, and my focus is to explain what the endocannabinoid system is, when it was discovered, and what it does in the body and brain. By understanding the endocannabinoid system, you will have a better grasp on how and why CBD works. It explains what cannabinoid receptors are (CB1 and CB2). I also explain what phytocannabinoids are and how they work within the endocannabinoid system.

Chapter 4, "The Connection between CBD and the Aging Process," explains how CBD may be beneficial for aging well. It provides a brief overview of the study of aging, how aging has changed over the past one hundred years, and the leading causes of death in the United States. Longevity and healthy aging are discussed, and a section on older adults using CBD as an anti-aging supplement is presented.

Chapter 5, "CBD and Arthritis, Cancer, Cardiovascular Disease, Diabetes, Endocrine Disorders, Fibromyalgia, and Gastrointestinal Disorders," presents research findings from medical and academic articles and books, written mainly by physicians, on the use of CBD and health outcomes. This chapter includes an overview of each condition, traditional treatments for them, and research findings on how CBD is effective in reducing negative symptoms of these disorders.

Chapter 6, "CBD and Headaches and Migraines, Lupus, Menopause, Pain, Respiratory Disorders, Seizures and Epilepsy, and Skin Conditions," provides a snapshot of each condition, current treatment options, and an overview of research findings on how CBD has successfully improved symptoms of these health issues.

Chapter 7, "CBD and Addiction, Anxiety, Depression, and Eating Disorders," gives the reader an introduction to each disorder and the use of psychological therapy, self-care, and psychiatric medications as well as research findings on the effectiveness of CBD in treating each emotional health condition.

Chapter 8, "CBD and Obsessive-Compulsive Disorder (OCD), Post-Traumatic Stress Disorder (PTSD), and Schizophrenia and Life-Onset Schizophrenia," provides an overview of each diagnosis and reviews how self-help methods, psychological therapy, and psychiatric medications are used to treat each disorder. The chapter also gives the reader a snapshot of recent research on CBD and its success in helping improve symptoms of each mental health condition.

Chapter 9, "CBD and Sleep Disorders," is dedicated specifically to some of the most common sleep problems. It examines insomnia and sleep apnea and provides information on natural solutions, therapy, and medications used to improve sleep. The chapter also offers numerous research findings on the effectiveness of CBD for sleep disorders.

Chapter 10, "CBD and Neurodegenerative Disorders," provides a snapshot of research findings on CBD and Alzheimer's disease, Parkinson's disease, Huntington's disease, multiple sclerosis, and amyotrophic lateral sclerosis (ALS). Traditional therapies, medical interventions, and medications are reviewed for each condition, as are positive research findings on the effectiveness of CBD for each neurodegenerative disease.

Chapter 11, "CBD and End-of-Life Care," examines what researchers are reporting about the use of CBD in palliative care and hospice. It gives the reader information concerning the potential effectiveness in treating end-of-life symptoms like nausea, vomiting, pain, anxiety, and depression.

Chapter 12, "Purchasing and Using CBD," gives the reader practical information for navigating the endless sources of CBD products online and in stores. Not all CBD products are created equal. These products come from various countries, and it may be difficult to find products that are of high quality. Some brands contain THC, while others do not. The reader will learn what to look for in a brand and what to avoid.

Chapter 13, "CBD for Your Pets," provides a snapshot of what experts are saying about the use of CBD for dogs and cats. Pets may suffer from a number of conditions like arthritis, pain, inflammation, fear of storms or loud noises, and separation anxiety. Research findings are reviewed on the use of CBD and pets.

Chapter 14, "The Future of CBD and Other Cannabinoids," examines what many thought leaders in the field are saying about the potential use and success of cannabidiol and other cannabis-related cannabinoids in medicine, psychiatry, and preventive health.

2

The Very Long and Fascinating History of Cannabis as Medicine

I like the dreams of the future better than the history of the past.
—Thomas Jefferson

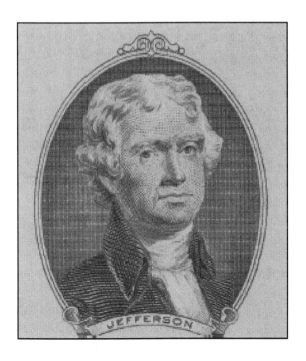

Introduction

Most people don't know that Thomas Jefferson was one of America's first hemp farmers, along with George Washington. While the future of hemp appears to be very bright, it's always good to go back and examine history. And the history of cannabis being used for health and the management of illness doesn't simply go back a mere couple hundred years, but instead, it goes thousands of years, deep into ancient times. Many ancient physicians, especially the Greeks, were known to mix cannabis with other plants, and physicians made sure they had it in their medication bags at all times, especially when they were visiting patients. As a matter of fact, the ancient Greeks so highly valued the cannabis plant that they used every part of it for medicinal purposes. The Greeks are the first known culture to use cannabis for their animals. Other cultures before the Greeks—including ancient China, ancient India, and ancient Egypt—knew of the healing properties of cannabis and hemp.

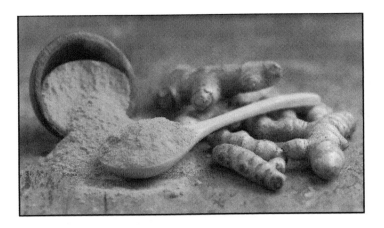

Turmeric in powder form and root

Throughout history, humans discovered the most effective medicinal uses of many plants, including the following:

- Aloe vera for burns, wounds, and other skin conditions
- Celery as an effective diuretic
- Cayenne to reduce pain, swelling, and cholesterol

- Chili to relief pain and soreness
- Eucalyptus as an analgesic and for cough
- Foxglove, the original source of digitalis used for cardiovascular health
- Garlic for antibiotic and antidepressant effects as well as cardiovascular health
- Ginkgo, used to treat asthma, bronchitis, and possibly Alzheimer's disease
- Turmeric, a spice from the ginger family that has been used for thousands of years for digestive and liver health, for pain, and for anti-inflammatory and antioxidant effects

The list of plants used for medicine throughout history would cover many chapters of this book. Don't forget about the use of flaxseed, chamomile, alfalfa, tree tea oil, peppermint, evening primrose, and oregano.

Traditional Chinese Medicine

The fascinating history of cannabis began millions of years ago in the Altai Mountains located in the high plateau of Central Asia. From there, it spread throughout China and Europe. The ancient Chinese have long been known to use natural, plant-based medicines for both physical and mental health. Fabric made from the plant dates back to over eleven thousand years ago. Seeds and oils from the cannabis plant were used for food eight thousand years ago. It is also believed that cannabis was used as medicine for injuries and health problems five thousand years ago. The Chinese discovered that cannabis could be effective to relieve pain and discomfort, rheumatism, gout, constipation, hair loss, and malaria. Ancient Chinese doctors treated their patients with a variety of methods, including acupuncture, massage, and herbal medicine. The main goal of Chinese medicine at the time was prevention. The primary principle was that it was far better to keep the body strong and healthy, thus preventing illness, rather than fighting diseases and health problems. The question remains, however, as to who exactly discovered the medicinal effects of cannabis. This is where the history of cannabis in ancient China becomes even more interesting.

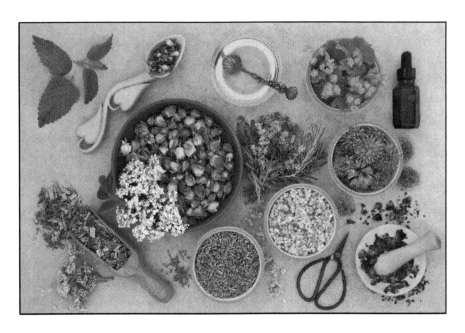

Various herbs used in traditional Chinese medicine

Shen Nung

Roughly forty-five hundred years ago, the Chinese Emperor Shen Nung practiced natural medicine, pharmacology, and agriculture and is known as the Founding Father of Chinese agriculture and herbal medicine. He was the first person in history to write about the health benefits of cannabis and recommended it for over one hundred illnesses and disorders. His writings in herbal medicine have also led to him being called the Father of Chinese Medicine. Obviously, he was an incredibly important historical figure.

Written in 2737 BC, his book, *The Herbal* is the earliest Chinese text about human consumption of herbs for medicinal purposes. He was a pharmacologist thousands of years before the term actually existed. Cannabis is one of the "fifty fundamental herbs" in traditional Chinese medicine. He recommended a tincture or tea made from the cannabis flowers and leaves, which he called *Ma'* and believed to be a healthy elixir. Shen Nung has been said to have digested hundreds of herbs and plants daily to examine what kinds of effects they had on him. He wore clothing made from hemp and leaves from various plants. One day, he experimented with different herbs and plants, turned green, and died, most likely from poisoning.

Hua Tuo

Another interesting early Chinese physician, Hua Tuo, who lived much later (AD 140–208), is credited for being the first person to use cannabis as an anesthetic. Interestingly, the Chinese word for "anesthesia" is *mazui*, which means "cannabis intoxication." He was a pioneer in developing new surgical techniques and the use of anesthesia. Hua Tuo created an anesthetic formula called *Ma Fei San*, and many scholars of Chinese medicine believe cannabis was the main ingredient. His formula consisted of cannabis that had been dried and made into a powder, which was mixed with wine. He used it both topically and internally during medical procedures and surgeries. *Ma Fei San* was essentially used as an anti-inflammatory and pain medication.

Pen Ts'ao Ching

This very old book on agriculture and medicinal plants goes by many names, including *Shennong Bencaojing, The Classic of Herbal Medicine*,[1] and *Shen-Nung Pen tsao Ching*. It was compiled in AD 1, based on the work and traditions of Shen Nung mentioned earlier. Experts believe the text is a compilation of oral traditions and was composed of three volumes containing 365 entries on plants and herbs used as medicine and is known as the oldest herbal reference book in written history. Cannabis is recommended for over one hundred different illnesses and diseases, including rheumatism, malaria, absentmindedness, and gout. The first volume described 120 drugs that have stimulating properties and are known as the "noble" or "upper" herbs. Cannabis is included in this volume with other herbs, including ginseng and Chinese cinnamon. Volume two explains 120 therapeutic substances used for treating the sick, but which also may have toxic side effects. Ginger and cucumber are examples. This volume contains what are called "human," "commoner," or "middle" herbs. The third and final volume contains 125 entries about substances that are poisonous and have negative effects on physiological functioning. Rhubarb and various pitted fruits are examples and herbs in this volume are referred to as "low" herbs.

Sun Simiao

Known as both the "Medicine God" and "King of Medicine," Sun Simiao (AD 581–683) was as famous alchemist and physician who continues to be hailed for his work in herbal medicine. He advocated the use of cannabis for treating severe pain from fractured bones. He wrote a famous thirty-volume work entitled *Prescriptions Worth a Thousand Gold*, which was printed in AD 652.[2] The book was so valuable and presented such numerous life-saving treatments that the saying "A life is worth more than a thousand gold coins" was incorporated in the title. He believed in searching for herbs and gathering them during the right seasons. Knowing exactly where the herbs came from was important to him as well. In his work, he described 519 medicinal materials from 133 countries.

Summary

Although this discussion was brief, cannabis has a long history of being used as medicine in ancient China. Many scholars believe that Chinese medicine is highly valued for its ancient healing properties, and much of it is remarkably still used today to treat a number of physical and mental conditions. Today, hemp seeds, known as *Huo Ma Ren*, are still used as a treatment for constipation. Just as modern physicians have high-tech tools and current pharmacotherapies, the ancient Chinese doctors had acupuncture, massage, herbal medicine, and cannabis.

The ancient Chinese realized how valuable the cannabis plant was and how it could be used to treat a number of human problems. It is documented that medical cannabis was used to treat depression, agitation, sleep difficulties, and hysteria. It is interesting that today a number of studies show potential benefits of cannabinoids such as CBD, in treating anxiety, post-traumatic stress disorder (PTSD), and obsessive-compulsive disorder (OCD).

Cannabis is also documented in Chinese medicine as being effective to treat seizures, muscle spasms, tics, and tremors. Currently, research on cannabis and cannabinoids is pointing to possible relief from symptoms associated with epilepsy, multiple sclerosis, and Parkinson's disease. It's amazing that cannabis has been used as a medicine for thousands of years and is experiencing a significant resurgence in Western medicine. CBD products are becoming increasingly popular throughout the world, and the research behind them is utterly amazing. It appears that medical marijuana and its many cannabinoids have truly come full circle.

Ancient India and Medical Cannabis

The long and interesting history of cannabis used as medicine doesn't stop in ancient China. In other parts of the world, people were using herbal medicine and cannabis in the treatment of many conditions, including ancient India, where it has been used for thousands of years. Physicians in the ninth and tenth centuries treated their patients with bhang, or cannabis, for a variety of health problems including pain, insomnia, gastrointestinal conditions, and headaches. It was specifically used to treat dysentery, which is an inflammatory bowel disease affecting the colon and intestines, producing diarrhea and abdominal pain. The ancient Indians knew that the plant could be used to treat digestion and appetite problems.

Medical cannabis has its roots in legend and religion. The earliest mention of cannabis is found in *The Vedas*, which are the sacred Hindu texts.[3] These writings go back as far as 2000 to 1400 BC. According to *The Vedas*, cannabis is one of the five sacred plants, and a guardian angel lives within the plant's leaves. The text states that cannabis is a source of happiness, liberation, and joy and that it was given to humans to help us attain delight and lose our fears. Interesting, modern research points to CBD's potential as an anxiolytic or anti-anxiety treatment as well as an antidepressant.

Traditional Indian medicine is deeply associated with Ayurveda, which is a five-thousand-year-old holistic healing system. It is based on the belief that health and wellness rely on a balance in mind, body, and spirit. Just like ancient Chinese medicine, the goal was to keep people healthy and strong versus fighting illness. In other words, it was preventive in nature. A belief in Ayurvedic medicine is that physical pain affects one's emotional state, which exacerbates the problem, leading to great stress. Pain can also influence a person's character, which can lead to significant imbalance and disequilibrium. Isn't it fascinating that the primary job of the endocannabinoid system—maintaining balance and equilibrium both physiologically and emotionally—wasn't discovered until the 1990s, but was understood in an early and primitive way by the ancient Indians?

There is an interesting story—or, perhaps better stated, a legend—behind Shiva, the god most associated with cannabis in India. Shiva is said to have had an argument with his family and then left, wandering off into the fields. Exhausted from the fight and blistering sun, he fell asleep under a leafy plant. Once he woke up, he ate some of the plant's leaves and felt instant relief and rejuvenation. Shiva made this plant his favorite thing to eat. He later became known as the Lord of Bhang, or cannabis.

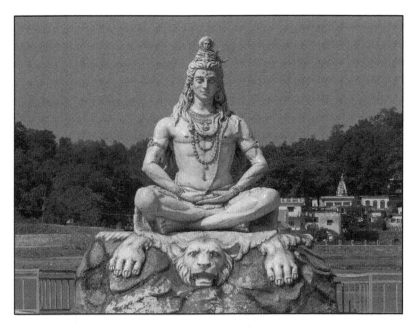

Shiva statue on the Ganges River, Rishikesh, India

During the Middle Ages, bhang was given to soldiers to drink before they entered battle. Cannabis maintained a strong religious connection throughout the years, and members of religious communities across the country would share bowls of bhang with one another. Today, Hindus use bhang to seek divinity. In the eighteenth century, the British conquered India. Later in colonial India, they became aware of the extensive use of cannabis and became very concerned that cannabis was deteriorating the Indian's health and making them mentally ill. As Western medicine became more popular in India, Ayurveda diminished for the most part, being practiced by only small pockets of the population. In 1947 India regained its independence, and Ayurvedic medicine made a strong comeback.

More recently, cannabis was added to the *Homeopathic Pharmacopoeia of India (HPI)* in 1971.[4] The book outlined some health benefits of medical cannabis. Among them are pain relief, the healing of wounds, and help with sleep. Cannabis can also be medically beneficial for people who suffer from rheumatoid arthritis, asthma, and migraines. India came under fire by the United States concerning its use of cannabis for any reason, recreational or medicinal. In 1985, Indian law shot down the use of the plant, which is illegal under the Narcotic Drugs and Psychotropic Substances Act, 1985, and Prevention of Illicit Trafficking in Narcotic Drugs and Psychotropic Substances Act, 1985.

Ancient Egypt

The use of cannabis was also well known in ancient Egypt. Egyptians made very good use of the plant, and Egyptologists have confirmed its uses in religious ceremonies, manufacturing (e.g., fabric and rope), and for treating various health conditions. Before the time of Christ, the Egyptians were making paper, textiles, sails, fine linen, and rope out of hemp. Writings on the walls of the pyramids and hemp in tombs are evidence of the Egyptian's relationship with this plant. There is even evidence that hemp was used to build pyramids.

Documentation dating back to 2000 BC indicates that cannabis was used medicinally for sore eyes and cataracts. Amazingly, it was also a treatment for cancer, which Egyptians get credit for first identifying. Egyptian women were given cannabis for sadness and "bad tempers." Written prescriptions for cannabis have been discovered throughout Egypt, providing further evidence the civilization understood the medical properties of cannabis. Evidence of a prescription for cannabis to treat inflammation can be found on the *Ebers Papyrus*, sometimes referred to as *Papyrus Ebers*, dating back to 1550 BC.[5] The *Ebers Papyrus* is an ancient medical document that provides the most comprehensive record of Egyptian medicine. Other conditions such as inflammation, glaucoma, excessive menstrual bleeding, and hemorrhoids were all treated with cannabis. Evidence that the ancient Egyptians ingested cannabis comes from mummies, including that of the Egyptian pharaoh Ramses the Great, who ruled in 1213 BC.

Ancient Greece

History shows us that Egypt (and Persia) influenced Greek culture in many ways, including the use of cannabis for medical problems. Ancient Greeks used it to treat inflammation, edema, and earache. They even used it to treat battle wounds on their horses and health problems of their livestock. Dressings were made from chopped cannabis leaves and mixed with other natural ingredients to heal the wounds of their animals. The ancient Greeks understood the veterinarian benefits of cannabis and used cannabis to treat back pain and tapeworms in animals.

The classic Greek term *cannabeizion* means to "smoke cannabis." This was usually done by mixing cannabis with myrrh, balsam, and frankincense and inhaling vapors from an incense burner. As mentioned earlier, Greek physicians were sure to carry cannabis plants and herbs in their medicine bags. They felt that every part of the plant had medicinal uses. Leaves were used to stop nosebleeds, and seeds were used to treat tapeworms, gastrointestinal problems, pain, and inflammation. The roots of the cannabis plant were applied to burns for relief and were also used to treat various types of tumors. Even the ash, once cannabis was burned, was used for the treatment of muscle soreness, pain, and inflammation. While the leaves and buds are considered the most popularly used parts of the plant today, the seeds were most valued by the ancient Greeks. Seeds would be soaked in various liquids, usually wine, and then pressed to create an ancient medicine used to treat earaches, pain, and inflammation.

The ancient Greek botanist and physician Pedanius Dioscorides (AD 40–90) wrote the famous five-volume medical text entitled *De Materia Medica*[6] and makes a very early reference to the medical use of cannabis. Dioscorides explains the use of around six hundred plants that were effective for treating many disorders. He also provided nine hundred recipes combining herbs and plants to be used for many ailments. He actually uses the term *Kannabis* and describes it as a plant that makes good rope and can be used to treat ear pain.

The historian and contemporary of Socrates Herodotus (450–420 BC) wrote of the medicinal and recreational use of cannabis. According to his writing, the ancient Scythians burned cannabis seeds on hot rocks in their bathhouses, which made them "shout for joy." It is also known that these ancient people used parts of the cannabis plant as offerings placed at the tombs and grave sites of royalty. According to these and many other historical references, the ancient Greeks had a firm idea about the medical uses of cannabis.

Summary

Ancient civilizations understood the medicinal benefits of cannabis for many physical and mental health conditions. It is actually quite surprising how well they knew and used the plant. Ancient physicians packed their medicine bags with various plants and herbs, including cannabis. Humans were not the only ones to be treated with cannabis, as there is historical evidence of the ancient Greeks practicing veterinary medicine on their horses and livestock. There is so much history that there simply is not enough room for it in this book. The ancient Chinese, Indians, Egyptians, and Greeks give us plenty of evidence that they had medical, practical, and religious bonds with the plant. These weren't the only ancient civilizations to use cannabis to heal their people. Evidence from Rome, Japan, Persia, Babylonia, Palestine, Mongolia, Siberia, Korea, the Netherlands, and the Islamic world suggests cannabis was used for a variety of reasons.

Medical Cannabis in the Modern World

The history of cannabis in ancient times is fascinating, and the story of this medicinal plant in modern times is quite interesting as well. It has been able to travel from country to country, impacting economics, politics, medicine, religion, and culture. Sometime in the 1500s, the Spanish brought cannabis to South America, where it spread across the continent. Hemp became the cash crop of the American colonies during the seventeenth century. England pressured the colonies to produce more hemp to be sent back to the motherland, and the colonies needed their own constant supply. The Virginia Company asked the colonists of Jamestown to grow a minimum of one hundred hemp plants to support England. Trade ships required sails and ropes. An interesting fact not known by most people is that the 1914 $10 bill was not only printed on hemp but had pictures of hemp on the back side of the bill. Later in the 1700s, hemp seeds and roots were being recommended in American medical journals to treat a variety of ailments, such as inflammation of the skin, venereal disease, and incontinence. There are other little-known facts about hemp's use in the colonies. The Declaration of Independence was written on hemp paper, and two of America's Founding Fathers, George Washington and Thomas Jefferson, were hemp farmers.

William Brooke O'Shaughnessy

The 1800s saw an expansion in the use of cannabis as medicine not only in the new world, but in other countries as well. Irish physician William Brooke O'Shaughnessy (1809–1889) has been hailed as the founding father of modern medical cannabis. He is also credited for reintroducing cannabis to the modern world. Dr. O'Shaughnessy was quite the thinker, as he was not only a physician but also an expert in underwater engineering. Regarding his work on medical cannabis, it is known that he delivered a speech to students and scholars at the Medical and Physical Society of Calcutta, India, in 1839. Medicines containing cannabis were already available in most American pharmacies at the time, but after the work of Dr. O'Shaughnessy, cannabis became even more available to treat a number of health conditions. He also did work in colonial India, where he was an assistant surgeon and professor of chemistry. He performed many experiments using cannabis on animals and then on humans. He created his own mixture of cannabis and other ingredients that was administered to his patients suffering from cholera, tetanus, rheumatism, and seizures. He also found hemp to be an effective anticonvulsive treatment.

He warned other physicians to use low doses of cannabis because delirium could be induced through the use of higher doses. His work can be said to have launched hundreds of medical studies on the medicinal uses of cannabinoids during his career.

Growth in Popularity of Cannabis-Based Medicines

During the mid- to late 1800s, cannabis products filled the shelves of pharmacies all over the United States and Europe. People used it as both an intoxicant to get high on and as a medicine for various medical and mental health problems. It was used for ailments including asthma, whooping cough, cholera, and gonorrhea. The main form of medicine was in the form of a tincture that was orally ingested. These tinctures were marketed as a pain relief product by large pharmaceutical companies both in the United States and Europe. Queen Victoria supposedly used cannabis tincture to relieve menstrual cramping. It is quite fascinating that the most popularly sold CBD product on the market today is in a similar tincture.

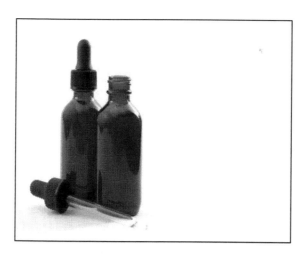

A typical tincture bottle of amber color

Just as the popularity of cannabis-based tincture exploded in the United States, state regulations attempted to legally handle mislabeling, adulteration, and the lack of ingredients on labels of so-called patent medicines. Potency, side effects, and efficacy of products varied immensely, and no one was sure that poisons weren't ingredients in these tinctures. During the late 1800s and early 1900s, "poison laws" and others were passed to regulate drug sales. Before the dawn of the twentieth century, over 280 manufacturers were making two thousand or more forms of cannabis-based medicines. It was only a matter of time before the government would step in and hand down heavy laws and regulations concerning both medical cannabis and hemp.

Mexico, Cannabis, and America

By the beginning of the 1900s, state laws restricted the use of cannabis products to prescription only. The times were changing once again in the United States as the masses began to change their minds about the use of cannabis, either recreationally or medicinally. Mexico had a central role in changing how Americans felt about cannabis. The early 1900s were also a time of heavy Mexican immigration into the United States. Mexican immigrants brought marijuana into the country, which increased the popularity of its recreational use. For the most part, cannabis arrived in the southwest parts of the United States from Mexico, with immigrants escaping the Mexican Revolution of 1910 and 1911. The dictatorship of General Porfirio Díaz created poverty and despair among Mexico's citizens, so many of them migrated north over the Rio Grande into Texas and New Mexico. The revolution that ousted Díaz increased the flow of immigrants and marijuana into the United States. Migrant workers spread out to other parts of the country and brought their customs and habits with them, including the use of marijuana. Racism, fear of marijuana, and many other misconceptions took hold and continued for decades.

Back in Mexico, marijuana grew wild in most parts of the country and was cultivated by peasants who would smoke it in their pipes. They also consumed it after mixing parts of the plant with chili peppers, sugarcane, and milk. Cannabis was used by witch doctors, or *curandero*, who practiced the old medical ways of Mexico. Eventually people would roll the leaves and flowers of the plant into cigarettes and smoke them. There are stories of the Mexican military using the slang phrase "Maria y Juana," or in English, "Mary and

Jane," referring to going to a brothel, finding some prostitutes, and enjoying some of the marijuana-filled cigarettes that were found there.

Scholars believe that the word "marijuana" itself most likely originated in Mexico. And just like flipping a switch, the majority of Americans saw cannabis as a social problem that led to worse troubles in life. People who smoked marijuana were seen as lowlifes, lower class, deviants, and even criminals. William Randolph Hearst did his best to do away with marijuana in the 1920s and 1930s. He was a successful businessman, politician, and media giant of his time and used all of his influence to create a direct connection between Mexicans and marijuana. During the Great Depression, Hearst was skillful at communicating to Americans that they were not only competing with Mexicans for scarce jobs, but that the country was in danger because of the drugs they were smuggling in.

Hearst was not alone in his quest to connect foreigners and people of color with marijuana. Harry Jacob Anslinger was the director of the newly formed Federal Bureau of Narcotics located in Washington, DC, and has gone down in history as the "godfather" of America's War on Drugs. Marijuana was not on Anslinger's radar until his bureau was falling apart. As tax revenues decreased during the Great Depression, funding for the bureau diminished, and his beloved Federal Bureau of Narcotics was about to become history. And then a light went off in Harry's mind. If he could tie marijuana to Mexicans and African Americans, he may be able to completely ban the substance. By stigmatizing a select group of people and marijuana, he could possibly get his way. And the rest, as they say, is history.

Cult Classic: *Reefer Madness*

If you have never seen this 1936 cult-classic propaganda movie, please do. The original title *Tell Your Children*, which later became known as *Reefer Madness*, is a government propaganda film about the evils of marijuana. It was part of a larger effort to ban hemp in the United States, which was competing with oil, lumber, and cotton. Remember, hemp was the largest crop in the United States for many years. It was big corporations and government that made it illegal in 1937. Interestingly, most of the actors in this movie were unknown, and it was financed by a church group.

The goal of the movie was to teach parents about the horrible outcomes associated with marijuana and depicts accidents, manslaughter, suicide, rape, and insanity that come with using marijuana. Anslinger painted a picture that marijuana made Mexican and African American men (the "degenerate races") have intense sexual desire for white women. While the film never made a significant impact and went largely ignored until the 1970s, when it became a comedic cult classic within the marijuana culture of America, its original intent was to assist federal prohibition of cannabis. The film is a good example of the intimate partnership between the government, mainstream media, and Hollywood. I guess some things never change.

Marijuana and the Law

The law that started it all is known as the Pure Food and Drug Act of 1906. This law, along with many other state laws, restricted any kind of habit-forming drugs. This law also brought the use of opium and morphine under the control of physicians treating patients who required these drugs. The Harrison Act of 1914 defined drug use as a crime for the first time in US history. Next is the Marijuana Tax Act of 1937. This act made the nonmedical possession and use of cannabis completely illegal within the United States. The act also imposed a tax on marijuana used for medical purposes. Criminal charges were brought on physicians who did not pay the tax. The American Medical Association (AMA) fought back against the law and believed that it would only get into the way of important medical research examining the health benefits of cannabis. They were indeed correct.

Later in 1938, the Federal Pure Food, Drug, and Cosmetic Act was instituted to regulate both prescription and nonprescription drugs. This old act is still being used today. Next, the Boggs Act of 1951 took a major step by adding cannabis sativa to the list of known narcotic drugs. One of the worst outcomes of these laws was the dramatic drop in medical research concerning the use of cannabis, cannabinoids, and other substances in the plant in the treatment of a number of physical and mental health problems.

The Comprehensive Drug Abuse Prevention and Control Act of 1970, under the Nixon administration, introduced a new classification system of drugs. This act placed all federal drug laws under one single statute. Some say that this ushered in the era of the "War on Drugs." Why was marijuana on Nixon's radar in the first place? The Vietnam War was raging on, and the country had become weary of it. Watching images of American soldiers fighting, dying, and being brought back home in body bags was unpleasant at best. The war was also associated with marijuana because the Asian nations where the war was fought had plenty of it to go around.

Cannabis was now classified as a Schedule 1 drug, which by definition has no medicinal value, has a high potential for addiction, and lacks acceptable safety measures under medical supervision. Drugs in this class include heroin, LSD, and ecstasy. This law essentially put a stake into the heart of research unless it was strictly approved by the federal government.

The Controlled Substances Act was passed as part of the Comprehensive Drug Abuse Prevention and Control Act of 1970. It made the possession or distribution of cannabis sativa a federal-level criminal act. This legislation led to the development of five different schedules of dangerous drugs. Schedule I drugs are those with no currently accepted medical use and possess a high potential for abuse. Examples include heroin, LSD, marijuana (cannabis), ecstasy, methaqualone, and peyote. Schedule II drugs have a high potential for abuse as well as the possibility of severe psychological or physical dependence. Examples include Vicodin, cocaine, methamphetamine, methadone, Dilaudid, Demerol, OxyContin, fentanyl, Dexedrine, Adderall, and Ritalin. Schedule III drugs have a moderate to low potential for dependence and have less abuse potential than Schedule I and II drugs but more than Schedule IV. Examples include codeine, Tylenol with codeine, ketamine, anabolic steroids, and testosterone. Schedule IV drugs are those with a low potential for abuse and dependence. Examples include Xanax, Soma, Darvon, Darvocet, Valium, Ativan, and Ambien. And last, Schedule V drugs have lower potential for abuse than Schedule IV and contain small quantities of certain narcotics. Schedule V drugs are commonly used as antidiarrheal, anticough, and analgesic medications. Examples include codeine and Robitussin C.

California and the Compassionate Care Act of 1996

Proposition 215, known as the Compassionate Care Act, was passed in 1996 despite a number of failed attempts, and California officially became the first state to legalize medical marijuana. The proposition was a statewide referendum that gave access to medical marijuana to qualified patients. In 2003, Senate Bill 420 opened the doors for growers, health care providers, and caregivers as well as an identification card system to obtain medical marijuana. Other states followed in the 1990s, including Alaska, Arizona, Colorado, New Mexico, Oregon, Vermont, Washington, and the District of Columbia.

The Cole Memo, drafted by US Attorney General James M. Cole in 2013, eased restrictions on the use of cannabis for medical purposes and gave individual states authority to make decisions regarding its use. Under the memo, law enforcement and prosecutors were instructed to focus on specific priorities regarding state-related cannabis operations. Among these were preventing distribution of marijuana to minors; preventing money made by cannabis sales from going to criminal enterprises, gangs, or cartels; preventing the movement of cannabis where it is legal across state lines to where it is not; and preventing state-authorized medical marijuana being used as a cover for drug trafficking. The Cole Memo also outlined prevention of violence through the use of firearms while cultivating or distributing cannabis, driving while using cannabis, and growing marijuana on public or federal land.

Changes in US Cannabis Laws

As states legalized cannabis either for recreational or medical use, the federal government had to respond. The US attorney general made a statement indicating that federal resources would not be used specifically to focus on the prosecution of seriously ill individuals or their caregivers who comply with state laws on medical marijuana. This, of course, was a major shift in ideology and policy regarding the use of cannabis for medical purposes as well as the power of the state. It was also made clear that no tolerance would be provided to drug traffickers who used medical marijuana as a front for illegal drug activity.

President Trump Signs the 2018 Farm Bill

History was made when President Donald J. Trump signed the 2018 Farm Bill into law legalizing hemp and its derivatives across the United States. This has been seen as a major victory for the American farmer and agriculture in general. President Trump was not alone. Senate Majority Leader Mitch McConnell strongly supported the comeback of hemp as a major crop in the United States. Some believe that without McConnell's leadership on this bill, it would never have seen the light of day. Not only did he have power as a Senate leader, but he also appointed himself to the conference committee that brought the House and Senate together to agree on the passage of the bill. Many thanks are owed to Senator Mitch McConnell and President Donald Trump in the world of hemp! McConnell is from Kentucky, as many of you know. Kentucky is one of the most ideal places for cultivating hemp in the world. He also knows that hemp doesn't get anyone high.

While the bill provides important agricultural and nutritional policy extensions for five years, some of the most interesting (and exciting) changes involve the cannabis plant. Marijuana and hemp belong to the family of plants known as cannabis. The major thing that sets them apart is the amount of THC in them. Traditionally, marijuana is grown with high levels of THC and is used for medical purposes and well as simply getting high. Hemp, on the other hand, is grown with less than 0.3% THC or less, and there are actually hemp plants being grown now with zero (0%) THC and high levels of CBD. For over eighty years, the federal government made no distinction between the two, and with the signing of the Marijuana Tax Act in 1937, both were effectively made illegal in the United States. In 1970, the Controlled Substances Act formally made both substances illegal and banned cannabis of any kind. Now, hemp policies have been changed drastically in the United States, and CBD is legal in all fifty states, as long as it comes from hemp containing either 0.3% or less THC. Anything above that level is still considered illegal by the federal government.

The 2018 Farm Bill allows hemp-derived products such as CBD, to be transferred across state lines for commercial and other purposes. There are also no restrictions on the sale, transport, or possession of hemp-derived products, which opens new markets and allows people to purchase CBD for their health and well-being without being afraid of breaking the law. It certainly has given thousands peace of mind and hope in seeking alternative ways to treat their own symptoms and ailments.

Section 7501 of the Farm Bill extends much-needed research on the uses of hemp by including it under the Critical Agricultural Materials Act. This provision acknowledges how important hemp is in research. Section 12619 removes any hemp-derived product from its former Schedule I status under the Controlled Substance Act. As long as cannabinoids, including CBD, come from legally grown and produced hemp, they are legal. Under this act, there will be an explosion in the types and numbers of CBD products brought to the market. This is a good thing for economic reasons, as well as for those seeking relief from aches and pains, depression and anxiety, and other ailments.

The bill also gives many farmers peace of mind in making annual decisions about their crops. It provides safety net programs and protects federal crop insurance, and maintains strong research initiatives and rural development. It promotes a massive shift back to farming in America, especially small family farms. The bill also offers assurances to the bankers and lenders behind farmers and ranchers, gives producers room to breathe as they get ready for a new year, and will surely stimulate the economy for years to come. Rural America can begin producing some of the safest and affordable food and fiber in the world, just as it did many years ago. In sum, the 2018 Farm Bill is nothing short of a miracle and blessing for countless people in the United States.

Summary

Throughout history, we have seen that many civilizations understood the medicinal uses of cannabis. From ancient China, Emperor Shen Nung wrote about the health benefits of cannabis for over one hundred illnesses and disorders. Chinese physician Hua Tuo used cannabis as an anesthetic. The oldest herbal reference book in written history, *Shennong Bencaojing*, recommended cannabis for over one hundred illnesses and diseases, including rheumatism, malaria, and gout. The "King of Medicine," Sun Simiao, advocated the use of cannabis for treating severe pain from fractured bones.

Physicians from ancient India treated patients with cannabis, or bhang, for a number of health conditions, including pain, insomnia, gastrointestinal problems, headaches, and inflammatory bowel disease. Ancient Hindu texts, *The Vedas*, consider cannabis one of the five sacred plants. Traditional

Indian medicine, which is deeply associated with Ayurveda, a five thousand-year-old holistic healing system, maintains that physiological and emotional balance are necessary for good health, as validated by the discovery of the endocannabinoid system in the 1990s. And as recently as 1971, the *Homeopathic Pharmacopoeia of India* outlined some of the benefits of cannabis, including pain relief, wound healing, and help with sleep. It also mentions cannabis as being beneficial for rheumatoid arthritis, asthma, and migraines.

The ancient Egyptians and Greeks also were known to understand and use cannabis in medicine. In ancient Egypt, it was used for sore eyes and cataracts, cancer, sadness, and tempers. The ancient document *Papyrus* recommended it for inflammation, glaucoma, excessive menstrual bleeding, and hemorrhoids. The Greeks used it for inflammation, edema, and earache. They treated their animals' wounds and health problems with cannabis. Greek physicians carried it in their medicine bags. Pedanius Dioscorides, an ancient Greek botanist and physician, made a very early reference to what he called *Kannabis*. And the historian Herodotus told the world that cannabis makes one "shout for joy."

Much later in history, around the year 1500, the Spanish brought cannabis to South America, where it spread like wildfire. Colonists at Jamestown were ordered by England to grow hemp, and George Washington and Thomas Jefferson were both hemp farmers. At the same time, American medical journals recommended hemp for inflammation of the skin, incontinence, and the treatment of venereal disease.

Later in the 1800s, Irish physician William Brooke O'Shaughnessy introduced cannabis to the modern world. He used it to treat cholera, tetanus, rheumatism, and seizures. He also found that cannabis had an anticonvulsive effect. It is believed that his work launched over one hundred medical reports on the medicinal properties of cannabinoids. Soon, cannabis-based products were on store shelves in the United States and Europe. People started to use them for mental and emotional problems. It has been said that Queen Victoria even used cannabis to treat her menstrual cramps.

The 1900s saw Mexico take center stage as immigrants brought cannabis into the United States, particularly the Southern states. They used it and taught others to use it recreationally. Competition for jobs during the Great Depression brought great conflict and animosity toward Mexican immigrants.

William Randolph Hearst had a large audience as a media giant of his time and used it to connect the problems created by marijuana and Mexican people. Harry Jacob Anslinger, the director of the newly formed Federal Bureau of Narcotics, became the godfather of America's War on Drugs. He did his best to connect marijuana with black Americans and Mexican immigrants. To some degree, this led to a cult-classic film, *Reefer Madness*, which was originally called *Tell Your Children*. It was a propaganda film urging Americans to stay away from marijuana and was a part of the effort to eventually ban marijuana and hemp in the United States.

In 1906, the Pure Food and Drug Act restricted any type of habit-forming drug, which was followed by the Marijuana Tax Act of 1937. Possession or use of nonmedical cannabis was now illegal. The American Medical Association fought back because they knew of the medical benefits of cannabis but lost the battle. Later in 1938, the Federal Pure Food, Drug, and Cosmetic Act was instituted to regulate both prescription and nonprescription drugs. The Boggs Act of 1951 added cannabis sativa to a list of narcotic drugs, which unfortunately lead to a halt in medical studies and research on the possible health and emotional benefits of cannabis or hemp-based substances. In 1970, the Comprehensive Drug Abuse Prevention and Control Act under President Richard Nixon created a new classification system, listing cannabis as a Schedule I drug, meaning it has no medical benefits and is highly addicting. This ushered in the War on Drugs, and possession or distribution of marijuana or hemp became criminal acts.

Fast-forward to 1996, and the Compassionate Care Act (Proposition 215) was passed in California, which became the first state to legalize medical marijuana. In 2003, Senate Bill 420 opened the door to doctors, growers, health care providers, and caregivers. Other states followed California's model, including Alaska, Arizona, Colorado, New Mexico, Oregon, Vermont, Washington, and the District of Columbia. The Cole Memo in 2013 eased restriction of medical marijuana and gave states the authority to decide how to use medical marijuana.

In December of 2018, President Donald J. Trump signed the 2018 Farm Bill led by Senator Mitch McConnell. Hemp and products derived from hemp were declassified from Schedule I drugs to nutritional supplements. As long as hemp contains 0.3% or less THC, it is completely legal to be grown and sold across state lines. Cannabidiol, or CBD, is one of the most sought-after supplements on the market, and numerous studies have examined its potential health and emotional benefits. From ancient China to President Trump, hemp's history has been long and interesting. What's even more intriguing is the future of hemp for health and wellness.

3

The Endocannabinoid System and Phytocannabinoids Explained

If you can't explain it simply, you don't understand it well enough.
—Albert Einstein

Introduction

The endocannabinoid system (ECS) was discovered not too long ago in the 1990s. The word *endo* means "internal," and it is the cannabinoid system that exists within all humans and animals, except for insects. Our endocannabinoid system is very important and is responsible for many functions in our bodies and brains. It plays a vital role in regulating disease and illness and consists of cannabinoid receptors, signaling molecules, and enzymes. This system is so important that we simply could not survive without it.

Endocannabinoid receptors CB1 and CB2 are found throughout the body and brain and influence, modulate, or regulate the function of cells, tissues, glands, organs, and systems. CB1 receptors are found mainly in the brain and central nervous system but are also present in the cardiovascular system, gastrointestinal tract, thalamus and hypothalamus, pancreas, bone, liver, adipose tissue, prostate, testes, and uterus. CB2 receptors are located in peripheral organs and cells associated with the immune system and are involved in both immunity and inflammation. Many tissues and organs have both CB1 and CB2 receptors, namely the skin, brain, liver, and bones.

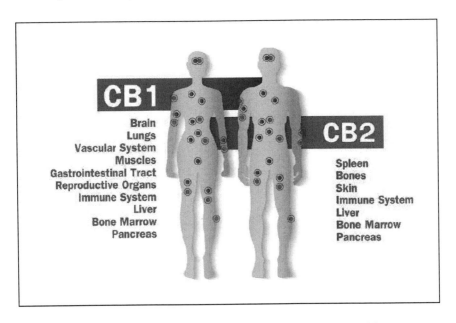

CB1 and CB2 receptors and where they are located in the body and brain

Taking CBD enhances or increases the levels of naturally occurring cannabinoids within our endocannabinoid system. While it does not possess the ability to directly interact with CB1 or CB2 receptors, it instead blocks an important enzyme that breaks down our natural cannabinoid, *anandamide*, or AEA. Another endocannabinoid is 2 arachidonoylglycerol, or 2-AG for short. Interestingly, the endocannabinoid system does not work solely within its own boundaries but strongly interacts with the immune system, endorphin system, and the vanilloid system, which is responsible for transforming acute pain into chronic pain. Once we put this picture together, it becomes clear that the endocannabinoid system regulates inflammation and pain, hormone balance, brain health, energy and mood, bone health, fat and sugar processing, and formation of new nerve cells.

Simply stated, this system is amazing; it's critical to good health and wellness—both physically and emotionally.

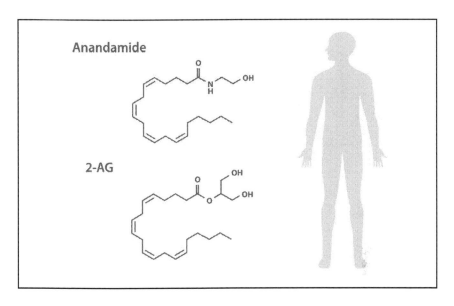

Molecular structures of anandamide and 2-AG

How CBD Works

If you went to high school or college when I did, you probably never heard about the endocannabinoid system. Other systems including the digestive, immune, pulmonary, nervous, circulatory, and endocrine systems were on the curriculum. The reason I didn't know anything about the endocannabinoid system is that it wasn't discovered yet! And while scientists have had three decades to study it, they are still unsure of all its components and functions. Here's where things get both interesting and, at times, somewhat complicated. To grasp how CBD and other cannabinoids work in the body and brain involves a quick lesson (or refresher) in neuroscience. Neurotransmitters are important to understand and are simply chemical messengers used by the brain to communicate vital information throughout the body. They relay signals between neurons, or nerve cells, in order to regulate the major systems of the body. Information relayed between neurons takes place throughout the entire nervous system, including the autonomic nervous system, central nervous system, and peripheral nervous system in the skin, spinal cord, and the brain.

> **Neuroscience**
>
> The study of the brain and how it impacts thoughts and behavior. It is also the study of the nervous system, how it develops, its structure, and what it does.

In 1992, Dr. Raphael Mechoulam discovered endocannabinoids, which are chemical compounds similar to the phytocannabinoids found in cannabis and hemp plants. He also found out that all animals and humans produce these naturally. Other researchers discovered two main cannabinoid receptors, CB1 and CB2, which both respond to endocannabinoids that naturally occur in the body, and phytocannabinoids that are found in hemp and cannabis. We have other receptor systems that use neurotransmitters for cellular communication, including serotonin, dopamine, histamine, and GABA. These play keys roles in health and wellness, both physically and psychologically.

Some writers have created the following analogy concerning how CBD works in the body: cannabinoids act as a key that fits into the lock of the endocannabinoid system and activates or unleashes its healing and balancing properties to a higher degree. The illustration below demonstrates how this process works.

There is, and has always been, an intimate relationship between humans and plants. Remember, endocannabinoids (AEA and 2-AG) are signaling molecules produced within the body. Cannabinoids, or phytocannabinoids, are molecules produced in plants like hemp and cannabis. They are very similar in structure to our naturally occurring endocannabinoids. By taking full spectrum CBD products, you are actually feeding your body and brain very powerful signaling molecules or cannabinoids, which will interact with your endocannabinoid system. This works with other systems throughout your body. CBD is the key that unlocks the health potential of our cannabinoid receptors, CB1 and CB2. More on this dynamic process below.

Living Longer and Stronger with CBD

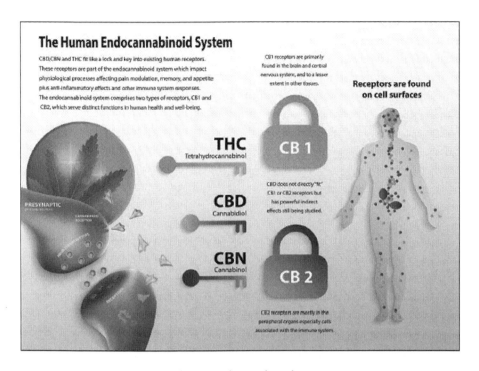

The human endocannabinoid system

Endocannabinoid System (ECS)

It makes sense to begin this section by discussing one of the greatest discoveries of our time—and the man behind it. Dr. Raphael Mechoulam has been a professor of medical chemistry and an organic chemist for decades. He is best known for his work in isolating THC from cannabis many years ago and his research concerning the medical uses of marijuana. Dr. Mechoulam is also the scientist who discovered the endocannabinoid system. Again, the ECS is a central regulatory system that affects many of the body's biological processes. This system modifies pleasure, energy, and overall well-being. It also attempts to keep the body in good health, even when disease and injury threaten to do damage.

Even though the ECS was discovered recently, it is believed to have evolved in human and animals over six hundred million years ago. Insects, interestingly enough, are the only creatures on earth that do not possess an ECS. It is a naturally occurring system that works throughout the body and brain.

The ECS regulates so many important functions that some experts say we simply would not exist without it. For instance, the ECS regulates our perception of pain, how well we sleep, our responses to stress, appetite, memory, and gastrointestinal motility. Without it, we might not sleep or eat and have no healthy ways to deal with stress. When specific systems in our body or brain are overheated by too many chemical messengers (e.g., serotonin), the ECS kicks into gear and releases its own chemical messengers to slow down the release of these messengers. And amazingly, the ECS does this "on demand" and only when a system in the body needs to "hit the break."

Two different chemical compounds—or, specifically, cannabinoid receptors—are important components of the endocannabinoid system. They were mentioned above and are cannabinoid receptor 1 (CB1) and cannabinoid receptor 2 (CB2). CB1 was only discovered in 1988, and CB2 was discovered in 1993, so these are also relatively new to science. Some researchers believe that they are close to discovering a third receptor, and there are probably more still to be discovered.

The endocannabinoid system also uses two different chemicals: arachidonoyl ethanolamide (AEA, or anandamide) and 2-arachidonoyl glycerol, or 2-AG. These two chemicals are called endocannabinoids and are the cannabinoids that are naturally made by the body. They do their work by attaching to a cannabinoid receptor on the cell. CBD does its work by entering the system, imitating the body's naturally occurring endocannabinoids, and giving the ECS a boost to do its job. Once the endocannabinoid is released (AEA or 2-AG), it is broken down by one of five enzymes. Just as ANA and 2-AG bind to CB1 and CB2, CBD and other phytocannabinoids do the same. All of them are considered the keys that unlock CB1 and CB2's medically therapeutic potential. When we use CBD, it provides higher quantities of cannabinoids than our bodies can make.

The endocannabinoid system consists of the following:

The Endocannabinoid System
Two cannabinoid receptors: • Cannabinoid-1 (CB1) • Cannabinoid-2 (CB2) **Two signaling molecules:** • Arachidonoyl ethanolamide (AEA or anandamide) • 2-arachidonoyl glycerol or 2-AG **Five enzymes:** • DAGL-a (for synthesizing 2-AG) • DAGL-B (for synthesizing 2-AG) • NAPE selective phospholipase-D (for synthesizing AEA) • MAGL (for breaking down 2-AG) • FAAH (for breaking down AEA)

It appears that the ECS does not work solely within its own confounds but rather interacts with other noncannabinoid systems in our body. It does this to further protect the body while maintaining balance and equilibrium in the face of illness or disease. To accomplish this, it interacts with the immune system, endorphin system, and the vanilloid system, which transforms acute pain to long-lasting, chronic pain. As the endocannabinoid system works with these systems, it helps to regulate inflammation, pain, mood, energy, hormone balance, brain health, bone health, the formation of new nerve cells, and fat and sugar processing. This system and how it works with others is so important that Pacher and Kunos state that "modulating endocannabinoid system activity must have therapeutic potential in almost all diseases affecting humans, including obesity/metabolic syndrome, diabetes and diabetic complication, neurodegenerative, inflammatory, cardiovascular, liver, gastrointestinal, skin diseases, pain, psychiatric disorders, cachexia, cancer, chemotherapy including nausea and vomiting, among many others."[1] It is therefore remarkable that this system has always been with us, working inside the body and brain, and was only recently discovered. Now that it has been, the research and medical potential on the endocannabinoid system seems endless. Can CBD and other cannabinoids like CBG and CBN be effective in managing symptoms of various health conditions? So far, it appears that they just may be.

Cannabinoid Receptors (CB1 and CB2)

As we have already discussed, two cannabinoid receptors have been discovered in the body and brain, and they are CB1 and CB2. Experts believe a third receptor will be identified soon and will be called CB-3. But let's focus on the ones we know about and review how important they are to our health and well-being. Both receptors are activated by the endocannabinoids that we have already discussed—AEA and 2-AG. CB1 receptors appear to be most abundant in the brain and central nervous system. In the brain, CB1 receptors are involved in nerve signaling, which involves both the structure and function of nerve cells. Nerve cells have many parts, including the nerve cell body, axons, and dendrites. Refer to the illustration below.

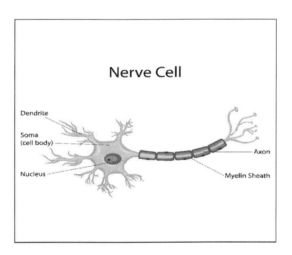

A human nerve cell

The axon of the nerve cell is coated with insulation called myelin (due to certain conditions, they are left uncoated). Nerves that are myelinated conduct electrical signals quicker than unmyelinated nerves, which impacts the speed at which electrical signals reach their target. All nerve cells are connected to each other at nerve endings where small gaps exist, and no signal can pass. Incoming electrical signals transform into chemicals released at the nerve terminals and pass between the space connecting cells. This chemical signal bonds to receptors on the nerve endings and creates a new electrical signal. The entire system enables nerves to transmit signals at various speeds, frequencies, and intensity, creating the movement of information throughout the brain. The brain then responds to this information and instructs the body how to respond.

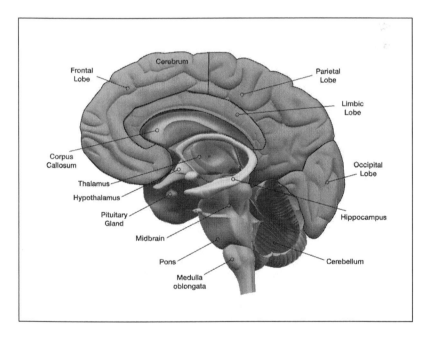

Parts of the human brain

CB1 receptors in the brain are found mainly in the hippocampus, which is important for learning, memory, and stress related to adverse memories (think about PTSD). It is also found in the hypothalamus, which regulates appetite; the limbic system, which moderates anxiety; and the cerebral cortex, which is responsible for higher cognitive functioning (e.g., abstract thought) and pain processing. Lastly, CB1 is also found in the brain's nucleus accumbens (regulates reward and addiction), basal ganglia (influences sleep and movement), and medulla (controls nausea and vomiting). CB1 is also found in the central nervous system, spinal cord, cerebellum, brain stem, olfactory bulb, thalamus, and pituitary.

CB1 receptors are found throughout the body, including the cardiovascular system, upper airways, gastrointestinal tract, pancreas, bone, liver, ovaries, uterus, prostate, testes, and adipose tissue. These receptors are important for regulating pain and anxiety, and work toward stabilizing mood and creating an overall sense of well-being. CB1 receptors also affect other systems in the brain by decreasing brain-based inflammation, changing energy metabolism, and diminishing cellular nerve firing. These receptors have also been found to be instrumental in bone formation and prevention of osteoporosis.

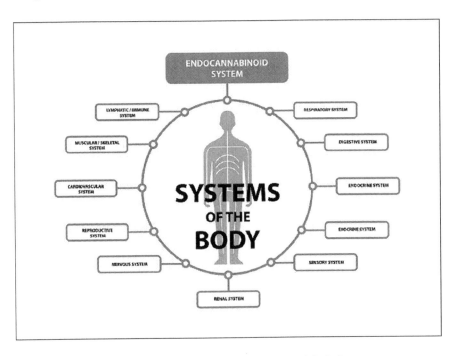

The endocannabinoid and others systems of the body

Phytocannabinoids

After reading about the endocannabinoid system, it should be easier to understand what phytocannabinoids are, why they are important, and how they work in the body. There is a lot of science behind how the two work together. Simply put, a phytocannabinoid is a molecule that is produced by plants, making it a plant-based cannabinoid. The plant that phytocannabinoids come from are marijuana and hemp. Currently, there are 113 known phytocannabinoids from these plants, the most sought after being CBD. The reason you're reading this book is because you've heard about this amazing nutraceutical and the many health and wellness benefits associated with it.

When cannabinoid receptors that already exist in our body interact with a cannabinoid, they transmit molecular messages to the cells, tissues, and organs throughout the body. Remember the lock and key analogy? Cannabinoids—either endocannabinoids or phytocannabinoids—unlock cannabinoid receptors by working together and initiating cellular changes that produce medicinal effects. Among the many phytocannabinoids in the cannabis plant, the main ones include THC, CBD, CBN, CBG, CBC, and THCV. How these all work together is amazing. Scientists like biologists and chemists continue to discover new information about how these interact and produce medical benefits for our bodies and brains. In general, it can be stated that this system maintains homeostasis and balance that becomes disrupted by genetics, environmental factors, and most especially, our lifestyles. In essence, it tries to restore the good when things go bad.

4

The Connection Between CBD and the Aging Process

In the end, it's not the years in your life that count. It's the life in your years.

—Abraham Lincoln

Introduction

This book is entitled *Living Longer and Stronger with CBD* for a very good reason. The vast majority of adults don't understand the connection between cannabidiol and how it may improve the quality of their lives throughout the aging process. For those who equate CBD with marijuana, it simply isn't the same at all.

Once again, CBD and marijuana are two completely different substances. Most CBD products now have *zero* THC, the substance commonly known to make people high. Most people, I assume, simply want relief from the pain, discomfort, and insomnia experienced throughout the aging process.

For centuries, CBD has been proven to be used as an effective anti-inflammatory, analgesic, antioxidant, and neuroprotective agent. Many older adults don't have the time or perhaps the opportunity to read hundreds of journal articles and books on the subject. Luckily, I do.

As a gerontologist, I have been fascinated with the aging process as well as the many factors that influence it, speed it up, or perhaps slow it down. Can we possibly slow the aging process? Is it possible to protect the brain from Alzheimer's disease? What about other neurodegenerative disorders like Parkinson's or Huntington's disease, multiple sclerosis, or amyotrophic lateral sclerosis (ALS)? With over three thousand research reports on CBD, it makes sense to investigate the relationship between CBD and aging and to examine specific age-related disorders and illnesses of the body and brain.

As a gerontologist, I have always been concerned with more than diseases and disorders related to aging. More so, I have been most interested in quality of life and wellness as we age. Having the ability to live independently, have one's mind intact, be in generally good health, have significant people in our lives, and have relative financial security are all important. Beyond these factors, living a meaningful life that is driven by purpose can lead to great satisfaction as we age. How is CBD related to any of this? I do not propose that CBD is a cure-all. Instead, I see it as a natural alternative that may help with a number of conditions, both physical and emotional, and with some assistance from nature, we may be able to maximize what we do, how long we do it and in essence, enhance our quality of life. When it comes to aging, it's not necessarily *what* you can do—it's *how long* you can do it.

We are all aging, and as we do, we will experience normal functions of the body and brain that naturally slow down or stop altogether. People will experience changes and losses in the senses such as eyesight, hearing, and taste. Changes take place in our muscles and bones. As we age, we also become more vulnerable to psychological issues like depression and anxiety. Some of us will develop sleep problems. According to the World Health Organization (WHO), around 20% of individuals sixty years of age and older will develop a neurological or psychological disorder. The most common will be depression, dementia, and anxiety.[1]

Our doctors may prescribe psychotropic medications including antidepressants, anti-anxiety drugs, and sleeping pills. Some people may do very well on prescription medications, and others may not. Some medications will cause unpleasant side effects, and others will be dangerous for the aging body and brain. Some medications cause death. It has been estimated that between 11.5% to

62.5% of older adults use medications inappropriately and are taking a minimum or one or two medications that are not needed at all.[2] It is well known that seniors are particularly vulnerable to adverse drug events or negative side effects of many medications, including those for psychological problems. Older adults may have multiple disorders, take a high number of medications, forget to take their medications, and miscalculate doses. This is one very good reason to find a safe and natural alternative to prescription drugs for seniors.

A Brief Introduction to the Study of Aging

I began studying aging in college in the 1980s, and we have come a long way in the science of aging since then. "Frailty" is now considered a major area of study and "refers to a state of increased risk compared with others of the same age."[3] Frailty is related to aging and the risk of adverse health outcomes (e.g., Alzheimer's, Parkinson's, arthritis) that occur with advanced age. As we age, we simply have less ability to fight back the many illnesses and disorders that might develop along the way. Our repair processes are less efficient as well, as evidenced by the time it takes elderly people to recover after injury or surgery. I wish that as we aged, we would have to deal with only one illness. The truth of the matter is that as we age, it's not that any given illness becomes more common—*all* illnesses become more prevalent with the aging process.

Over the past few decades, many specialized fields in the study of aging have developed, including gerontology, geriatrics, geropsychiatry, and geroscience. Briefly, gerontology is the scientific study of the aging process and old age and is one of my specialty areas. It examines age-specific social, economic, and health-related problems of aging. Geriatrics, on the other hand, is a specialized branch of medicine and social science dealing with health concerns associated with aging and caring for older adults. Gerospsychiatry is a subspecialty in psychiatry that deals with the study and treatment of various mental and emotional disorders among elderly individuals. I spent seven wonderful years managing a group of geropsychiatrists, working side by side with them, performing psychological tests, and assisting with medication reviews. And lastly, geroscience is a new and exciting field in the study of aging that combines the biology of diseases (e.g., heart disease, cancer, Alzheimer's disease) with the biology of aging (e.g., inflammation, genetics, stress response, cellular damage). This makes a lot of sense since there is a close relationship between aging biology and the risk for age-related chronic illnesses. Geroscience strives to understand the relationship between aging and age-related disorders and disabilities. The goal of any treatment must involve the management of multiple illnesses, frailty, and psychosocial problems, as they are all more common with aging. One of the many questions I strive to answer in this book is this: *Can CBD be an effective form of treatment by itself or as an adjunct alongside other interventions?* Keep reading to find out!

Aging Then and Aging Now

Bob Dylan wrote "The Times They Are A-Changin'" in 1964, one year before I was born. Mr. Dylan was right then and is even more correct now. Decades ago, the most common cause of death in the United States was due to infectious diseases like pneumonia and tuberculosis. Americans were lucky to make it into their forties or fifties in the 1800s and 1900s. Many infants and children died and never made it to adulthood. The Industrial Revolution brought better living conditions, increased food distribution, improved hygiene, pasteurization, and vaccination.

In the second half of the twentieth century, life expectancy increased dramatically due to improvements in sanitation, food safety, and medicine. This began the "graying" of the United States population, and this trend has continued. We no longer die of infectious diseases as often as chronic, long-lasting illnesses like cardiovascular disease, cancer, Alzheimer's disease, and diabetes. While the elderly population is growing, it is the oldest of the old—the eighty-five-plus population—that is growing the fastest. There is also a boom in the number of centenarians in the United States and around the postindustrialized world, as well as an increase in "supercentenarians," or those living to 110 years or older.

Most of us will live well into our senior years, but with this comes the risk for developing chronic diseases that are related to the aging process. Such diseases include atherosclerosis, diabetes, and kidney disease, and if we live long enough, we run the risk of developing Alzheimer's disease and other neurodegenerative disorders. Some researchers believe that the maximum human life span for women is 120, and for men it is 113. Do you remember Jeanne Calment, the French woman who in died in 1997 at the age of 122? Look it up. It's true!

Leading Causes of Death

Let's quickly take a look at some of the leading causes of death to get a better picture of how far we've come in terms of longevity and aging. Heart disease is currently still the number one cause of death, but it is on the decline due to wonderful advances in rapid cardiac catheterization, coronary artery bypass graft surgery, rapid anticoagulation of stroke victims, new drugs, fewer people smoking, and healthier behaviors.

Cancer is the second cause of death but is expected to become the leading cause of death within the next few years, not only in the United States but also in many developed nations worldwide. While overall mortality from cancer is expected to increase, there should be a decrease in deaths from malignant diseases. This is due to advancements in genome sequencing, tumor cell genome sequencing, virus therapy that will target and kill specific tumor cells, and micro-RNA whose dysregulation is implicated in the development of many cancers. These may all be used to treat cancer in the near future.

Lung disease is the third leading cause of death and has surpassed stroke, which until recently, was the third leading cause of death. While smoking has declined significantly over the past forty years, the popularity of electronic cigarettes and legalization of marijuana raise many questions about the rise of lung disease again in the United States. It seems like we did away with one problem, only to see a new issue cause another health problem. It is not clear how these will impact chronic obstructive pulmonary disease or COPD.

Alzheimer's disease is the sixth leading cause of dementia-related death, but two other dementias, Lewy body dementia and frontotemporal dementia, are becoming more common. Until a drug is developed that will either prevent dementia, slow down the progress of deterioration, or cure it altogether, there is great urgency to find a treatment that will make life easier while living with Alzheimer's or Lewy body or frontotemporal dementias. It is truly upsetting to know that billions of dollars have been spent searching for drugs that can help, and nothing has yet been found.

Coming in at number seven is diabetes. Some researchers believe that many people are prediabetic and don't know. People who are prediabetic may benefit from diet control and exercise. Obesity is a major problem in the United States and is the biggest risk factor for developing type 2 diabetes. Unfortunately, until the obesity crisis is effectively dealt with in our population, diabetes will continue to be a problem in the future.

Other significant causes of death include stroke, accidents, kidney disease, influenza, pneumonia, and suicide. Among the infectious diseases, some experts fear the potential for massive viral epidemics from mutations in influenza, Middle East respiratory syndrome coronavirus (MERS-CoV), Ebola, and Marburg viruses. We have all seen the devastation that epidemics and pandemics can bring, as evidenced recently by COVID-19.

Longevity and Healthy Aging

We are living longer than ever before, and while there has been an increase in life expectancy, scientists have become more focused on "health expectancy" in life later. In other words, you may live to be ninety but start to become ill in your late seventies and experience loss in quality of life. Although we may live longer, can we have good quality to life and health? Life expectancy simply does not equate to health. It is therefore important to continue seeking medicines and natural supplements that can not only keep us alive longer but also improve our health while we are alive. This is another reason I wrote this book. I believe that CBD may be a key that unlocks better health and wellness, particularly in our later years.

There is an old joke that goes like this: "Aging is inevitable, but maturing is optional." Let's stay as physically healthy and youthful in mind and spirit as we age. Lifestyle matters. To achieve longevity and healthy aging, smoking is simply not beneficial for any reason whatsoever. It is related to a wide range of health problems, including lung disease, heart disease, a number of cancers, and death. Maintaining a healthy weight for your body frame is just as important to longevity and healthy aging. Exercise, strength training, and balance might prevent falls in the future. Maintaining an active social lifestyle, living with purpose and meaning, being a part of your community, volunteering, and engaging in spiritual practices can all help us age with grace and vitality.

I'd like to make it clear at this point of the book that as a gerontologist, I firmly believe that living a long and healthy life takes some work and may not come easily to everyone. I should add that having some resources (e.g., savings, investments, low debt, the ability to enjoy hobbies and travel) are important pieces of the aging puzzle. It is also critical for me to stress that CBD is not a cure-all; as a matter of fact, I'm not sure it cures anything at all. But, according to over three thousand studies and counting, cannabidiol does appear to have some benefits for a number of illnesses and disorders. What you're about to read is a scientific overview of the many health benefits of CBD.

CBD and Older Adults

I hear more and more that older adults are trying CBD products of all kinds—tincture, gel capsules, gummies, and topical creams and salves—for a number of physical and emotional issues. They are incorporating these products into their everyday routines, much like taking vitamins or supplements. It is important to stress that cannabidiol is just that—a nutritional supplement that can be taken every day. In a recent issue of *Forbes* magazine, it was reported that seniors take CBD, primarily oil-based tinctures, to help with pain, improve sleep, reduce anxiety, relieve stress, improve mood and cognitive functioning, increase appetite, and lower blood pressure. Of those who tried CBD, over 65% reported positive results. Most of these adults said they would recommend CBD to friends and family for health-related problems.[4] Most seniors have not tried CBD, so we'll have to see what happens in the future, but for now it seems that CBD could be a safe and effective supplement for them.

CBD and Anti-Aging

Growing old is a natural part of the life course and is mainly a biological process. Intrinsic and extrinsic aging are behind age-related changes that take place in our bodies and brains. Let's use the skin as an example of an age-associated change. The signs of aging are all over our bodies. The skin is our largest organ and goes through many changes. It becomes less firm, has a greater number of lines and wrinkles over time, and produces less collagen beginning after our twentieth birthdays. Our skin becomes thinner and more delicate and is increasingly vulnerable to tears, bruising, and tissue damage. Oil glands in the skin don't function at capacity, and the skin becomes drier. Elastin levels decrease, and the skin becomes less efficient at healing itself. All of these changes in the skin are examples of intrinsic aging. Slowly and over time, the skin changes and ages due to age-related biological processes.

Extrinsic aging, on the other hand, involves environmental conditions and factors such as pollution, exposure to the sun, and lifestyles choices like smoking that affect how the skin ages and appears. These factors add to the loss of both elastin and collagen, which in turn leads to more wrinkles, deep lines, marks on the skin, fragility, and sunspots. Experts believe that extrinsic aging is responsible for 90% of how the skin ages. I have mentioned that CBD is a powerful antioxidant, but it may actually be more powerful than both vitamins C and E. Antioxidants are important for many reasons, but they may, in fact, slow down the aging process by reducing free radicals and their damage to the skin. Collagen, for instance, breaks down faster due to free radicals. Antioxidants slow down the process of collagen loss, which helps our skin look younger, even at older ages.

The endocannabinoid system is active in sebaceous glands, which excrete oil in the skin. It appears that endocannabinoids are responsible for the production of oil, so it may actually help our skin with dryness, psoriasis, or eczema. CBD also has anti-inflammatory properties that help the skin to relax. This can make lines and wrinkles less apparent. All of this, if you stop and think about it, is nothing new. Humans have used plants as natural treatments for centuries. Even Cleopatra used hemp oil as a natural beauty product!

5

CBD and Arthritis, Cancer, Cardiovascular Disease, Diabetes, Endocrine Disorders, Fibromyalgia, and Gastrointestinal Disorders

The part can never be well unless the whole is well.

—Plato

Introduction
This chapter is dedicated to presenting as many research-based findings as I have discovered in the scientific literature. I have tried to review some of the most common diseases and disorders and provide you with an overview, traditional treatments currently used, and research findings for each disorder. There will be some diseases that won't be in this chapter. The reason for that is I couldn't find any research on those specific illnesses. Some sections will be longer and will contain more detail than others; this is related to how much information I could find in the literature.

In an attempt to organize the information in this and some of the following chapters, I have created sections for each disease or disorder. In each area, you will find an introduction, an overview of the disease, a review of traditional therapies and treatments, research findings between cannabidiol and each disease, and finally, a summary of the previous sections. My goal is to provide as many facts as possible, provide some treatment options other than CBD, and provide research findings that many people will not search for; in doing so, I hope to create a better flow of content as you read on. Some of the language will be a bit technical, particularly in the "Research Findings" sections of this and the following five chapters.

Arthritis

Introduction
Inflammation—Can't live with it; can't live without it. On one hand, inflammation is a natural and necessary response to injury, so it is required to heal the body. When the body encounters an unwelcome invader, exposure to environmental toxins, or simply impaired or injured cells, inflammation responds to begin the healing process. On the other hand, if it persists chronically, it can lead to a variety of diseases and disorders, including asthma, rheumatoid arthritis, lupus, multiple sclerosis, psoriasis, diabetes, and inflammatory bowel syndrome (IBS).

Overview of Arthritis
"Arthritis" refers to the acute or chronic inflammation of one or more joints causing pain and discomfort. According to the Arthritis Foundation, there are currently over one hundred known types of arthritis. Regardless of the type of arthritis, they all share similar symptoms in common, including pain and swelling in the tissues surrounding the joints, stiffness, decreased range of motion, and structural changes of the joints. Arthritis can attack any joint in the body. Some individuals may experience symptom severity that can range from mild to severe, and even debilitating at times. The worst outcomes associated with any arthritic condition, besides pain, include a reduction in activity as

well as a reduced quality of life. In fact, there are plenty of cases in which the pain experienced by arthritis sufferers is life changing.

Arthritis is an extremely common condition, affecting almost fifty-five million adults and three hundred thousand children in the United States. It has become a leading cause of disability in the United States, and the disease does not discriminate who it affects. People of all ages, genders, and races are diagnosed with some form of arthritis. It is well known that arthritis is an age-related disease, meaning that risk for developing it increases as we get older. Arthritis can be a major burden to older adults, due to the combination of pain and functional impairment it presents. Many adults report that arthritis limits their ability to work or engage in leisure activities.

There are two major types of arthritis: osteoarthritis and rheumatoid arthritis. The most common type of arthritis is osteoarthritis, which is a degenerative joint disease that develops due to the wearing down of protective cartilage on the ends of our bones. It is known as the "wear-and-tear" type of arthritis. Some experts describe it as a multifactorial joint disease, which includes joint degeneration, recurrent inflammation, and peripheral neuropathy. Osteoarthritis of the knees is one of the top five leading causes of disability among older adults.

Rheumatoid arthritis is another common type of arthritis. This develops as the body's immune system erroneously attacks healthy cells, including the synovium that lines the joints. This type of arthritis can occur at any time throughout life, from early childhood to much later. Women are three times more likely to develop rheumatoid arthritis than their male counterparts. Women may develop rheumatoid arthritis between the ages of thirty to sixty, while men typically develop it later in life. Around 1.5 million people in the United States have this type of arthritis.

Other types of arthritis include gout, caused by a buildup of uric acid; juvenile arthritis, which develops earlier in life; psoriatic arthritis, which affects individuals who have psoriasis; and infectious arthritis, which is caused by infection that spreads to joints. Currently, there are no cures for any of the arthritic diseases, and individuals must engage in self-care to manage their symptoms. Some types of arthritis may have a genetic basis and be passed from parents to children.

Traditional Therapies for Arthritis

Very practical interventions for arthritis include healthy eating, regular exercise, and weight loss. Seeing a chiropractor, getting regular massage therapy, swimming, and the use of medications may also help with symptoms. The most commonly used medications include analgesics, which help to reduce pain but have no effect on the inflammation causing it. Some may be over-the-counter, like Tylenol, while others may require a prescription like the opioid OxyContin. It is widely known that opioids carry a high risk for abuse, misuse, and addiction. Another class of medications used are the nonsteroidal anti-inflammatory drugs, or NSAIDS. These help to reduce pain as well as inflammation. These medications carry risks and side effects, including stomach irritation and the risk for heart attack or stroke. Many experts agree that long-term use is not advisable due to the adverse cardiovascular and gastrointestinal issues they cause, and because the more they are used, the less effective they continue to be. This isn't new information. In 1999 it was stated that "each year 41,000 older adults are hospitalized, and 3,300 of them die from ulcers caused by NSAIDs. Thousands of younger adults are hospitalized."[1]

Other treatments include counterirritants, which are topical products that contain menthol or capsaicin, the natural ingredient that makes hot peppers spicy. Disease-modifying antirheumatic drugs, or DMARDs, are used to treat rheumatoid arthritis and slow or stop the immune system from attacking the joints. Examples of these drugs are Trexall and Plaquenil. Biologic response modifiers are usually prescribed in addition to DMARDs and are genetically engineered medicines that target various protein molecules involved in the immune response. Examples are Enbrel and Remicade. Commonly used medications also include corticosteroids like prednisone and cortisone. These reduce inflammation while suppressing the immune system.

Beyond medications, physical therapy can be helpful in reducing pain and discomfort and help keep the body moving as much as possible. Therapy might focus on range of motion and strengthening muscles around joints. Devices like splints or braces may be recommended by the physical therapist.

In some cases, when medication and therapy are no longer effective, surgery may be necessary. Various types of surgeries for arthritis include joint repair, joint replacement, or joint fusion, depending upon the severity of the disease and how disabled the individual has become. But what about the potential effectives of CBD for arthritis?

Research Findings on CBD and Arthritis

We know that arthritis is a disease of inflammation, and CBD is an anti-inflammatory agent. Studies have shown CBD to reduce inflammation and prevent joint damage. CBD may be effective in reducing pain, discomfort, stiffness, and swelling. Let's examine what research has found.

In a preclinical or animal trial, CBD was shown to block the progression of arthritis. The same study found that CBD protected joints against serious damage and offered a powerful anti-arthritic effect.[2] Another study found that CBD has both powerful anti-inflammatory and immunosuppressive effects on joint damage in osteoarthritic mice.[3] You may be asking, "How does CBD produce these kinds of positive results on arthritis?" The answer is this: CBD activates the two main cannabinoid receptors we discussed earlier in the book—CB1 and CB2—both part of the endocannabinoid system. These two receptors regulate the release of neurotransmitters and immune cells in the central nervous system that work at reducing pain.[4] One study showed that by CBD activating the CB1 receptor, lab rats experienced a reduction in pain in osteoarthritic knees.[5] I don't think lab rats are able to lie or fake recovery! Another study looked at the quality of sleep once pain was controlled by the artificial cannabinoid Sativex.[6] Some researchers come right out and say that the endocannabinoid system is intimately involved in reducing pain and inflammation associated with arthritis.[7]

It has been stated in the literature for quite some time that cannabinoids had positive outcomes on pain, cancer, and multiple sclerosis as well as rheumatoid arthritis. A 2018 study showed that cannabinoids had potential benefits in treating rheumatic diseases in general and specifically rheumatoid arthritis.[8] In 2017, a government sponsored committee in the United States concluded that "there is substantial evidence supporting cannabis' ability to reduce chronic pain."[9] Another group of researchers agrees that cannabinoids might be an appropriate treatment for rheumatoid arthritis and found that cannabinoids reduce pain by activating central and peripheral CB1 and CB2 receptors as well as CBD-sensitive noncannabinoid receptor targets.[10] One study concludes the following: "Local CBD administration inhibited pain and peripheral sensation in established OA [osteoarthritis]" and "CBD may be a safe therapeutic to treat OA pain locally as well as block the acute inflammatory flares that drive disease progression and joint neuropathy."[11]

Summary

Arthritis is a group of over one hundred diseases that cause mild to debilitating pain and sometimes a change in lifestyle and diminishment in quality of life. Men and women at almost any age can be diagnosed with an arthritic disorder, but the vast majority of cases are age related. While there are many things an individual can do to help with pain and discomfort, including therapy and dietary changes, medications used for arthritis come with various side effects, some being very dangerous. Numerous studies have been performed on animals, mainly mice or rats, and some on humans. Most show some level of positive outcome. Can CBD and other cannabinoids be used to prevent or successfully treat arthritic disorders?

Cancer

Introduction

It seems that we all know someone in our family, in our circle of friends, or perhaps a colleague or coworker who currently has cancer, or who has passed away from some form of it. My wife's sister, Minerva, was diagnosed with an aggressive form of colon cancer, and after a trip to the hospital for stomach pain, she was diagnosed with stage 4 colon cancer and was given roughly a year to live. At the time, she was married with two very young daughters. She received traditional chemotherapy, and after receiving little to no benefit from it, she sought out alternative medicine. Once that option yielded no positive outcomes, she returned home with her family until her last breath on one cold February morning. My wife, Anabel, regrets that she wasn't aware that either medical cannabis or cannabidiol may have provided relief for many of her cancer-related symptoms, including her lack of appetite and pain. To this day, Anabel says that if she knew then what she knows now about cannabis, she would have found it and provided it to her sister. I know my wife's story isn't the only one like this. We all share a common bond around cancer and those lives that it takes from us. Because of experiences like Minerva's, shouldn't we strive for more remedies for people's pain and suffering?

Overview of Cancer

The term "cancer" encompasses many diseases in which abnormal cells divide uncontrollably and invade and destroy body tissue. These cells grow abnormally and then have the capability to spread through the blood and lymph system to other parts of the body. While there are actually over one hundred types of cancer, some of the more common ones include carcinoma (skin cancer), sarcoma (bone, cartilage, blood vessels), leukemia (bone marrow), lymphoma and multiple myeloma (immune system), and central nervous system cancer that begins in the tissues of the brain and spinal cord. Lung, breast, prostate, and colon/rectal cancers are also common in the Western world.

Today, cancer is ranked as one of the leading causes of death around the world. Each year, over twelve million people learn that they have cancer, and seven million die. In the United States, it has been estimated that over three hundred thousand lives could be saved annually if lifestyle changes were made like quitting smoking, eating healthier diets, and exercising regularly.

Traditional Therapies for Cancer

Everyday practices may help to manage symptoms of cancer including exercise, massage, meditation and stress management, music therapy, tai chi, and yoga. Most cancer patients will try a number of things that might help to preserve their quality of life. Nobody wants to suffer. Trying these techniques can make the individual feel they have some control over their disease and help them physically and emotionally. It is always important to work with your doctor when adding any new regimen.

Some people gain benefits from acupuncture, such as relief from nausea and pain. Aromatherapy may be helpful to provide calming effects and stress reduction. Hypnosis may be an alternative for some people and can be helpful in controlling breathing, pain, stress, and anxiety. It can also help to prevent anticipatory nausea and vomiting. There are also various relaxation techniques that can be helpful, including visualization exercises and progressive muscle relaxation. Some of these techniques work well together.

Cancer treatments include surgery, medications, radiation therapy, and chemotherapy and are used to shrink tumors, stop the progression of cancer, or cure it altogether. The goal of any treatment is to allow the individual to live symptom free for as long as possible and return to their previous quality of life. The type of treatment depends largely on the type of cancer and how severe it has become. It is important to note that cancer researchers are seeking new ways to cure or at the very least abate cancer for as long as possible. Because you or someone you know has a cancer-related diagnosis, it is not the end of the fight. Actually, it's only the beginning.

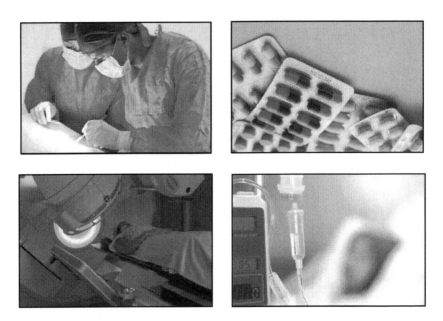

Current traditional treatments for cancer: Surgery, medication, radiation, and chemotherapy

In general, there are three main categories of treatment for cancer: primary, adjuvant, and palliative. The goal of primary treatment is to completely clear cancer from an individual's body and to make sure all cancer cells have been destroyed. The most common forms of primary treatment are surgery and chemotherapy. Adjuvant treatment aims to kill any remaining cancer cells after primary treatment is completed. Examples include chemotherapy, radiation therapy, and hormone therapy. Palliative treatment attempts to relieve any pain or discomfort associated with cancer or the side effects from the treatment itself. Medications are commonly used in the palliative treatment of cancer.

As stated earlier in this book, cancer will surpass heart disease and become the leading cause of death in the United States within a few short years. Surgery, chemotherapy (the use of drugs to destroy cancer cells), radiation therapy (the use of x-rays or protons to kill cancer cells), bone marrow transplants, immunotherapy (a.k.a. biological therapy; using the body's immune system to fight cancer), hormone therapy (removing or blocking hormones that fuel cancer cells in certain types of cancer like breast and prostate cancer), targeted drug therapy (focusing on specific abnormalities in cancer cells that allow them to survive), cryoblation (using cold to freeze and kill cancer cells), radiofrequency ablation (using electrical energy to heat cancer cells and kill them), and clinical trials (taking part in studies to investigate new ways to destroy cancer cells) are all options, but they can be rather intense and come with mild to serious side effects.

The lists of drugs for specific types of cancer and for conditions related to cancer are far too long to cover in this book. The National Cancer Institute provides comprehensive lists for both cancers and cancer-related conditions. Some individuals will be prescribed several types of medications. Various conditions that occur with cancer are anemia, cardiac problems, constipation, bleeding in the bladder, high blood calcium, nausea and vomiting, loss of bone density, kidney problems, and dry mouth.

Research Findings on CBD and Cancer
Cannabinoids have been used for palliative effects for quite some time. They have shown varying degrees of benefit for symptoms, including nausea, vomiting, appetite, sleep, pain, and mood. Research shows cannabinoids to possess antitumor properties, inhibit growth of new cancer cells, and prevent of metastases. Some studies have demonstrated the regression of different types of

cancer. A landmark study in 1975 demonstrated that cannabinoids inhibited malignant tumor growth in thin tissue in mice.[12]

According to the Cannabis Health Index (CHI), cannabinoids may be helpful for symptoms of bone, bladder, and nonmelanoma skin cancer.[13] It also shows moderate benefits in cases of brain and kidney cancer. According to the CHI, other cancers and their related health issues that may be assisted by cannabinoids are breast cancer, cervical cancer, colon cancer, gastric cancer, leukemia, liver and lung cancer, lymphoma, pancreatic cancer, prostate cancer, skin cancer (melanoma), and thyroid cancer. An in-vitro study showed that cannabidiol induces programmed cell death in breast cancer cells.[14] Another study showed that CBD had a "chemoprotective effect" in a mouse model of colon cancer.[15]

The activation of cannabinoid receptors CB1 and CB2 might impair cancer development, and endocannabinoid signaling can stop the formation of tumors. This occurs when endocannabinoid-degrading enzymes increase in cancer cells and tumors, leading to a decrease in tumor growth. This has been shown in a study examining pancreatic lesions in a mouse colon[16] and prostate cancer cells.[17] One study found that CBD is effective is stopping the spread of new cancer cells.[18] Another study reported that CBD may actually prevent cancer caused by smoking tobacco products. This type of cancer is linked to the protein cytochrome P450, which is harmless in low levels but dangerous in elevated amounts. CBD was shown to bind to cytochrome P450 and stop it from increasing to higher levels.[19] Researchers have shown that cannabinoids induce the process of autophagy in specific cancer lines, including glioma (brain), melanoma (skin), hepatic (liver), and pancreatic cancer.[20, 21, 22]

Pancreatic cancer is one of the most feared cancers because it carries a five-year survival rate of less than 5%, making it one of the deadliest cancers of our time. Lung cancer is also very common and is a leading cause of death in the United States. One study showed that combining cannabinoids and radiation treatments proved effective in treating pancreatic and lung cancers. In-vitro (test tube, culture dish) studies confirmed greater effective tumor cell killing when CBD is combined with radiation therapy. In-vivo (within a living organism) studies revealed major increases in survival when smart biomaterials (materials designed to be sensitive to specific stimuli, like a tumor microenvironment) are used to deliver CBD directly to tumor cells.[23] Another study showed effective results when cannabinoids were synergistically used with radiation therapy for brain tumors.[24]

According to Leinow and Birnbaum, "cannabinoids are known to have palliative effects in oncology, including relief of chemotherapy-related nausea and vomiting, appetite stimulation, pain relief, mood elevation, and sleep in cancer patients."[25] Currently, two FDA-approved drugs that are cannabinoid-based are dronabinol (Marinol) and nabilone. They are prescribed for appetite stimulation, chemotherapy-induced nausea and vomiting, and sleep apnea. The national Comprehensive Cancer Network Guidelines recommend cannabinoids as a "breakthrough" treatment for chemotherapy-induced nausea and vomiting.[26] The American Society for Clinical Oncology (ASCO) antiemetic guidelines recommend that dronabinol or nabilone be prescribed for nausea and vomiting that might be resistant to other antiemetic medications.[27]

Summary

It has been a well-known fact that cannabinoids offer relief of many cancer-related symptoms including pain, nausea, and poor appetite. Cannabinoids work by inhibiting the spread of cancer cells and promoting autophagy (when cells remove unnecessary or dysfunctional components; the degradation or recycling of cellular components) and apoptosis (normal death of cells). They also have shown the ability to inhibit the development of new blood vessels that would feed a cancerous growth and stop metastasis or the secondary malignant growth of a primary site of cancer.

It has been shown that cannabidiol has antitumor effects and antiemetic effects, helps with appetite stimulation, relieves pain, helps with anxiety and sleep, and is an anti-inflammatory and antioxidant. Despite what is currently understood about the relationship between cannabinoids and cancer, much is unknown, and we are only in the infant stages of incorporating cannabis-derived products into everyday clinical care. So many questions regarding the best ways to administer cannabinoids, the appropriate dosages for certain conditions, how cannabinoids interact with other medications, and assess negative side effects remain unanswered. Some studies show that combining cannabinoids with traditional treatments like radiation therapy can be effective for treating certain cancers like pancreatic, lung, and brain cancer.

Cardiovascular Disease

A Personal Story

Heart health is very important to me. My father, Jim, was a tall fellow with blue eyes and silver hair. I am not tall; I have brown hair and brown eyes. A running joke in the family was, "Mom, are you sure Dad is my real father?" Turns out, he was. Jim was an electrician and a WWII vet. He had a very stressful career, ate poorly, smoked daily, and was a regular consumer of adult beverages. He ended up having symptoms of a heart attack one weekend back in 1993. We took him to our local hospital, where he was admitted on the cardiac floor. My mother, my sisters, a dear friend, and I were in the family waiting room as we heard on the intercom system, "Code blue, code blue." That was the staff's signal that a heart attack was taking place, and we knew it was Dad. "Code blue" was heard several times that weekend, and finally Dad was taken in for heart surgery, where he lost around 60% or more of his heart muscle.

After surgery, the surgeon came out to speak with us and said that my father would be in a coma or semivegetative state most likely for the remainder of his natural life. He was on life support, and that was the only thing keeping him alive. The doctor also gave us the option of forgoing life support and allowing my father to die naturally, because he simply would never function normally again. In other words, his life, for all practical purposes, was over.

My dad reminded me of the iconic actor John Wayne—tall, strong, and didn't take any shit from anyone. He was in the war, came back to the United States, and became an electrical engineer and a foreman for two large companies that supplied electronics to the automobile industry. He worked with his mind and hands and almost always had a cigarette dangling out of the right corner of his mouth, eyeglasses on the tip of his nose.

My mother was in no emotional condition to make the decision to end life support. They were both looking forward to retirement, and now her husband was going to die. My sisters also found it far too difficult to make the decision. So at the tender age of twenty-one, I told the cardiovascular surgeon, "My dad was like John Wayne. He would not want to live this way," and then made the decision and persuaded my family to pull the plug. Before I did, I told Dad, while he was in a coma and hooked up to machines, wires, and whistles, that it was time for him to go. I promised to take care of Mom for the rest of her life and that he had nothing to worry about. I kissed him on the cheek and said goodbye.

Overview of Cardiovascular Disease
The heart is so small, about the size of a fist, compared to the big things it does for the body and brain. It has four chambers that regulate how blood moves throughout our body. It beats around seventy times a minute and one hundred thousand times a day. It feeds around one trillion cells and gets its own nourishment from three coronary arteries. The human heart is a magnificent and miraculous machine. Despite this, the heart is also vulnerable and fragile. When one of the coronary arteries becomes blocked—for instance, by a blood clot—or when it gradually narrows due to a buildup of plaques, like in the case of atherosclerosis, the heart begins to feel pressure and pain. If the pain is ignored and nothing is done, tissue death can occur and lead to myocardial infarction or heart attack.

The heart is also vulnerable to a whole host of factors, including high blood pressure; high blood cholesterol levels; obesity and a poor diet; maintaining a stressful lifestyle (especially chronic stress); a buildup of toxins such as lead or mercury; metabolic syndrome or insulin resistance; street drugs like cocaine, crack, and methamphetamines; prescription medications; mineral imbalances; and degeneration from overexposure to free radicals. Each one of these threats has a common denominator: a lack of oxygen. Our heart cannot thrive or survive without oxygen, and each of these threats decreases or eliminates oxygen from the heart, causing damage or death.

Age is the leading risk factor for heart disease, but there are plenty more. Gender is a factor, and men are at greater risk for heart disease than are women. Your family history can be a risk factor for many reasons, including genetics, lifestyle, and learned behavior. Smoking is a heart killer. Nicotine constricts the blood vessels, and carbon monoxide damages the inner lining of the vessels. People who smoke regularly have an increased risk for heart disease and heart attack. Diabetes, lack of physical activity, certain types of chemotherapy drugs and radiation drugs for cancer, and poor hygiene can all lead to heart problems.

I use "heart disease" to encompass multiple conditions of the heart. It's a catchall term that includes coronary artery disease, which is caused by atherosclerosis (heart disease of the blood vessels), heart arrhythmias (abnormal heart beats), congenital heart defects that one may have been born with, dilated cardiomyopathy or weakened heart muscle, endocarditis or heart infections, and valvular heart disease. In a 2018 article, the *Journal of the American Heart Association* reported that a total of 92.1 million US citizens currently have one or more forms of cardiovascular disease and predict that the numbers will only increase to 43.9% of the US population by the year 2030.[28]

Around 24% of people in the United States have hypertension or high blood pressure.[29] There is no cure for this disorder of the heart, and science still does not have a clear understanding of how hypertension begins. What is known is that it can range from being damaging to deadly and can lead to other complications like stroke, heart attack, blindness, kidney failure, and brain aneurisms. Currently, normal blood pressure is 120/80, but optimal pressure is not so clearly defined. In other words, some people run higher or lower numbers and are quite healthy and happy.

A stroke is another form of heart disease and is also known as cerebrovascular accident or CVA. It literally means a loss of brain function. The two types of stroke are ischemic and hemorrhagic. In an ischemic stroke, some type of obstruction like a thrombosis or embolism prevents blood from reaching brain cells. It blocks the necessary supply of oxygen and can cause either tissue damage or death. A hemorrhagic stroke is the result of a ruptured blood vessel causing a leakage of blood. A stroke can, depending upon the size and location, cause loss of certain brain functions that may be limiting and self-correcting, as in a transient ischemic stroke or TIA, or it can cause massive damage, as in a CVA, which may result in a major loss of motor function. The greatest risk factor for stroke is high blood pressure. A stroke taking place in the lower part of the brain, which regulates heartbeat and breathing, can cause instant death. With stroke and other cardiovascular diseases, response time is crucial, and the quicker the person gets medical attention, the better the outcome.

Not long ago, atherosclerosis was considered a disease that develops due to a buildup of plaque, and while this is partially true, it's not the complete picture. The obstruction or plaque is actually a response to injuries inside the arterial wall's lining. Some things that cause injuries inside the wall's lining are high blood pressure, excess presence of homocysteine, and infectious microbes. An interesting relationship exists between atherosclerotic lesions and inflammation. Studies have shown that inflammatory molecules stimulate events that lead to the development of atherosclerotic lesions, making atherosclerosis "nature's Band-Aid" to deal with an injury or inflammation within the arterial wall's lining. If the Band-Aid becomes too thick or breaks off, the tissue becomes oxygen deprived, and strokes or heart attacks are the result. Like other cardiovascular diseases, atherosclerosis takes many years to develop, and the individual may experience few to no symptoms whatsoever.

Traditional Therapies for Cardiovascular Disease

Although heredity plays a part in some of these disorders, there are many things you can do to reduce your risk of developing cardiovascular diseases. We hear about these preventive measures all the time, but it takes commitment to follow through on them. For instance, eating a healthy diet is a good place to start, and remember this—what is healthy for the heart is also healthy for the brain, and what is not good for the heart or brain, either limit or eliminate it! Add more foods high in antioxidants and fiber and those that are heart smart, like dark chocolate, red wine, coconut, garlic, ginger, rosemary, saffron, and turmeric. Many experts suggest a plant-based diet for good heart health. Eat foods low in saturated fats and trans fats, limit salt and sugar intake, and stay away from fast or processed foods as much as possible. I like to make sure I have at least one raw food for each meal.

The "Use it or lose it" theory is appropriate for heart health. Incorporate some regular physical activity into your daily or weekly routine. You don't have to run a marathon, but taking a brisk walk three times a week reduces your risk for heart disease. It helps to maintain a healthy weight and can lower blood pressure, cholesterol, and sugar levels in the body.

I am a big fan of wine, so much so that I became a sommelier. I can find good health reasons to drink wine, but for the life of me, I find no reasons to smoke. There are absolutely no health benefits to smoking. In fact, smoking tobacco significantly increases your risk for heart disease. If you do smoke, try to stop. I know it's tough, and I am not preaching. I'm not fond of people who preach about such things. If you don't smoke, don't start. Instead, drink wine! And since we're on the topic of wine, drinking in moderation has been shown to be healthy, but overdrinking is not. By "moderation," I am referring to two glasses of wine per day.

If you already have a heart condition, high blood pressure, high cholesterol, or diabetes, there are many things you can do to maintain good health. See your doctor regularly, and be very honest during your visits. What your doctor doesn't know can hurt you. Get your cholesterol and blood pressure checked as often as your doctor recommends. Manage any symptoms of diabetes. Be medication compliant, and follow the regimen your doctor prescribes. And lastly, do your own research, and engage in self-care.

Other options for treating heart disease include CPR, stents, angioplasty, heart bypass surgery, a pacemaker, and as a last resort, a heart transplant. There are numerous medications that can help, including ACE inhibitors, antiarrhythmics, antiplatelet therapy, aspirin therapy, beta-blocker therapy, calcium-channel blocker drugs, clot buster drugs, digoxin, diuretics, nitrates, and blood thinners.

Research Findings on CBD and Cardiovascular Disease
One study in 2010 found that CBD exerts a positive pharmacological impact in ischemic stroke, and CBD can be an effective cerebroprotective agent.[30] An earlier study reported that cannabidiol (CBD) protects against myocardial ischemic reperfusion injury and may become a promising new treatment for myocardial ischemia.[31] A study in 2017 concluded that "preclinical studies show CBD has numerous cardiovascular benefits, including a reduced blood pressure (BP) response to stress."[32] The same study goes on to say that CBD has numerous advantageous effects on the cardiovascular system, including weakening high-glucose-induced, pro-inflammatory changes in coronary artery endothelial cells (cells that line the interior surface of blood vessels).

Researchers in Montreal made some very important discoveries about the effectiveness of the endocannabinoid system and its association with cardiovascular health, especially protecting the heart from damage. They found that endocannabinoid receptors CB1 and CB2 reside inside heart tissue. The internal "cardiac cannabinoid system" is involved in numerous phenomena associated with cardioprotective effects such as reduction in the size of infarct (small, localized area of dead tissue after a heart attack) after induced ischemia (inadequate supply of blood and oxygen to the heart). They also found that cannabinoids exert direct cardioprotective effects both in vivo and in vitro. The researchers conclude by stating, "The endogenous cardia cannabinoid system, through activation of CB2 receptors appears to be an important mechanism of protection against myocardial (heart muscle) ischemia."[33]

A study in 2007 revealed that cannabinoids have a positive effect in terms of cardiac protection, vasodilation, progression of atherosclerosis, inhibition of endothelial inflammation, and the baroreceptor reflex (a mechanism that keeps blood pressure steady) in the control of systolic blood pressure.[34] Two years later, another study showed that CBD calms autonomic responses to stress, like a rapid heartbeat, by interacting with serotonin, which results in a calming effect.[35] The same year, another study showed that CB2 receptors protect ischemic heart cells during angina or heart attack.[36]

It is also important to know that besides studies like these, the US government issued itself a patent (patent 6,630,507) titled, "Cannabinoids as antioxidants and neuroprotectants," which was issued on October 7, 2003, to the United States as represented by the Department of Health and Human Services. The patent finds cannabinoids

> useful in the treatment and prophylaxis of a wide variety of oxidation-associated diseases, such as ischemic, age-related, inflammatory, and autoimmune diseases. Cannabinoids have popular application as neuroprotectants, for example in limiting neurological damage following ischemic insults, such as stroke and trauma, or in the treatment of neurodegenerative diseases, such Alzheimer's disease, Parkinson's disease, and HIV dementia.[37]

It is a baffling question why the US government would patent cannabinoids based on their usefulness in health conditions, yet research on these important molecules and their ability to treat symptoms of disorders could not move forward because of the stigma, politics, legality, and other issues surrounding cannabis and hemp.

An important study by Japanese researchers examined the effects of CBD on stroke-induced rats and found that cannabidiol provides "potent and long-lasting neuroprotection through an anti-inflammatory CB1 receptor-independent mechanism, suggesting that cannabidiol will have a palliative action and open new therapeutic possibilities for treating cerebrovascular disorders."[38] Uwe Blesching, in his book *The Cannabis Index*, believes that if these results can be applied to humans, cannabinoids, and especially CBD, can be used as an effective neuroprotective for persons at risk for stroke and as a medication used after the stroke has taken place.[39]

Summary

Heart disease is the leading causes of death in the United States and carries a heavy personal as well as a financial burden on our health care system. There remains a need to find out exactly how these diseases develop and search for better alternatives for both prevention and treatment. Because the endocannabinoid system is intimately involved with cardiovascular disease, it seems to be a therapeutic target for treating cardiovascular diseases. You can see by reading the results of the studies above that science is taking a serious stand on the effectiveness of CBD and other cannabinoids for heart health. Many experienced researchers believe that CBD may be a promising new treatment for heart diseases. We have seen that CBD in an inflammatory and cardioprotective agent and the endocannabinoid system and cardiovascular system have a unique relationship.

Diabetes

Introduction

Let's start with some interesting information about diabetes. The word *diabetes* is Greek in origin and means "fountain," as in the frequent stream of urine that ancient Greek physicians noted of their patents with this disease. Frequent urination is the body's way of eliminating excess sugar, which ants in ancient Greece seemed to enjoy collecting around for consumption.

Apparently, diabetic urine is sweet due to the high levels of sugar in it. The word *mellitus* is Greek for "honey" and that is where the diagnostic term *diabetes mellitus* comes from.

On a more serious note, millions of people throughout the world have diabetes, and many more are prediabetic. According to the CDC National Diabetes Statistics Report (2017),[40] the percentage of American seniors, either diagnosed or undiagnosed, remains high at twelve million, or 25.2% of the population. Diabetes is the seventh leading cause of death in the United States, and despite this, it may be underreported as a cause of death. Studies have found that only 35% to 40% of people who died with diabetes actually had diabetes listed anywhere on their death certificate, and only 10% to 15% had it listed as an underlying cause of death. There are roughly 1.5 million new cases diagnosed each year, and many people (around 84 million) may be prediabetic and unaware.

It seems like we all know someone with diabetes, and I know of at least five family members or friends who have been diagnosed with the disease. Lives can be changed, lifestyles interrupted, and sometimes quality of life can suffer in a number of ways. Not only is diabetes a difficult disorder to deal with, but it also can lead to other conditions, some of which may already be present. Cardiovascular problems are associated with diabetes, as are kidney disorders, eye disease, ulcers of the legs and feet, nerve damage, and depression.

Overview of Diabetes

Diabetes is a disease in which the body becomes incapable of properly using and storing glucose, which is a form of sugar. Excess glucose backs up in the bloodstream, causing blood glucose or blood sugar to increase at high levels. The pancreas plays a role in diabetes and is an organ that produces hormones like insulin and glucagon and other digestive enzymes that break down the food we eat into basic sugar molecules that provide energy to cells in the body. The pancreas works with two different organ systems, the endocrine system and the exocrine system. The endocrine system includes the hypothalamus, pituitary, thyroid and parathyroid, adrenals, and reproductive organs, which produce hormones that help regulate growth, mood, metabolism, and reproduction. Insulin is an important hormone that helps to regulate blood glucose levels and is produced by the pancreas. It also assists transporting glucose through the blood into other cells in the body.

The exocrine system consists of hormones and glands including the salivary and sweat glands, as well as many glands in the digestive system. This system secretes substances outside of the body, whereas the endocrine system secretes within the body. The exocrine system aids in maintaining body temperature, lubrication, digestion, and reproduction.

There are two major types of diabetes, type 1 and type 2. Type 1 diabetes used to be called "juvenile" diabetes because it occurred earlier in childhood and adolescence. In type 1 diabetes, the body completely stops making insulin, which is necessary for survival because it enables the body to use the glucose in food as a source of energy. People with type 1 diabetes have to take daily shots of insulin to live. Type 2 diabetes, formerly known as "adult-onset" or "insulin-dependent" diabetes, is the most common form of the disease. It is the result of insulin resistance or the body's inability to produce enough or use insulin properly. Another type, gestational diabetes, can occur during pregnancy and usually corrects itself after the baby is born. Hormonal changes during pregnancy may cause a temporary insulin resistance, which leads to higher blood glucose levels.

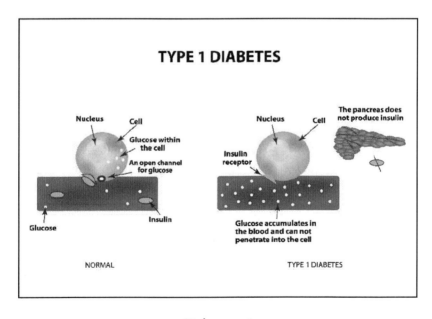

Diabetes type 1

Living Longer and Stronger with CBD

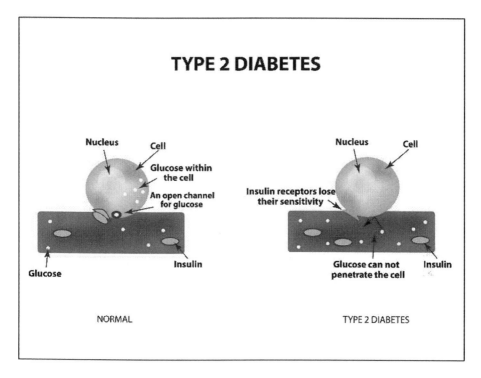

Diabetes type 2

While people who are older than forty and overweight are at a higher risk of developing type 2 diabetes, we are seeing much younger people develop this disease. There is also a genetic component to the disease, and those with close relatives who have diabetes are more likely to develop it. People with high cholesterol or high blood pressure, or who experience physical inactivity, are also at a higher risk. The risk also increases as people age.

In some cases, people have no signs or symptoms of diabetes, especially with type 2. They can live for months and even years without knowing they have the disease. Common symptoms include frequent urination, thirst, sweet-smelling urine, increased hunger, blurry vision, irritability, a tingling sensation in the hands or feet, wounds that don't easily heal, fatigue, and frequent skin, bladder, or gum infections. As the disease progresses, the symptoms become worse and can include heart disease, stroke, sepsis, loss of vision, diabetic coma, kidney problems, skin ulcers, neuropathies, and loss of consciousness.

Traditional Therapies for Diabetes

Today there are many options when it comes to managing diabetes. Let's start by looking at natural or alternative treatments, including herbs and supplements, diet and exercise, and stress management. One of the main goals of managing diabetes is maintaining healthy blood sugar levels. Keep in mind that the FDA doesn't consider herbs and supplements "medicine," and they are not regulated. Always talk with your physician before starting any herbal treatment, along with prescribed medications.

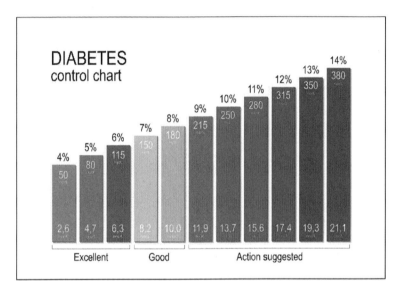

Blood sugar levels

Some people believe in the power of aloe vera for a number of health conditions, including diabetes, due to its ability to lower fasting blood sugar. But be careful! When aloe vera is taken orally, it can have a strong laxative effect! Getting alpha-lipoic acid, an antioxidant, in your diet from spinach, potatoes, and broccoli may be helpful to reduce nerve damage or diabetic neuropathy. Cinnamon is another natural source that seems to improve glucose metabolism, so much so that it is being studied as a potential antidiabetic medication. Cayenne is also being examined as a potential medication for diabetes because of its fat- and sugar-balancing effects.

Researchers conducted a study examining the effects of powered garlic tablets on diabetic type 2 patients and found that garlic improved metabolic control due to lowered blood glucose and triglyceride levels.[41] Garlic helps make glucose and fat metabolism more efficient, which may also contribute to prevention of other related conditions like heart disease. Another preclinical study found that ginger could lower blood glucose, cholesterol, and triglyceride levels.[42]

Other natural sources that may be helpful in managing diabetes include cacao, caraway, clove, cumin, nutmeg, oregano, rosemary, and turmeric. Since some people with low magnesium levels may be more likely to develop diabetes, a diet including whole grains, nuts, and green leafy vegetables may be helpful. Getting omega-3 fatty acids or "good fats" into your diet can also help manage diabetes, including foods like salmon, walnuts, and soybeans.

While eating well is beneficial for everyone, people with diabetes may struggle with other conditions, such as high blood pressure and depression, that can interfere with nutrition. Mind and body techniques can help manage both diabetic symptoms and related problems. Going back to the basics and finding things that reduce stress is a good first step. Aromatherapy, relaxation techniques, meditation, prayer, and exercise may be helpful. Seeking treatments like acupuncture or acupressure may also relieve symptoms and increase well-being.

Beyond diet, exercise, stress management, and other treatments, there are medications that help control diabetic symptoms and improve quality of life. Taking insulin has been shown to be effective in most cases. The medicine will vary according to your type of diabetes and how well it controls blood glucose levels. Several types of insulin are available, and each works at a different speed (onset) and lasts a different amount of time (duration). Each type of insulin reaches a peak in strength and effectiveness and then wears off over a few hours. Methods for taking insulin include pills, needle and syringe, pen, insulin pump, inhaler, injection port, or jet injector.

Research Findings on CBD and Diabetes

Researchers reported in *The American Journal of Pathology* the following:

Oxidative stress and inflammation play critical roles in the development of diabetes and its complications. Recent studies provide compelling evidence that the newly discovered lipid signaling system (i.e., the endocannabinoid system) may significantly influence reactive oxygen species production, inflammation, and subsequent tissue injury, in addition to its well-known metabolic effects and functions. The modulation of the activity of this system holds tremendous therapeutic potential in a wide range of diseases, ranging from cancer, pain, neurodegenerative, and cardiovascular diseases, to obesity and metabolic syndrome, diabetes and diabetic complications.[43]

The same study stresses the importance of the endocannabinoid system and its protective, antidiabetic effects on diabetic cardiovascular dysfunction, neuropathy, retinopathy, and nephropathy. It also reminds us how powerful CBD is as an anti-inflammatory and antioxidant.

One study found that cannabinoids eased diabetic neuropathies or nerve pain,[44] while another found that synthetic cannabinoids may have the ability to grow nerve extensions in a glucose-rich environment.[45] This might actually form a solid basis for a novel neuroprotective drug for diabetes. A group of scientists from Israel showed a link between endocannabinoid receptors and diabetes, suggesting that CBD might have the potential to become a new treatment option for type 1 diabetes.[46]

Summary

Some researchers believe that CBD can be a preventive supplement for improved fasting insulin, cholesterol, and insulin resistance levels. One of the greatest benefits of CBD, then, may be prevention of diabetes in the first place. Various studies show a connection between chronic inflammation and insulin resistance, and we know of CBD's powerful anti-inflammatory benefits. Research also shows that hemp has been linked to smaller waist circumference, lower BMI (body mass index), and decreased obesity levels. CBD may be related to weight management and appetite suppression and might also relieve pain from neuropathy and speed skin healing.

Endocrine Disorders

Introduction
The endocrine system consists of a number of glands including the thyroid, hypothalamus, pituitary, parathyroid, adrenals, pineal body, ovaries, and testes. Each of these glands is responsible for producing and distributing hormones throughout the body, which in turn regulate numerous bodily functions like the ability to turn calories into energy. Maintaining good endocrine health is essential for reducing the risk of certain endocrine disorders like diabetes, thyroid disease, mood disorders, growth disorders, and sexual dysfunctions.

Overview of Endocrine Disorders
Some people express that they are exhausted a lot or all the time and don't know why. Perhaps their endocrine system is not working properly. Some outcomes of a poorly balanced endocrine system are stress, weight gain, and weak bones. Age brings many changes to the endocrine system including a slower metabolism that can lead to weight gain. Hormones also change and can lead to problems like heart disease, diabetes, and osteoporosis. Infections, stress, genetics, and lifestyle can all negatively affect the endocrine system.

According to the American Thyroid Association, over 12% of the population in the United States will develop thyroid disorders sometime in their lives. Twenty million Americans currently have a thyroid disorder, and 60% of them are not aware they have a condition. Women are far more likely to develop thyroid problems. It is still unknown why these disorders begin.[47]

Two forms of thyroid disorders include hyperthyroidism and hypothyroidism. Hyperthyroidism is caused by an overproduction of thyroid hormones and can occur as Graves' disease, toxic adenomas, subacute thyroiditis, and pituitary gland malfunctions or cancerous growths in the thyroid gland. Hypothyroidism, on the other hand, is due to the underproduction of thyroid hormones, which is associated with lower energy levels that many people complain about. The causes of hypothyroidism include Hashimoto's thyroiditis, removal of the thyroid gland, and exposure to excessive amounts of iodine.

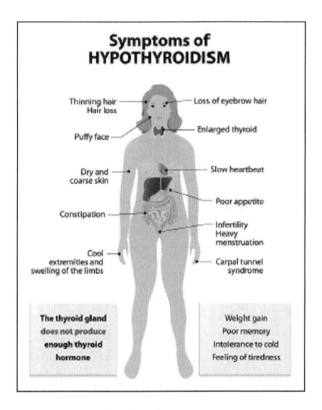

Hypothyroidism symptoms

Mood disorders are associated with endocrine disorders and can be expressed as anxiety or depression. Either one can interfere with normal daily living and quality of life. Some examples of depressive disorders from the fifth edition of the *Diagnostic and Statistical Manual of Mental Disorders*, published by the American Psychiatric Association, include disruptive mood dysregulation disorder; major depressive disorder; dysthymia, or persistent depressive disorder; premenstrual dysphoric disorder; substance- or medication-induced depressive disorder; and depressive disorder due to another medical condition.[48] Some mood conditions may be the result of hormone imbalances.

Growth disorders may also be associated with dysfunction of the endocrine system and can affect both children and adults. Growth disorders among children prevent normal height, weight, sexual maturity, and other conditions. Either very fast or slow growth can be indicative of gland problems.

People who have too much growth hormone may develop a condition called gigantism, and adults may experience acromegaly, a condition which makes one's hands, feet, and face much larger than normal.

Sexual dysfunctions may also be associated with the endocrine system. In particular, the sexual response cycle—excitement (desire and arousal), plateau, orgasm, and resolution—may be interrupted by problems in the endocrine system. Sexual dysfunction is common in both men and women, many of whom may not wish to talk about it. They may have less interest in sex than they used to, have trouble becoming aroused, have problems with orgasm, and experience pain during intercourse.

Traditional Therapies for Endocrine Disorders

There are many options for people seeking treatment of endocrine problems, depending upon the type and severity of the disorder. Medications such as synthetic hormones may be helpful, and in some cases, chemotherapy mat be used to treat a cancerous or noncancerous endocrine gland. Surgery may be necessary to remove both cancerous and noncancerous tumors, and radiation treatment may also resolve endocrine disorders.

There are also plenty of things you can do to manage symptoms of endocrine disorders and stay as healthy as possible. Think about the conditions associated with endocrine dysfunction—diabetes, hyper- and hypothyroidism, mood disorders like anxiety and depression, growth disorders, obesity, and sexual dysfunctions. What would be some of the best ways to handle these conditions? First of all, eating healthily and getting adequate amounts of protein at each meal is important because protein influences the release of hormones that control appetite and food intake. Eating protein reduces the hunger hormone, ghrelin, and stimulates the production of hormones that make you feel full.

Engaging is regular exercise is also important because it can strengthen hormonal health by reducing insulin levels and increasing insulin sensitivity. High insulin levels are associated with inflammation, diabetes, cancer, and heart disease. While you're at it, staying away from too much sugar and too many refined carbohydrates is also a smart move to maintain or improve endocrine health. Sugars increase insulin levels and promote insulin resistance.

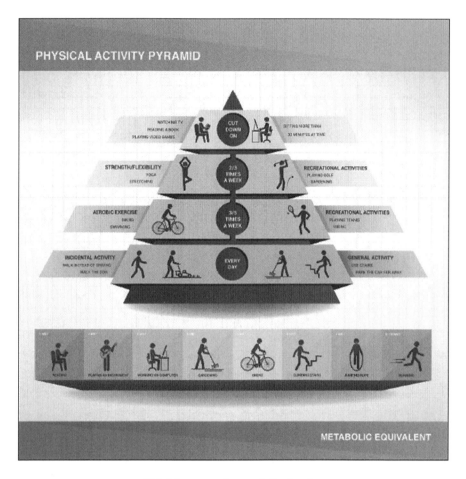

Helpful exercises for metabolic disorders

White bread and foods made with white flour also promote insulin resistance, so try to limit or eliminate them from your diet. Eat healthy fats because they can reduce insulin resistance. Get medium-chain triglycerides (MCTs) in your diet, as they are taken up immediately by the liver and are used as energy. These are found in foods like coconut oil, palm oil, and pure MCT oil. Try not to under- or overeat, because both interfere with insulin levels. Drink green tea for its antioxidant properties and metabolism-boosting caffeine effects. Eat fatty fish to get long-chain omega-3 fatty acids in your diet. These have unique anti-inflammatory effects on the body.

An endocrine-friendly diet should include lots of soluble fiber because it increases insulin sensitivity and stimulates production of hormones that give you that full feeling. It's also smart to stay clear of too many sugary drinks because liquid sugars may be the worst for your health. They contribute to insulin resistance, increase blood sugar levels, and decrease insulin sensitivity, which all contribute to increased belly fat. Don't be afraid to add more eggs to your diet. They affect hormones in a good way by lowering levels of insulin and ghrelin, and they also make you feel full.

Stress management is critical because study after study has shown the relationship between stress and two major hormones: cortisol and adrenaline. Cortisol is the stress hormone that helps us cope with stress, and adrenaline is the "fight or flight" hormone that gives us energy in times of danger. Chronic stress can elevate cortisol to unhealthy levels leading to overeating and obesity and, in particular, belly fat. When adrenaline levels run high for too long, they, too, produce very unhealthy effects on the body and its endocrine system, like high blood pressure, anxiety, and rapid heartbeat. Stress management can reduce levels of cortisol, so engaging in meditation, prayer, yoga, massage therapy, and anything else that relaxes you is good for your endocrine system.

We have all heard about the importance of sleep, and getting consistently good sleep is healthy for overall well-being and endocrine health. On the other hand, poor sleep is associated with hormonal imbalances, in particular, insulin, leptin, cortisol, growth hormone, and ghrelin. Sleep is one of those things that require both quality and quantity, so try to get at least seven solid hours of sleep at night to maintain healthy hormonal balance.

Research Findings on CBD and Endocrine Disorders

Researchers in 2006 found an important relationship between the endocannabinoid system, endocrine regulation, and energy balance. They believed that the endocannabinoid system may possess the ability to restore the endocrine system and restore balance to it. They also reported that cannabinoids affect the secretion of pituitary hormones, and through the endocannabinoid system, hormonal balance and regulation can occur. The use of dietary hemp, or CBD, can be an effective way to boost endocannabinoid signaling, which improves the regulation of the hypothalamic pituitary adrenal (HPA) axis. CBD can also naturally increase endocannabinoid system tone, leading to balance throughout the HPA axis.[49]

A study in 2008 found that endocannabinoids have antitumor affects in the endocrine system and are able to inhibit cell growth, invasion, and metastasis of thyroid, breast, and prostate tumors.[50] In 2011, researchers found that the endocannabinoid system plays an important role in food intake, energy homeostasis, and regulation of the endocrine pancreas. They also reported that pathological overstimulation of the endocannabinoid system can lead to weight gain, glucose intolerance, and reduced sensitivity to insulin. On the other hand, blocking CB1 receptors reduces body weight through increased secretion of anorectic (appetite reducing) signals and improved insulin.[51]

Researchers reported that the endocannabinoid system has been found to interact with peripheral signals, like insulin, leptin, ghrelin, and satiety hormones and affect energy balance and obesity. They also state that dysregulation of the endocannabinoid system can lead to high levels of fats and cholesterol in the blood, glucose intolerance, and obesity.[52] A more recent study confirmed that endogenous cannabinoids participate with the regulation of food intake and energy homeostasis of the body and have a significant impact on the endocrine system. This includes activity of the pituitary gland, adrenal cortex, thyroid gland, pancreas, and gonads. The authors agree that the relationship between the endocannabinoid system and endocrine system may become a therapeutic target for drugs that can treat obesity, diabetes, and prevent diseases of the cardiovascular system.[53]

Summary

The endocrine system consists of many glands that control important functions of the body. When it is healthy, we generally experience no problems, but when it becomes imbalanced, we can experience health problems like diabetes, mood disorders, growth problems, sexual dysfunctions, and thyroid disease. Science is exploring the relationship between the endocannabinoid system and the endocrine system, and so far, it seems that they have an important relationship together. The endocannabinoid system may actually help to maintain health and balance in the endocrine system and reduce the risk of developing diseases and disorders. CBD might play a central role in boosting the endocannabinoid system by regulating food intake and energy balance and preventing proliferation of endocrine cancer cells, all being functions of the endocrine system.

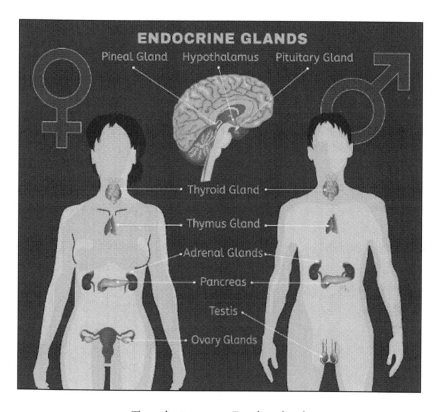

The endocrine system: Female and male

Fibromyalgia

Introduction

Fibromyalgia is a chronic condition characterized by widespread pain that co-occurs with other problems, including sleeping difficulties, fatigue, and depression. This disorder, which affects more women—specifically, middle-aged women—than men can occur at any age and is associated with high rates of disability and decreased quality of life. It is estimated that over three million Americans are affected by fibromyalgia every year. Around 2% of the population (around four million) in the United States[54] suffer from fibromyalgia, roughly between six and twelve million people, and there is no cure.

Overview of Fibromyalgia

Fibromyalgia is a serious condition that causes pain in muscles and connective tissues, especially in highly sensitive pressure points of the body. The disease also causes joint stiffness, weakness, fatigue, insomnia, anxiety, and depression, making it both a physiological and psychiatric condition. There is no specific test to diagnosis fibromyalgia, and it closely resembles other diseases like rheumatoid arthritis and osteoporosis. Diagnosing fibromyalgia becomes a process of ruling out or eliminating other diseases. The key symptoms for a diagnosis include diffuse and chronic pain for three months or longer that exists throughout the entire body, as well as the presence of pain in eleven of eighteen specific trigger pain points (lower neck in front, knee, hip bone, edge of upper breast, et cetera). Other symptoms include fatigue, joint stiffness, tension headaches, pelvic pain, sleeping difficulties, cognitive problems, anxiety, depression, bowel and bladder problems, and migraines.

Risk factors for developing fibromyalgia include genetics, infections, trauma, and psychosocial stress. The pain caused by the disorder may be a function of the brain lowering the pain threshold, which changes the person's perception of pain. It may also originate from receptors and nerves in the body becoming more sensitive to stimulation, which may cause overexaggerated pain. Unfortunately, fibromyalgia is chronic, and most people who are diagnosed will live with it for the rest of their lives.

Traditional Therapies for Fibromyalgia

Since there is no cure for the disorder, treatment focuses on pain management and improving one's quality of life. Like many other health conditions, self-care can make a big difference in one's life. No one will care for you like you can care for yourself. Getting some exercise, especially hydrotherapy, and being mindful of any aches or pains during physical activity is important for general health, and especially for cardiovascular health. Engaging in stress management and relaxation therapies like meditation, prayer, yoga, or deep breathing exercises may help to manage symptoms of pain, anxiety, and depression.

Some people like to join support groups and be with others who have the same condition. They can talk to each other and discover new ways to manage symptoms and find relief. Other will seek help from professionals who practice biofeedback, psychotherapy, counseling, massage therapy, or acupuncture. Chiropractic medicine can also be helpful to reduce pain or discomfort.

Sometimes prescription medication may be necessary, depending upon the severity of symptoms. Nerve pain medications, muscle relaxants, and antidepressants are sometimes prescribed for fibromyalgia. Over-the-counter solutions like analgesics and NSAIDS can be helpful, although they come with negative side effects if used for long periods of time.

Dr. Ethan Russo
Board-certified neurologist and a research pioneer in psychopharmacology. He is the past president of the International Cannabinoid Research Society and former chairman of the International Association for Cannabinoid Medicines.

Research Findings on CBD and Fibromyalgia

The work of Dr. Ethan Russo has made a profound impact in the research world of cannabinoids and health. He believes that some conditions, like fibromyalgia, are the result of an endocannabinoid deficiency and can only be reversed by using cannabis-based or cannabinoid products, like CBD. The analogies that depression is associated with serotonin deficiency, Parkinson's disease is related to dopamine deficiency, and Alzheimer's disease is due to the destruction of acetylcholine is in the same line of thinking with chronic endocannabinoid deficiency. The body simply lacks sufficient amounts of cannabinoids and requires them to boost the endocannabinoid system. It is only then that the body will achieve maximum functioning and equilibrium. We have seen that cannabidiol may help with pain, sleep problems, depression, and anxiety, all coexisting conditions of fibromyalgia.

The Cochrane Library published a document entitled "Cannabinoids for Fibromyalgia (Review)" in 2016.[55] It in, the authors remind us that cannabis has a long history of treating pain and emotional problems. It also points out that current medical treatment provides only modest benefits for the majority of people diagnosed with fibromyalgia, and sometimes the side effects of medications simply outweigh the benefits of taking them. There is a need to seek out and find new alternatives to treat this disorder. The authors state, "The frontal-limbic distribution of cannabinoid receptors in the brain suggests that cannabinoids may preferentially target the affective qualities of pain, believed to have an important contribution to the suffering of people with fibromyalgia." Cannabis has also been shown to reduce inflammation and buffer stress. Some researchers believe that fibromyalgia is a stress-induced disorder, and cannabidiol may be effective at reducing stress as well as pain: "Therefore, taking into consideration the complexity of symptom expression and the absence of an ideal treatment, the potential for manipulation of the cannabinoid system as a therapeutic modality is attractive."

A study in 2018 examining the use of cannabinoids for fibromyalgia stressed that people who experience negative side effects from prescription medications may be less compliant with those medications, which completely defeats the purpose for taking them. Among people taking cannabis for fibromyalgia, 94% reported pain relief and better sleep. In the same study, 85% of people stopped taking other pain medication or reduced the dosage. The authors state, "This reflects the advantage of cannabis over other meds in alleviating pain in addition to its favorable effects on sleep and mood."[56] The same study reported that 81% of people reported improvement in their ability to carry out activities of daily living, and 64% went back to their part- or full-time jobs. An earlier study in 2011 showed that after two hours of cannabis use, people in the study reported a reduction in pain and stiffness, enhanced relaxation, and feelings of general well-being.[57]

Researchers have examined the effects of nabilone, a synthetic cannabinoid, on quality of life and pain associated with fibromyalgia. They concluded that nabilone was beneficial and well tolerated, and improved pain and functionality.[58] Another study found that nabilone was superior to prescription medications concerning insomnia, which is experienced by some people with fibromyalgia.[59] A meta-analysis found that cannabinoids show anti-inflammatory action and reduce pain from inflammation experienced by people with rheumatism, rheumatoid arthritis, chronic neuropathic pain, and fibromyalgia.[60]

Summary

While there are not numerous studies specifically on cannabidiol and fibromyalgia, there is a theory that chronic endocannabinoid deficiency may be behind the disorder, and treating people with CBD may provide relief of the symptoms most associated with fibromyalgia, like pain and depression. Clearly there is a need for more research, but the question remains: Can CBD be a better treatment option than pain medications that have potentially negative side effects? Another question: If CBD works, will people remain compliant and take it regularly because there are few to no side effects? Again, time and more research will hopefully answer these and many other questions.

Gastrointestinal Disorders

Introduction

Millions of people suffer from digestive and gastrointestinal distress every day, and the symptoms range from unpleasant and irritating to painful and life threatening. According to the American Nutrition Association, seventy million people experience symptoms associated with GERD (gastro esophageal disorder), irritable bowel syndrome (IBS), abdominal pain, indigestion, constipation, and diarrhea.[61] Many people live fast-paced lives and don't necessarily eat as healthy as possible. Factors such as getting little to no exercise, eating too much dairy, experiencing stress, overusing laxatives and antibiotics, and eating a diet low in fiber all contribute to these disorders.

Gastrointestinal disorders are very expensive and cost the US economy around $136 billion in 2018. This is a huge amount of money, and when you compare the expenses associated with heart disease ($113 billion), trauma ($103 billion), or mental health ($99 billion), they rank as the most expensive disorders in the United States.[62] The same source reports that abdominal pain is the main symptom for visits to doctors' office, three million hospitalizations occur due to GI problems, eighteen million endoscopic procedures are performed, and the highest risk is for adults between the ages of fifty to seventy-five.

Overview of Gastrointestinal Disorders

The gastrointestinal system is amazingly complicated and is the largest system that exists in the human body. It consists of a collection of organs that break down food into smaller, absorbable nutrients like carbohydrates, proteins, and fats, and any of their accompanying vitamins, minerals, and other elements. The majority of digestion and absorption takes place in the small intestine, which runs around twenty-five feet in length. The colon, or large intestine, provides water reabsorption and the release of nonabsorbable food and waste and is five feet long.

Many disorders and diseases of the gastrointestinal system afflict millions of people. Two of the most common problems affecting the gastrointestinal system are constipation and irritable bowel syndrome, or IBS. These are sometimes referred to as functional disorders because the GI tract looks normal but doesn't work properly. On the other hand, there are structural disorders of the GI tract, in which the bowel appears abnormal and doesn't work properly. These disorders include inflammatory bowel disease, colon cancer, colon polyps, hemorrhoids, and diverticular disease. Inflammatory bowel disease can be further broken down into two specific disorders: Crohn's disease and ulcerative colitis.

While Crohn's disease can cause widespread problems throughout the entire gastrointestinal tract, it mainly impacts the terminal ileum, or where the small intestine meets the large intestine. Inflammation is involved in this disease and extends deep into the lining of the GI tract. Acute inflammation causes swelling and ulceration, which in turn may cause symptoms like diarrhea, fever, weight loss, vitamin deficiency, abdominal pain, and bleeding with anemia. Chronic inflammation, on the other hand, can scar the GI tract, leading to bowel obstruction or perforation.

Ulcerative colitis is also a disease caused by inflammation of the large intestine or the colon. Acute inflammation causes swelling and ulceration, which produces symptoms like abdominal pain, fever, diarrhea, GI bleeding, and urgency to eliminate the bowels. Chronic inflammation can lead to atrophy of the colon and the formation of strictures and pseudopolyps.

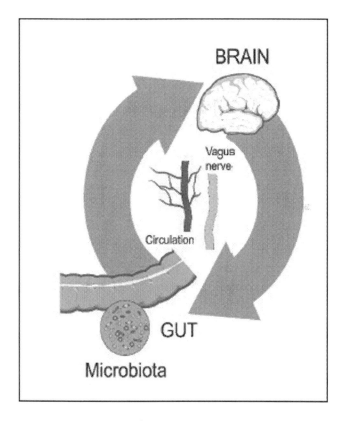

The brain-gut axis

Inflammatory bowel disease can affect organ systems outside of the GI tract, including the skeletal, cutaneous (skin), ocular (eyes or vision), hepatobiliary (liver and gallbladder), renal (kidneys), and hematologic (blood-forming organs) systems. IBD affects one out of every one thousand to three thousand people in the United States and is diagnosed either earlier in life between the ages of ten and twenty or later in life, around sixty to seventy years of age. There are many risk factors involved in developing IBD. A family history is one of the most important risk factors. A habit of smoking, the overuse of NSAIDS, oral contraception, and antibiotics during childhood can all increase the risk of IBD. Diet is crucial, and not being breastfed during infancy can increase the risk of the disease.

One last disorder deserves attention: irritable bowel syndrome, or IBS. This is sometimes called "spastic colon" or "nervous stomach," both of which capture the essence of IBS. It is a functional disorder of the GI system, meaning that the GI system is not damaged whatsoever, but symptoms still present themselves. It is believed that the "brain-gut axis," which is a signaling system between the brain and gut, sends abnormal signals that result in irregular motility and sensation, which then lead to distressful symptoms. The brain-gut axis is also influenced by stress, emotions, and a balance of good and bad bacterial flora in the gut. Currently in science and medicine, the gut is being called the "second brain" due to its significant impact and influence on all other systems in the body.

Around 20% of the adult population in the United States experiences irritable bowel syndrome. It affects women more than men and is occurring more commonly than before in the younger population. Symptoms of IBS are like those of other GI disorders, including celiac disease, chronic pancreatitis, IBD, and food intolerance or food allergies. Some people with IBS experience migraines, chronic fatigue, insomnia, chronic pelvic pain, depression, and anxiety.

Traditional Therapies for Gastrointestinal Disorders
While I cannot go into specific treatments for each GI disorder, there are some common practices and remedies widely used to manage symptoms of these conditions. The first line of action is see your doctor and have him or her rule out other serious gastrointestinal diseases or disorders. Having a solid

diagnosis moving forward can guide how your symptoms are treated. Since the brain-gut axis is becoming more researched, it's important to look at psychological stressors in your life and determine whether they are behind your GI distress. Practices that involve stress management like meditation, prayer, yoga, exercise, and restful sleep may be helpful. Seeing a mental health professional can also help to manage symptoms, and the use of hypnosis or cognitive behavioral therapy may help you reduce negative emotions and bring balance back to your life. Perhaps antidepressants or anti-anxiety medications might also be helpful.

Keeping the brain-gut axis healthy also involves getting good nutrition, eating cleaner, and getting more uncooked and raw foods in your diet that promote growth of good gut bacteria. An anti-inflammatory diet can also help to reduce unpleasant symptoms and keep your GI tract less inflamed. Some experts stress that digestive enzymes and probiotics are good for the gut. Consuming less caffeine, monitoring foods that trigger symptoms, and taking prescribed medications may all be a part of your treatment of GI disorders. Lastly, bowel-modifying agents such as fibers, laxatives, antidiarrheals (IMODIUM, Pepto-Bismol), antispasmodics (Bentyl, Levsin), and upper prokinetic agents (Reglan, Cisapride) may be recommended by your health care provider and can help in managing symptoms of many GI disorders.

Research Findings on CBD and Gastrointestinal Disorders

While researching the benefits of cannabinoids for gastrointestinal disorders, I came across an interesting theory contending that "clinical endocannabinoid deficiency," or CED, is behind not only GI problems, but other physical health problems like migraines, fibromyalgia, and post-traumatic stress disorder. According to Russo, "The theory of CED was based on the concept that many brain disorders are associated with neurotransmitter deficiencies, affecting acetylcholine in Alzheimer's disease, dopamine in parkinsonian syndromes, serotonin and norepinephrine in depression and that a comparable deficiency in endocannabinoid levels might be manifest similarly in certain disorders that display predictable clinical features as sequelae of this deficiency."[63]

A study examining cannabinoids and colitis in mice found that an orally active cannabis extract that is high in CBD reduced intestinal hypermotility and inflammation.[64] An earlier study also found that CBD prevents colitis in mice.[65] Some researchers examining intestinal inflammation have stated that CBD can be a new therapeutic treatment for inflammatory bowel diseases.[66] A year earlier, researchers made the claim that since endocannabinoids are found throughout the gut and are involved in many GI functions such as the regulation of food intake, gastroprotection, nausea and vomiting, GI motility, and intestinal inflammation, cannabinoids may be helpful in treating GI disorders.[67]

In 2012, researchers believed that CBD could become a promising treatment for inflammatory bowel disease and could either be taken alone or in combination with other conventional anti-IBD drugs.[68] Two years later a paper was published concluding that cannabidiol and cannabigerol (CBG) both have proven anti-inflammatory effects and might be promising in the treatment of IBD.[69] The same study stresses the point that this finding isn't exactly new. During ancient times, people used the cannabis plant to treat a wide variety of human ailments, including gastrointestinal disturbances. The difference is that today, we know some of the science behind how CBD and other cannabinoids work within the body. One such piece of knowledge is that the wall of the gastrointestinal tract houses the endocannabinoid system, and consuming CBD can help to restore balance and health to the GI system.

Another research study supports this line of thinking and states that "modulation of the endocannabinoid system, which regulates various functions in the body and has been shown to play a key role in the pathogenesis of IBD, has a therapeutic effect in mouse colitis."[70] As this book is being written, there are clinical trials being conducted on cannabidiol's ability to treat symptoms of irritable bowel syndrome. Earlier, researchers found that CB1 and CB2 receptors found in the gut could reduce the increase in GI motility brought on by inflammation and believe that cannabinoids might become a useful therapeutic treatment for disorders of gastrointestinal motility.[71]

Many other studies provide evidence that CBD can be effective for treating gastrointestinal disorders. CBD has antioxidant effects that could be helpful for good gut health.[72] CBD can also have a positive effect on muscle contraction, which creates pain and absorption of water in the stool and leads to either diarrhea or constipation.[73] The same author writes, "The high prevalence of CB2 receptors in the intestinal tract also means that CBD will turn down the inflammatory processes that cause colitis and Crohn's disease."

Summary

Cannabidiol used medicinally for bowel problems goes back to ancient times. As you can see, disorders of the gastrointestinal system are common, distressing, and sometimes very dangerous. They are also rather common in the United States and around the world. Numerous studies support the use of CBD for multiple GI disorders, including inflammatory bowel disease (IBD), inflammatory bowel syndrome (IBS), ulcerative colitis, Crohn's disease, and others. The research into the effectiveness of CBD continues with clinical trials around the world. Conventional treatment has not always been successful and comes with potential side effects, sometimes worse that the disorders themselves. When medications produce unattractive side effects, people are less likely to continue taking them. It is therefore worthwhile to continue researching how CBD can help millions of people with gastrointestinal disorders.

6

CBD and Headaches and Migraines, Lupus, Menopause, Pain, Respiratory Disorders, Seizures and Epilepsy, and Skin Conditions

Pain is inevitable, suffering is optional.

—Buddha

Headaches and Migraines

Introduction

My wife comes from a family of ten children, and around half of them have experienced migraines. According to experts, genetics and family history can be contributing factors for developing migraines. Interestingly, Anabel's sisters have the headaches and not her brothers. It seems that women are three times more likely to experience migraine headaches than are men. Beyond Anabel's family, headache is a huge problem in the United States, as around 50% of the US population experiences headaches, migraines, and other related ailments.

Migraines affect one billion people around the world and thirty-eight million in the United States. Migraines are the third most prevalent illness and the sixth most disabling disorder in the world.

Overview of Headaches and Migraines

Migraines are specific forms of headache. The condition is characterized by recurrent headaches that range from moderate to severe. The headache often affects only one side of a person's head and has a pulsing sensation. Some migraines last for hours, and others can span over the course of days. Symptoms associated with migraines can be mild, moderate, or completely debilitating. Nausea and vomiting are common, and it is now understood that they occur mainly due to the brain-gut axis. Extreme sensitivity to light, sound, smell, and touch often occur. Some people report a tingling sensation or a dull, numb feeling in their extremities or faces. Some people also experience an "aura" or a visual experience (flashes of light) that precedes a migraine. Other symptoms reported by individuals who have experienced migraines include general weakness and fatigue, stiff necks, and vision changes.

Migraines can impair daily living, keep people home in bed with all lights turned off and shades down, with no noises and little movement. Physical activity can actually make these headaches worse. Some people also experience depression, anxiety, and sleep disturbances due to migraines. People report off work, cancel social engagements, and completely shut down until the migraine passes.

While the underlying mechanisms of migraines are not fully understood, they are believed to involve the nerves and blood vessels in the brain. Some experts believe that they can also be associated with dysfunctions in the cervical spine. The majority of symptoms caused by the headaches are caused by excitation of the trigeminovascular pathway (a system of neurons in the trigeminal nerve that supply cerebral blood vessels), which results in dilated blood vessels and neural inflammation. The neurotransmitter glutamate may also be involved in these headaches as the agent causing the aura that some people experience.

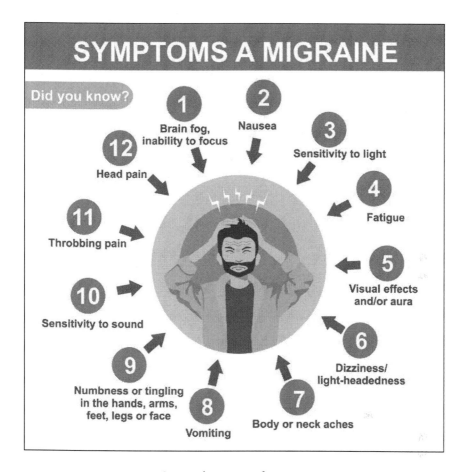

Signs and symptoms of migraines

Traditional Therapies for Migraines and Headaches

The most common method to reduce the risk of migraine or control symptoms when one starts is the use of various medications. Such medications are categorized into two groups: pain relievers or preventive medications. Individuals will be prescribed or recommended certain drugs based on their symptoms, frequency and duration of headaches, severity, and other co-occurring medical conditions one may have.

Medications for relief will work best when they are taken at the first sign of an oncoming headache. These medications include pain relievers like aspirin or ibuprofen. If these are taken over an extended period of time, they can produce negative health outcomes, including medication-overuse headaches, stomach ulcers, and GI bleeding. Migraine medications that combine caffeine, aspirin, and acetaminophen, such as Excedrin Migraine, may help.

A physician may prescribe a triptan, which is a class of medication that is used to stop cluster headaches and migraines. Some examples include Imitrex, Maxalt, Frova, Relpax, and Zomig. They work by blocking pain pathways in the brain and are taken as pills, shots, or nasal sprays. They seem to be effective at relieving many symptoms of migraine but are not recommended for people who are at risk for a heart attack or stroke.

Dihydroergotamines, such as DHE 45 and Migranal, are available as either nasal sprays or injections and can be very effective if taken as soon as migraine symptoms begin. They are generally prescribed for people who have long-lasting migraines (twenty-four hours or longer) but carry negative side effects such as the worsening of migraine-induced nausea and vomiting. People who have coronary artery disease, high blood pressure, and kidney or liver diseases should not take these medications.

The next line of treatment is the use of opioids when all other treatments have failed, but these drugs also carry significantly dangerous side effects, including addiction, overdose, and death. These are narcotic opioid drugs and usually contain codeine and, when used appropriately, can provide relief for many migraine symptoms.

Antinausea medications can also help people manage some of the most distressing symptoms of migraine and severe headaches—vomiting and nausea, especially when the migraine is accompanied by an aura. These medications are sometimes prescribed along with pain medications and include chlorpromazine (Thorazine), metoclopramide (Reglan), and prochlorperazine (Compro).

The other category of migraine medications, preventive drugs, are those that are generally taken every day for people who experience frequent, long-lasting, or severe headaches that don't respond well to other treatments. The goal of these medications is to reduce the risk of developing a migraine in the first place or reduce the severity of the headache once it develops. Medications including blood-pressure-lowering drugs (Inderal and Lopressor), as well as calcium-channel blockers such as Calan and Verelan, can help to prevent migraines with auras.

Antidepressants might be recommended or prescribed by your doctor, because some of them (amitriptyline) can prevent migraines. Some people don't like the side effects of these types of antidepressants because they can cause unwanted weight gain and excessive fatigue. Antiseizure medications like Depacon and Topamax may help people who have fewer migraines. However, they can also cause side effects including nausea, weight changes, and dizziness. Again, if people don't care for the side effects, they may stop taking the medication and end up with more severe symptoms.

A newer line of migraine prevention involves Botox injections around every three months. And the latest drugs for migraines at the writing of this book are calcitonin gene-related peptide (CGRP) monoclonal antibodies. Aimovig, Ajovy, and Emgality are examples of such drugs approved by the FDA for the treatment of migraines. These drugs are delivered as monthly shots, and so far, the most noticeable side effect is a little skin irritation at the site of the injection.

Beyond medications, there are lifestyle modifications and natural remedies for migraines and severe headaches. Stress management and relaxation techniques are good places to start. Getting adequate rest and eating healthy foods could also be beneficial. Staying hydrated, maintaining a migraine or headache diary, and getting some exercise are all healthy ways to prevent or handle migraines. Some people believe in acupuncture, hypnosis, and biofeedback. Others turn to psychotherapy, psychiatry, and counseling. Taking supplements, herbs, vitamins, and minerals can also be helpful in reducing risk for headaches. Magnesium, vitamin B_2, and Coenzyme Q10 have shown some promise in relieving or preventing headaches.

Research Findings on CBD, Headaches, and Migraines

Cannabis has a long history of being used as medicine and treating multiple disorders, including migraines and headaches. Studies have looked at CBD activating the CB1 and CB2 receptors, inhibiting responses of the trigeminovascular system, and restricting inflammation that causes migraine pain.[1, 2, 3] Another study found that CBD decreased the frequency of migraines.[4] In 2015, a group of researchers found that cannabis is effective at providing pain relief caused by chronic neuropathic conditions that are treatment resistant.[5] Four years earlier, researchers concluded that the activation of CB1 and CB2 receptors could correct the problems of a dysfunctional endocannabinoid system, thereby alleviating symptoms of migraine-induced pain.[6] The same researches stated that "the study confirms that a dysfunction of the endocannabinoid system may contribute to the development of migraine attacks and a pharmacological modulation of CB receptors can be useful for the treatment of migraine pain."

A very important meta-analysis of cannabis and migraine treatment comes from Ethan Russo, one of the founding scientists of cannabinoid medicine. It reviews the modern biochemical discoveries of the plant's potential to treat a number of human ailments, including migraines. He suggests that the components of the cannabis plant work through "anti-inflammatory, serotonergic, and dopaminergic mechanisms, as well as by interaction with NMDA and endogenous opioid systems."[7] Later, Russo stated that certain conditions, including migraines, "display common clinical, biochemical and pathophysiological patterns that suggest an underlying clinical endocannabinoid deficiency that may be suitably treated with cannabinoid medicines."[8] According to Russo's theory, increasing the amount of naturally occurring cannabinoids by using CBD can improve symptoms or reduce the frequency or severity of migraines.

Summary

Migraines and severe headaches are common problems that impact millions of people's daily activities and quality of life. It seems like we all know someone who suffers from terrible headaches, whether they are cluster headaches or migraines. While there are numerous over-the-counter remedies and prescription medications, they all come with side effects and other complications. There are some studies that show promising results of CBD for such ailments. Of course, we will need more studies and evidence to become more confident in this natural element from the hemp plant. Will there one day be a CBD-based migraine or headache solution on every store shelf? I, for one, think there will be. Only time will tell.

Lupus

Introduction
It is estimated by the Lupus Foundation of America that around 1.5 million Americans and 5 million people around the world have some form of lupus.[9] While men, children, and teens can develop lupus, it mainly affects women, especially those of childbearing years. If an individual will develop the disorder, it is usually between the ages of fifteen through forty-four. The Centers for Disease Control and Prevention (CDC) estimate that there are sixteen thousand new cases of lupus annually in the United States.[10] Lupus is a devastating and life-altering disease that has no cure.

Overview of Lupus
Lupus is a chronic and systemic autoimmune disease that occurs when the body's immune system attacks its own tissues and organs. The primary characteristic of lupus is inflammation, which can damage many systems of the body, including the joints, skin, kidneys, blood cells, brain, heart, and lungs. Some experts identify lupus as an inflammatory disease. There are four different forms of lupus. Systemic lupus accounts for 70% of cases and affects the heart, lungs, kidneys, or brain. Cutaneous lupus affects another 10% of people and only impacts the skin. Drug-induced lupus accounts for another 10% of cases and is caused by high doses of certain medications, including Pronestyl, Apresoline, and Quinaglute, which are used for cardiac conditions. When these medications are discontinued, the issue usually resolves itself. Neonatal lupus is rare and occurs when the mother's antibodies affect the fetus. When the baby is born, he or she may have skin rashes, low blood counts, or liver problems. Thankfully, these symptoms subside after six months or so without any lasting effects on the baby.

Symptoms of lupus include pain throughout the body, but especially in the muscles and chest while breathing, achy and swollen joints, rashes on the skin, hair loss, fatigue, unexplained fever, and a butterfly-shaped rash on the cheeks and nose. Other symptoms can include depression, anxiety, headaches, sensitivity to light, water retention, and weight loss. While between 10% to

15% of people with lupus will die earlier than normal due to lupus-associated complications, most people will live their full lives due to improved diagnostics and treatments. There are times when people have lupus but experience no symptoms.

Lupus may run in families and have a genetic component. Genes have been identified and impact who develops lupus and how severe it can become. If the family has other autoimmune disorders, there can be a risk of developing lupus. While the cause of lupus is still unknown, it might be triggered by certain factors like sunlight, infections, and certain medications. Lupus affects more non-Caucasian people, especially African Americans, Hispanics, and Asian Americans. Lupus can also cause a number of health complications, such as kidney damage, anemia or bleeding, inflammation of the heart and lungs, increased risk of cancer, infections, and bone tissue death. Lupus can also cause complications during pregnancy.

Traditional Therapies for Lupus

Generally, lupus is treated with medications that target and manage inflammation. Unfortunately, most medications cause unwanted side effects. Symptoms of lupus tend to appear and then disappear, so medication use will vary. Nonsteroidal anti-inflammatory drugs (NSAIDS), antimalarial drugs, immunosuppressants, and corticosteroids may be recommended.

Self-care is important for those who are living with lupus. Getting exercise and eating right is always recommended. Keeping a good relationship with your physician can be helpful. Avoiding excessive sun exposure and smoking, as well as joining a lupus support group, may help in managing the disease. Calcium, vitamin D, dehydroepiandrosterone (DHEA), and fish oil containing omega-3 fatty acids may also be recommended.

Research Findings on CBD and Lupus

As I write this book, there is only one study on the effects of CBD for symptoms of lupus. It is examining the synthetic, endocannabinoidlike drug Lenabasum, by Corbus Pharmaceuticals.[11] Scientists are hopeful that it will be effective in reducing inflammation associated with lupus. This drug binds to cannabinoid receptor 2 (CB2) and triggers the production of anti-inflammatory mediators, reducing inflammation. Lenabasum may be able to "turn off the switch" that causes chronic inflammation and stop tissue thickening and scarring. By reducing inflammation, Lenabasum might help prevent permanent tissue damage in the lungs.

Beyond this study, CBD has been shown in research to have anti-inflammatory properties and may be helpful to manage symptoms of pain and inflammation. In other studies, CBD has also shown to help with mood and emotions. Research is greatly needed on the effects of cannabidiol on symptoms of lupus.

Summary

To date, there is only one study examining a drug that mimics the body's natural endocannabinoid system, but at least it's a start. Hopefully, there will be more interest among scientists in successfully treating this disorder and helping people manage their symptoms of lupus and improve their quality of life.

Menopause

Introduction

My wife, Anabel, allowed me to use her testimonial about CBD and menopausal symptoms. She initially began taking CBD oil for sleep, not menopause, but as her sleep improved, she also noticed that her hot flashes reduced significantly—in her words, "by 85%." She has had issues with insomnia for many years, and after taking over-the-counter remedies, she found that CBD worked much better and with no negative side effects. She also commented that with no hot flashes, flipping the pillow over to the cooler side, and removing sheets all night, she began to sleep more soundly. Anabel also said that it has been many years since she has been able to dream, a result of deep sleep, but that while taking CBD, she actually dreams again and quite a bit. I have heard similar results from numerous people. Apparently, Anabel isn't the only person benefiting from CBD concerning sleep and menopause-induced hormonal changes.

Overview of Menopause

Menopause is a natural physiological process that occurs once a woman has not had a menstrual period for twelve months and marks the end of her menstrual cycles. It can happen between the ages of forty to fifty-five, but women who smoke or are underweight or anorexic may experience symptoms much sooner. The average age for women in the United States to become menopausal is fifty-one. Biologically, the body's production of estrogen and progesterone—two hormones produced by the ovaries—varies to a large degree. These hormonal changes bring on a number of unpleasant symptoms, such as night sweats, insomnia, fatigue, irritability, and mood swings. Sexual intercourse may become painful, and some woman experience depression. These hormones also play an important role in bone health, and during menopause, bones become less dense, increasing the risk of falls and fractures. Fat cells change and weight gain can occur.

After menopause, women enter postmenopause and become more vulnerable to other health conditions like heart disease, diabetes, and osteoporosis. Some women may experience new aches and joint pain. Others may encounter sexual health problems, bladder control issues, and memory loss. Everyone is different, and women will experience symptoms and effects of menopause in different ways. Some will experience mild to moderate symptoms, while others will experience severe menopausal issues. It can be a very stressful time in a woman's life. How long this period of time lasts is important, and it can range between two to ten years, and sometimes a little longer.

Traditional Therapies for Menopause

Experts seem to agree that there are many lifestyle changes and alternative means of decreasing the severity and discomfort of menopausal symptoms. Basic healthy habits like getting enough sleep, eating a well-balanced diet, and getting some exercise may provide relief. Drinking alcohol (red wine) or caffeine in moderation, staying hydrated, and taking vitamins B, C, D, and E may also be beneficial during this time. Cooling down the hot flashes, like Anabel does by placing her wrists on something cold (an ice bucket), seems to help. It can also be helpful to practice stress management and relaxation techniques. Some women may choose hypnosis, acupuncture, or yoga as methods to manage their symptoms.

Beyond these solutions, estrogen therapy has shown to be effective at treating menopausal hot flashes. There are benefits as well as risks with hormone therapy, so it is always advisable to talk to you doctor about your options. Some women have turned to antidepressants to help with depressive symptoms and hot flashes. Your doctor may recommend medications to prevent or treat osteoporosis. Neurontin (used for seizure disorders) and Catapres (used to treat high blood pressure) have also been prescribed for women who have moderate to severe hot flashes and seem to provide relief.

Research Findings on CBD and Menopause

Some researchers believe that the biological mechanisms behind menopause stem from endocannabinoid deficiency. Some evidence for this comes from reports made by women who use cannabis or cannabinoids to treat their symptoms. An early study examining the effects of Sativex, a cannabis-based medicine, found it relieved menopause-related insomnia.[12] According to a more recent study, estrogen helps the endocannabinoid system to regulate emotional response and relieves anxiety and depression. When estrogen levels are lower, as in menopause, the endocannabinoid system is less activated and cannot manage these emotions as effectively.[13] Cannabis has been known to lower body temperature naturally and therefore can be effective at reducing hot flashes.

While there is not a lot of research specifically on CBD and menopause, much has been done on the associated conditions, including pain, anxiety, depression, diabetes, and sleep disturbance. Menopause triggers inflammation and changes in the brain, which lead to many symptoms that might be helped by CBD. As estrogen levels decrease, the body produces more inflammatory molecules, which lead to discomfort, pain, and increased arthritic symptoms. If CBD reduces inflammation, it could help with these conditions. As you will read soon, CBD is also effective in alleviating mood disturbances like depression and anxiety. CBD has been shown to activate serotonin receptors, which help regulate mood and hot flashes. The anti-inflammatory effects of CBD may also help with symptoms of osteoporosis. In a later chapter, you will also see studies that report CBD's effectiveness for sleeping problems.

Summary

Menopause is a natural part of the aging process and is experienced by millions of women. It can bring on mild to moderate biochemical changes, or it can become a very difficult period of time during a woman's life. There seems to be more anecdotal evidence than research-based facts, but many people, including my wife, researchers, and physicians, believe CBD can be effective to help with the negative symptoms associated with menopause. More research is needed in this area, and hopefully we will see it soon.

Pain

Introduction

Who among us has not experienced some kind of pain? People throughout the ages have felt pain brought on by many conditions, and cannabinoids have been widely used to help manage their symptoms. Sir John Russell Reynolds, Queen Victoria's personal physician, in 1859 said, "For the relief of certain kinds of pain, I believe there is no more useful medicine than Cannabis within our reach."[14] The main reason most people go to the doctor is for symptoms of pain. If an individual experiences pain for more than one hundred days, it is considered chronic pain, and over seventy million Americans live with it every day.

Although some chronic pain begins without any specific cause, most people will experience it after an injury or surgery, or due to health problems like arthritis, migraines, back problems, or infections. Pain can range from mild to moderate, and severe to debilitating. Some people will experience pain continually to some degree. Other types of pain will come and go.

While there are various types, sources, and causes of pain, one thing is true about them all: no one likes pain. It can interfere with things that we like to do, interrupt our daily lives, and impair quality of living. And pain doesn't just affect the body; it also causes emotional and psychological upset and makes symptoms of other disorders we may have even worse. Pain can cause depression, anger, anxiety, and frustration. Pain that causes depression can be further worsened by symptoms of depression, creating a vicious cycle. Pain can be spiritual and take away joy and well-being. Everyone experiences it differently and has significantly different thresholds to pain, making it highly subjective.

Overview of Pain

There is no shortage of research, literature, books, or magazines that address one of the biggest health problems on the planet: pain. It can be daunting trying to figure out which kind of pain you are experiencing and then find the words to describe it to your doctor. Where exactly is your pain? When did it start? Is it sharp, dull, or tingling? Does it stay in one spot on your body, or does it travel? Are you experiencing only one type of pain or multiple types of pain? There is much to learn about pain and how to treat it. Read on to discover more about pain and how to more effectively manage it.

Throughout the literature, there are numerous types and categories of pain described. I'd like to present four different types of pain that are experienced by most people. First, there is "acute" pain, which is short term and starts suddenly. It has a specific cause like a tissue injury and will usually go away once it's properly treated. Acute pain starts out with sharp or intense sensations and then gradually improves. Some causes of acute pain are cuts, burns, dental problems, surgery, labor and childbirth, and broken bones.

The second type of pain is "chronic" pain and usually lasts from three to six months after an injury has occurred somewhere in the body. Chronic pain can last for years or a lifetime, and the severity can range from mild to severe on any given day. This type of pain is common in the United States and affects millions of people. Sometimes there's a specific cause for the pain, and other times there's no apparent cause. If untreated, chronic pain can diminish one's quality of life and lead to further complications like depression and anxiety. Symptoms accompanying chronic pain include lack of energy, tense muscles, limited mobility, lower back pain, pain from arthritis and fibromyalgia, nerve damage pain, and frequent headaches.

"Nociceptive" pain is another category and happens to be the most common type of pain. It is caused by stimulation of nociceptors, which are pain receptors located throughout the body. When you experience a cut, your nociceptors send electrical signals to the brain, causing you to feel the pain from the cut. Nociceptive pain can be either acute or chronic and is further classified as *visceral* or *somatic*.

"Visceral" pain is associated with injuries and damage to internal organs and can be felt in the abdomen, pelvis, and chest. This type of pain is sometimes difficult to pinpoint and can be described as cramping, pressure, squeezing, and aching. Other pain-related symptoms may include nausea and vomiting, as well as changes in heart rate, blood pressure, and body temperature. Visceral pain can be caused by conditions including irritable bowel syndrome (IBS), gallstones, and appendicitis.

"Somatic" pain starts in the pain receptors of tissues (skin, muscles, joints, connective tissues, and bones) rather than in the organs. It may be easier to pinpoint the area of pain compared to visceral pain and usually feels like a constant aching sensation. Somatic pain may be deep or superficial. Deep somatic pain can be felt in your joints, tendons, muscle, and bone and is an aching feeling. Superficial somatic pain, on the other hand, is felt in the skin and mucus membranes and feels sharp or throbbing. Many athletic injuries, like tearing a tendon, will cause deep somatic pain, while an ingrown hair on the face will cause superficial somatic pain.

Last, there is "neuropathic" pain, which is the result of damage to or dysfunctions of the central nervous system and leads to damaged nerves that misfire pain signals throughout the body. This type of pain seems to come out of nowhere and is not the result of injury. People with neuropathic pain may feel painful sensations doing things that would normally not cause any pain whatsoever. Cold air and even clothing against your skin can be irritating and painful. It is a very troublesome and devastating type of pain. People describe neuropathic pain in terms of electrical shocks, tingling sensations, numbness, freezing, burning, shooting, or stabbing. While diabetes is one of the most common causes of neuropathic pain, other conditions including shingles, Parkinson's disease, multiple sclerosis, carpel tunnel syndrome, Bell's palsy, infections, accidents, and chronic alcohol consumption, can all result in this type of pain.

While these are the four major types of pain, others do exist and are worth mentioning. "Breakthrough" pain usually takes place in between regularly scheduled pain treatments. "Bone" pain is generally associated with cancer. "Referred" pain is when pain from one area is felt in another location in the body. "Phantom" pain is associated with amputation of limbs. And "total" pain is very wide ranging and includes emotional, behavioral, social, and spiritual areas affecting the person's experience of pain.

Traditional Therapies for Pain

The first line of treatment for most types of pain are over-the-counter and prescription medications. Common analgesics include acetaminophen, nonsteroidal anti-inflammatory drugs (NSAIDS), and opioids. Acetaminophen (Tylenol) works on the brain to reduce pain and is broken down in the liver. This happens to be the most dangerous issue with acetaminophen, because it can cause liver damage. Overdosing on acetaminophen is associated with many negative events, such as ending up in the emergency room and even dying. NSAIDS work on pain by reducing fever and inflammation. Ibuprofen is the most commonly purchased NSAID on the market and includes brands like Advil and Motrin. Unfortunately, there are dangerous side effects associated with NSAIDS, including stomach and gastrointestinal ulcers, bleeding, stroke and heart attack, and renal or liver failure. Overuse of NSAIDs is associated highly with bleeding stomach ulcers and hospitalization. Some people die due to bleeding ulcers.

Opioids seem to be in our national headlines frequently and are associated with addiction, misuse, and abuse. They are also a leading cause of death in the United States. Despite this, they are effective in treating many kinds of pain. They do so by binding to the body's opioid receptors in the nervous system, thereby stopping the pain. Opioids are derived from the poppy plant and have been around for centuries. They also come with a long list of side effects, including sedation, mood alteration, constipation, constricted pupils, and reduction in respiration. While short-term use of opioids can be effective in treating pain, long-term use is highly associated with addiction. Two prescription opioid medications, oxycodone and fentanyl, are responsible for thousands of deaths every year in the United States.

General Uses for Tylenol	**General Uses for NSAIDS**
• Mild to moderate pain • Headaches • Muscle aches • Menstrual periods • Colds and sore throats • Toothaches • Backaches • Fever	• Conditions that cause inflammation • Mild to moderate pain • Fever • Headaches • Coughs and colds • Sports injuries • Arthritis • Menstrual cramps

Beyond medications, many people find relief by engaging in many self-care activities. Reducing stress and finding relaxation techniques that work can take the edge off. Some find relief in meditation, prayer, yoga, and exercise. Finding a good chiropractor or massage therapist can also be helpful. Acupuncture or physical therapy, or seeing a counselor, are healthy ways to deal with pain. Biofeedback and electrical stimulation (TENS unit) may be effective as well. The use of gel packs for hot or cold therapy may relieve certain types of muscular pain. Pet and art therapy can be good distractions and ways to express oneself throughout the pain process. And finally, surgery may be necessary to correct whatever is causing pain in the body.

Research Findings on CBD and Pain

As you have read in this book, cannabis and cannabinoids have been used for thousands of years to relieve various kinds of pain. The ancient Chinese, Indians, Greeks and Romans all used it to treat both humans and animals. Physicians regularly carried it in their medical bags and treated countless patients with cannabis around the world. It was widely used in the Western world for pain relief, anti-inflammation, and relaxation. Historically, it was viewed as an acceptable, safe, and effective means of treating symptoms of pain.

One of the most common areas in research on cannabinoids and health conditions is for the treatment of pain. Behind most of this work is the body's endocannabinoid system and how it regulates pain. The endocannabinoid system is made up of cannabinoid receptors (CB1 and CB2 and, maybe soon, CB3) and cannabinoids. This system acts like a signaling network that functions to regulate many processes throughout the body, including the stimulation of nerve cells that increase or decrease pain. This is some of the science behind the benefits of CBD and pain management.

Cannabinoids have been found to be synthesized in the body on demand. They then act upon cannabinoid receptors located in the peripheral and central nervous systems to either increase or reduce pain signals. If the endocannabinoid system is healthy and working properly, nerve cells are stimulated when there is an actual injury. Once the injury is healed, the system kicks in again to reduce the sensations of pain. If the endocannabinoid system isn't healthy, as in the case of chronic endocannabinoid deficiency, pain signals may be activated when there is no injury or other cause for pain to occur. Scientist Ethan Russo believes this process is behind many chronic health conditions like fibromyalgia and migraines. If the body cannot produce enough cannabinoids for the endocannabinoid system to work properly, pain and inflammation will likely be the result. It is believed that CBD can supplement the deficiency within the endocannabinoid system and help to regulate pain and maintain overall balance in the body. In other words, CBD might help with endocannabinoid deficiency and improve both pain and wellness. CBD may also be a safer alternative to the pain-relieving medications commonly used. Let's look at some research findings.

In 2006, researchers reported that cannabinoids are useful in treating diverse diseases, including those associated with acute and chronic pain. They also stated that cannabinoids can be superior to opioids in treating intractable pathologic pain syndromes: "Medications prepared with cannabinoid receptor agonists or with drugs that enhance endocannabinoid function (by either increasing release or diminishing reuptake of endocannabinoids) may afford the novel therapeutic approaches demanded by disorders in which pain is the prominent symptom."[15] The types of pain they examined were postoperative pain, chronic pain associated with multiple sclerosis, neuropathic pain, cancer pain, fibromyalgia, migraine, and phantom limb syndrome.

A year later in 2007, researchers concluded that targeting the cannabinoid receptor system in the body's connective tissue may provide relief of pain and inflammation from osteoarthritis and rheumatoid arthritis.[16] In 2008, Ethan Russo wrote an important paper on cannabinoids and their role in managing pain, focusing for perhaps the first time on the aging population. He states that while up to 80% of nursing home residents experience pain, it is often treated inadequately by opiates, anticonvulsants, and antidepressants. He firmly believes that cannabinoid medicines may provide an effective approach to treating pain experienced by older adults.[17] Russo also believes that an endocannabinoid deficiency is behind many sources of chronic pain.

Researchers in 2009 examined potential analgesic properties of cannabinoids and declared that they might be a greatly needed alternative to the use of opioids. They stress that opioids are the only medication for the treatment of chronic or severe pain, but that they come with a host of negative side effects. After prolonged use of opioids, they tend to lose their effectiveness over time, possibly leading to tolerance, dependency, or becoming more sensitive to pain than before taking these medications. They found evidence in animal studies that cannabinoids can help with neuropathic pain, inflammatory pain, and cancer pain. Cannabinoids also showed to be an effective treatment for nausea and vomiting as well as an appetite stimulant. They also state that cannabinoids may be helpful in treating pain, spasticity, tremor, nocturia (waking up in the middle of the night to urinate), and improved general well-being. In particular, endocannabinoids and CB2 agonists may be effective at protecting neuro-inflammation associated with multiple sclerosis.[18]

A study in the *European Journal of Pain* found that CBD is effective at reducing pain without side effects. Using a topical transdermal application avoids gastrointestinal or liver processing because it does not reach the bloodstream. In this study, test subjects were provided with a transdermal CBD gel, which significantly reduced joint swelling, leading the researchers to state that CBD has the potential to treat arthritis pain and inflammation with no side effects.[19] In 2018, researchers examined the effectiveness of cannabinoids for osteoarthritis and found that in animal studies, they did reduce osteoarthritis pain, inflammation, and nerve damage. They state:

> There is a growing body of scientific evidence which supports the analgesic potential of cannabinoids to treat OA (osteoporosis) pain. OA pain manifests as a combination of inflammatory, nociceptive, and neuropathic pain, each requiring modality-specific analgesics. The body's innate endocannabinoid system (ECS) has been shown to ameliorate all of these pain subtypes.[20]

Authors of a position paper written by the European Pain Federation state, "The quantity and quality of evidence are such that cannabinoid-based medicines may be reasonably considered for chronic neuropathic pain. For all other chronic pain conditions (cancer, non-neuropathic pain, non-cancer pain), the use of cannabis medicines should be regarded as an individual therapeutic trial." They go on to say that they "expect the quantity and quality of evidence as well as the clinical experience of physicians, medical cannabis and cannabis-based medicines for chronic pain will substantially improve within the next three years."[21] This sheds some light on how European pain researchers and physicians feel about cannabinoids used for the treatment of pain. They seem to believe that more research will not only continue, but that it will yield positive results.

Summary

Cannabinoids have been used to treat pain for thousands of years, and now modern science is confirming what ancient people knew about the healing powers of cannabinoid-based medicine. Hundreds of studies examining the effectiveness of CBD have shown promising results in the treatment of many kinds of pain. Everyday use of CBD for arthritis may improve a person's pain level and mobility, allowing them to enjoy life and maximize quality of living. Despite the type of pain, it appears that CBD may be an effective and safe alternative to other types of medicines used for pain, which all come with negative and sometimes dangerous side effects.

Respiratory Disorders

Introduction

Respiratory, or breathing, disorders are common in the United States and include asthma, chronic obstructive pulmonary disease (COPD), chronic bronchitis, emphysema, lung cancer, and pneumonia, among others. While some individuals are genetically prone to develop these disorders, others who are exposed to environmental toxins may end up with some type of breathing disorder. It is well established that smoking puts an individual at a high risk for developing a respiratory disease.

Disorders of the respiratory system generally belong to four different groups. Obstructive conditions include emphysema, bronchitis, and asthma attacks. Restrictive conditions include fibrosis, pleural effusion, sarcoidosis, and alveolar damage. Vascular diseases include pulmonary edema, pulmonary embolism, and pulmonary hypertension. And lastly, infectious, environmental, and other diseases include pneumonia, tuberculosis, asbestosis, and particulate pollutants.

Overview of Respiratory Disorders

While there are other breathing disorders to consider, I'd like to focus on two of the most common in the United States: asthma and COPD. Asthma is a chronic respiratory disease that affects around three hundred million people around the world and, according to the Centers for Disease Control (CDC), twenty-six million people in the United States.[22] This is around 8.3% of the adult population. It appears that asthma occurs more commonly in women than men, but it is unknown why. Children and older adults, especially elderly people, are more vulnerable to asthma and asthmatic attacks. Over eleven million visits to the doctor's office occurs annually because of this breathing disorder, and ten Americans die each day from asthma.

In asthma, the airways contract either spontaneously or in response to multiple factors in the environment and within the body, leading to a range of mild breathing problems to life-threatening emergencies. The responsiveness of the airways is accompanied by inflammation, seen in many human diseases and conditions. Airways contract and narrow during asthmatic attacks, leaving less air for the lungs to work with. Some symptoms include coughing, wheezing, shortness of breath, and tightness in the chest. There may be a significant connection between environmental allergies and asthma.

Chronic obstructive pulmonary disease, or COPD, is a progressive inflammatory lung disease that obstructs airflow to the lungs, making it very difficult to breathe. According to the American Lung Association, COPD is the third leading cause of death in the United States.[23] COPD is most usually associated with the development of both emphysema and chronic bronchitis. In emphysema, the lung tissues weaken, and the walls of the air sacs (alveoli) break down. The end result is that less oxygen passes into the blood.

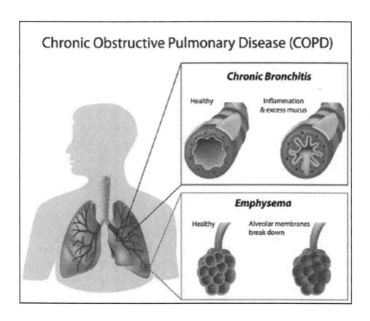

COPD and emphysema

In COPD, less air flows in and out of the airways due to the loss of elasticity or the accumulation of mucus, which can cause the airways to become congested or blocked up. People with COPD have ongoing inflammation of the bronchial tubes, which carry air into and out of the lungs. Irritation caused by this inflammation leads to the growth of cells that make too much mucus, and it leads to coughing. The irritation causes airway walls to thicken and develop scars, furthering limited airflow.

Chronic bronchitis and emphysema are two conditions that form COPD. Chronic bronchitis is one type of COPD in which inflamed bronchial tubes overproduce mucus, which leads to coughing and breathing difficulties. Emphysema is another form of COPD commonly accompanied by chronic bronchitis. Both develop due to chronic exposure to irritants, but the most common cause of these diseases is smoking. COPD develops gradually over time, and symptoms become worse and include shortness of breath, coughing, wheezing, and tightness in the chest. Symptoms may not appear until there is damage to the lungs. This disease can significantly impair activities of daily living and quality of life.

COPD is usually diagnosed in middle-aged and older adults. While it is a difficult disease on its own, it is also highly associated with other diseases, such as lung cancer, high blood pressure, heart problems, respiratory infections, and depression. To date, there is no cure for chronic obstructive pulmonary disease, and damage to the airways is irreversible. Thankfully, there are treatments that can help people control their symptoms and make breathing easier in most cases. Medications can also reduce the risk for developing complications and exacerbation of symptoms.

Traditional Treatments for Respiratory Disorders

Medication and prevention are the key ingredients to prevent asthmatic attacks before they begin. For any respiratory disease, it is important that you are aware of triggers in the environment, avoid them as much as possible, and track your breathing to ensure your medications or treatments are working. Treatments for asthma include long-term asthma control medications, including inhaled corticosteroids, leukotriene modifiers, long-acting beta agonists, combination inhalers, and theophylline. These are usually taken daily and form the basis of traditional medical asthma treatment. Long-term asthma control medications are meant to keep asthma symptoms under control and reduce the risk of an asthma attack.

Quick-relief or rescue medications, on the other hand, are used when needed for fast relief of symptoms that occur during an asthma attack. Some people need to take these medications before any physically active events, like exercise. Medications including albuterol and levalbuterol are short-acting beta agonists that are commonly prescribed. Ipratropium is a bronchodilator that acts immediately to relax the airways, making it easier to breathe. Other quick-relief beta agonists include oral and intravenous corticosteroids, such as prednisone and methylprednisolone, which relieve airway inflammation caused by severe asthma.

Allergy medications may also be recommended to help with symptoms of asthma. Some people take over-the-counter allergy medications, and others receive allergy shots, which is called immunotherapy. It is believed that over time, allergy shots reduce the immune system's reactions to specific allergens. Omalizumab, or Xolair, is given as a shot every two to four weeks and is meant for people who have both allergies and severe asthma. It works by altering an individual's immune system.

People with asthma can also become more engaged in self-care. This includes activities like getting regular exercise, which can strengthen the lungs and heart, and this in turn can relieve symptoms. Maintaining a healthy weight can be effective in reducing breathing problems. Adding weight can make asthma symptoms worse. Controlling heartburn and gastroesophageal reflux disease, or GERD, may help with symptoms of asthma. It is believed that acid reflux, which causes heartburn, can damage lung airways and make asthma symptoms worse.

Some people believe in alternative treatments and incorporate them with their usual medical therapies. It is important to note that alternative medicine should never replace prescribed medical treatment, and it's always important to talk to your doctor when starting any new type of self-care. Stress management, breathing exercises, and herbal remedies may be effective for some people. Caffeine, anise, cacao, and turmeric may help manage symptoms. Practicing effective coping and maintaining a supportive network can also improve quality of life.

Medications for COPD can help to reduce inflammation and open your airways, making breathing easier. Short-acting bronchodilators, like albuterol, may be prescribed by your physician for emergency situations and fast relief of symptoms. These are taken using an inhaler or nebulizer. Corticosteroids are also used to reduce inflammation in the body, making air flow easier in the lungs. Some corticosteroids include Flovent, Pulmicort, and prednisolone. Methylaxanthines are used for severe COPD and when fast-acting bronchodilators and corticosteroids do not work. Long-acting bronchodilators are used over a long period of time and are usually used once or twice a day using inhalers or nebulizers. These drugs work gradually and are not meant to use as rescue medications or in emergency situations. Combination medications are used for people with COPD and are combinations of either two long-acting bronchodilators or an inhaled corticosteroid and a long-acting bronchodilator.

Research Findings on CBD and Respiratory Disorders
There are several studies that have examined the effects of CBD on COPD. They all conclude that it potentially may be of therapeutic value for managing acute attacks of constricted airways caused by inflammation. CBD may actually be a preventive measure for people who have COPD by reducing inflammation and managing inflamed airways.[24, 25, 26] An early study in the 1970s reported that CBD has bronchodilatory effects. This means that it can decrease resistance in the respiratory airway and increase airflow to the lungs.[27] In another study, researchers discovered that when cannabinoids activate the CB1 receptor, it inhibits contraction of the smooth muscle that surrounds the lungs and dilates the bronchial tubes to further open up the airways.[28]

A 2014 study showed that CBD has potent anti-inflammatory effects and improves lung functions in mice.[29] Earlier in 2012, another study found that cannabinoids have bronchodilator effects and may help with airway hyperactivity and asthma.[30] In 2015, researchers reported that cannabis has a bronchodilator, anti-inflammatory, and antitussive effect on the airways.[31] Another study in 2015 reported that "CBD seems to be a potential new drug to modulate inflammatory response in asthma."[32]

Other anecdotal evidence exists from various sources. According to one group of family physicians, CBD not only helps with breathing-related symptoms associated with asthma, but it also helps to reduce asthma-induced anxiety. Asthma and anxiety go hand in hand, and one tends to worsen the other, so if CBD can reduce both sets of symptoms, that would be a great treatment option for people with asthma and anxiety. Another source reports that CBD is effective as a bronchodilator, anti-inflammatory, immunosuppressive, and antispasmodic, making it ideal for people with breathing problems associated with asthma. Beyond the anecdotal findings, drug companies are now working to develop respiratory inhalers that deliver cannabinoids to the person's lungs.

Summary

As we can see, respiratory problems are extremely common and make life difficult for millions of people in the United States and around the world. Some of the most dangerous breathing disorders are asthma, chronic obstructive pulmonary disease (COPD), and lung cancer. But others, like chronic bronchitis, emphysema, cystic fibrosis, and pneumonia, are troubling breathing disorders that can impair quality of living for many people. While there are a number of medical treatments available, most come with unpleasant side effects. There are not many studies on the effects of CBD on breathing disorders, but results of the few that have been completed seem to be fairly impressive. Most respiratory disorders are responses to internal or external stimuli that produce inflammation. If CBD reduces inflammation, acts like an antitussive, bronchodilator, immunosuppressive, and antispasmodic and reduces anxiety, it may become a useful therapeutic treatment for respiratory disorders.

Seizures and Epilepsy

Introduction

According to the Centers for Disease Control and Prevention (CDC), a few short years ago, around 1.2% of the US population had epilepsy. Of those, around 3.4 million were adults, and 470,000 were children.[33] It is estimated that one in twenty-six people in the United States will eventually develop epilepsy sometime during their lives. Having two or more seizures may lead to a diagnosis of epilepsy, and each year, there are 150,000 newly diagnosed cases. Thankfully, most people are treated with medications that help to manage their symptoms.

Overview of Seizures and Epilepsy

Seizures take place when there are abnormal electrical changes or discharges in the brain: "Brain cells inhibit or excite other brain cells from sending messages and while there is usually a balance of these cells, during a seizure there is too much or too little activity, causing an imbalance."[34] This imbalance may lead to chemical changes in the brain, causing an electrical surge that results in a seizure. While seizures are not a disease or disorder by themselves, they are symptoms of other disorders of the brain. Some seizures will be noticeable, and others will be undetectable or silent.

According to the Epilepsy Foundation, there are three main groups of seizures. Generalized onset seizures are those affecting both sides of the brain, as well as groups of cells on both sides of the brain at the same time. There may or may not be motor symptoms involved with these types of seizures. If there are motor symptoms, they include jerking movements, muscle weakness or rigidity, muscle twitching, and epileptic spasms. If there are nonmotor symptoms, the person may stare for a while or have minor twitching in a body part or an eyelid.

"Focal onset seizures" refer to the location the seizure has taken place in the brain. They generally begin in one area or group of cells on only one side of the brain. There are two subsets of focal onset seizures: focal onset awareness seizures, in which the individual is awake and aware that he or she is having a seizure, and focal onset impaired awareness, in which there is confusion and lack of awareness. These may present with motor or nonmotor symptoms. When motor symptoms are present, they may include jerking movements, muscles becoming limp or weak, tenseness or rigidity of muscles, brief twitching of muscles, or epileptic spams. In nonmotor events, the person may experience changes in sensation, thinking, or emotions. They may feel sensations in their gastrointestinal system or feelings like heat, cold, or a racing heart. Sometimes they may experience a complete lack of movement, referred to as "behavioral arrest."

Lastly, there are unknown onset seizures, in which the start of the seizure is neither known nor witnessed. These types of seizures may occur at night or in people who live alone, and no one sees the seizure taking place. These include motor seizures and nonmotor seizures, in which the individual makes no movement whatsoever. While many people possess a 10% chance of having some type of seizure, the risk increases for those who have suffered a stroke or some type of brain injury. Having a single seizure does not qualify for a diagnosis of epilepsy.[35]

Epilepsy, on the other hand, is a seizure and neurological disorder affecting the nervous system. Epilepsy is diagnosed after the individual experiences at least two seizures or after one seizure with a very high risk of experiencing more. These types of seizures are generally not caused by medication side effects or another medical condition that the physician is aware of. Epileptic seizures may have a genetic component and run in families, or they may be associated with some type of brain injury or trauma, sometimes referred to as "adult-onset seizure disorder." Unfortunately, most of the time, the origin of the seizure is unknown.

Traditional Treatments for Seizures and Epilepsy

According to the literature, seizures and epilepsy symptoms can be controlled through the use of medications, referred to as antiepileptic drugs (AEDs), and antiseizure or anticonvulsant medications. There are numerous prescription medications available depending on the person's condition (types of seizure, age, gender, other medical conditions), and experts report that at least seven out of ten people will benefit from their medication. Most medications come with side effects. Mild side effects include fatigue, light-headedness, weight gain, compromised bone integrity, rashes, clumsiness, and trouble talking, remembering, and thinking. The more serious side effects may include depression, inflamed liver, and severe skin conditions.

Beyond medications, many experts suggest dietary changes, including adding the ketogenic, medium-chain triglyceride (MCT) diet to one's lifestyle, and the low glycemic index treatment, or (LGIT), and consuming more carbohydrates that are low on the glycemic scale. Some individuals may be candidates for nerve stimulation or surgery. There are two kinds of nerve stimulation: vagus nerve stimulation and responsive neurostimulation. The vagus nerve begins in the chest and abdomen and runs through the neck and to the lower part of the brain. It is responsible for controlling automatic functions like heartbeat. The procedure involves inserting a small vagus nerve stimulator under the skin of the chest and connecting it to the nerve. The device then sends bursts of electricity through the nerve to the brain, helping to control seizure activity. Responsive neurostimulation involves the use of a neurostimulator that is inserted into the scalp. It searches for patterns of potential seizure activity in the brain and send impulses to stop them. A last resort may be surgery, which can be either resective or disconnective. Resective surgery involves removing the part of the brain causing seizures, and disconnective surgery is a procedure in which the surgeon cuts nerve pathways in the brain that are involved in the individual's seizures.

There are many natural methods and lifestyle changes that can reduce risk for seizure activity and help manage epileptic symptoms. First and foremost, being compliant with medications is a must. Take your medications as your doctor has prescribed, and do not veer off course. Get good and restful sleep. Lack of sleep is one of the triggers that can lead to seizures. If you are epileptic and have regular seizures, be sure to always wear your medical alert bracelet. Emergency professionals will be able to provide help faster and more accurately if you wear it. Get regular exercise, eat a healthy and well-balanced diet, and drink lots of water.

Education is the best weapon when dealing with any disease or disorder. The more you know about your condition, the better you can engage in self-care. Let your family and friends know about your disorder, what they may expect, and how they can effectively respond to a seizure. Don't let others get under your skin if they react inappropriately—it's your life. Find a great doctor, and stick with him or her. One thing that many people with seizure disorders or epilepsy think about a lot, or even sometimes obsess over, is having another event. This is just like having one panic attack and then obsessively thinking over and over about having another one. What do you think will come of this? Another panic attack! So try not to think about it. Lastly, finding a good support group in your town or city can be very liberating and healing. Always remember, you're not the first or the last person to suffer from seizures or epilepsy. Many people do, and they probably want to talk with others who share similar experiences. You just might be the one who helps someone else today.

Research Findings on CBD and Seizures and Epilepsy

Leinow and Birnbaum (2017) state in their book *CBD: A Patient's Guide to Medical Cannabis*, "Out of all of the many medical uses of CBD, using it for seizure control has shown some of the most spectacular and well-publicized results."[36] They also report that many patients experience a reduction in frequency, intensity, or duration of seizures, or they stop completely after using CBD. And equally as important, prescription drugs used for such disorders can cause serious side effects, like sedation and cognitive impairment or dependency. Some people have to take many medications at the same time, also known as polypharmacy, which can also be dangerous. CBD, on the other hand, is well tolerated and has few to no side effects.

Smith joins the chorus and reminds us that in over 30% of cases, even multiple medications do not adequately control seizures or manage symptoms. Sometimes the side effects are so bad that people stop taking their medications altogether. Smith also reports that "CBD has been shown to be somewhat to highly effective as significantly reducing frequency and severity of seizures."[37] EPIDIOLEX is a patented pharmaceutical made from cannabidiol and is prescribed for Lennox-Gastaut syndrome (a severe form of infant and childhood epilepsy) and for Dravet syndrome, also known as severe myoclonic epilepsy of infancy (SMEI), a rare and devastating form of intractable epilepsy beginning in infancy, in patients who are two years of age and older. Sativex, another CBD-based medication, is being prescribed for multiple-sclerosis-related spasticity.

In 2014, Dr. Cilio stressed that epilepsy can be very harmful to the brain during development and is associated with other problems such as cognitive, behavioral, and psychiatric conditions that can significantly impair quality of life. She found that CBD is an ideal therapeutic solution for treatment-resistant epilepsy.[38] Researchers in 2016 proposed that CBD is able to manage epilepsy in children and adults who suffer refractory seizures, and with few to no side effects.[39] A more recent meta-analysis reviewing 199 scientific papers found that CBD has been described as a therapeutic agent for seizures as far back as the 1980s, and since then, many other studies agree.[40]

One paper reported that "CBD use resulted in a significant reduction in seizure frequency" and that "adverse effects of CBD overall appear to be benign." The same researchers revealed that "in most of the trials, CBD is used in adjunct with epilepsy medications, therefore it remains to be determined whether CBD is itself antiepileptic or a potentiator of traditional antiepileptic medications." The authors also stress that there is a great need to develop a cannabis-based treatment for drug-resistant epilepsy to hopefully decrease death rates associated with this type of epilepsy.[41]

An earlier paper presented similar findings: "CBD shows a better-defined anticonvulsant profile in animal models considered to be predictive of efficacy against focal and generalized seizures."[42] Another important statement from this paper is this: "One of the reasons for the utilization of cannabis products to have become so popular among patients and their caregivers is that the products are generally regarded as causing fewer adverse effects compared with traditional AEDs." AEDs are antiepileptic drugs, and many of them have moderate to severe side effects, which CBD does not have. This seems to be a theme in the literature on CBD and seizure disorders.

Summary

Seizure disorders, and epilepsy in particular, affect many people around the world and in the United States. While there are alternative treatments and prescription medications for such disorders, CBD has been shown in studies to be effective and safe. One of the greatest advantages of CBD is that it has few to no unpleasant side effects that prescription medications can have. Once individuals experience side effects that they find disturbing or negative, they are less likely to stay on their medications, which can interfere with progress and symptom management. Can CBD help these people remain compliant with treatment, manage symptoms, and lead better-quality lives?

Skin Conditions

Introduction

The skin is the largest organ of our body, weighing up to twenty pounds, and is composed of three layers. The epidermis is the outermost layer, which is waterproof; the dermis is the next layer, composed of tougher connective tissue, glands, and hair follicles; and the innermost layer is the hypodermis, which is mostly fat and connective tissue that maintains the skin's structure and connects it to muscles. Our skin is the only thing between us and the elements and has many important functions. It protects us from microbes, pathogens, chemicals, and ultraviolet light. It also produces moisture and regulates body temperature.

The skin is a smart organ, too, as the hypodermis is constantly generating new skin cells, which take around four weeks to rise to the epidermis. Once there, they do their job, grow tougher, and shed off, and this takes place an amazing one thousand times during a lifetime. We've been told that it's a good thing to have "thick skin," especially in times of trouble and change, but thickness of skin really depends on many factors, including age, gender, and lifestyle habits like smoking. These can all change the skin's elasticity and cause us to perhaps look older than we are.

Overview of Skin Conditions

While the skin may be a tough defender of the elements, it is also vulnerable to many diseases and disorders. Skin diseases are generally those that affect the skin, hair, and nails. Some of the most common disorders of the skin include acne, dermatitis (eczema), unwanted hair growth (hirsutism), hair loss or baldness, itching (pruritus), psoriasis, seborrhea, and systemic sclerosis. To get a better idea of how cannabidiol can help with symptoms of skin conditions, let's take a quick look at some of these conditions.

Acne is a common skin condition, which is the result of increased sebum (a lipid-enriched, oily exocrine product) production and inflammation of the sebaceous glands. Experts believe that acne can be induced and aggravated by stress, immune and inflammatory factors, endocrine conditions, bacteria, and diet. Acne usually occurs earlier in life but does affect older adults as well. While there are plenty of drugstore remedies, treatments, and prescription medications for acne, there is no cure for it.

Dermatitis is a general term that describes inflammation or swelling of the skin. Dermatitis can be induced by many factors, including allergens and infections. Atopic dermatitis is also known as eczema and is a condition that makes the skin red and itchy. People who have atopic dermatitis may experience periods of relief and flare-ups. Contact dermatitis is a red and itchy rash that forms in response to something coming into contact with the skin, such as poison ivy, soaps, fragrances, lotions, cosmetics, and jewelry. The rash is red in color and usually burns, stings, or itches with the possibility of blistering. Another type, seborrheic dermatitis, produces scales, reddened skin, and dandruff. It usually affects the face, back, and chest. This condition may subside and then flare up.

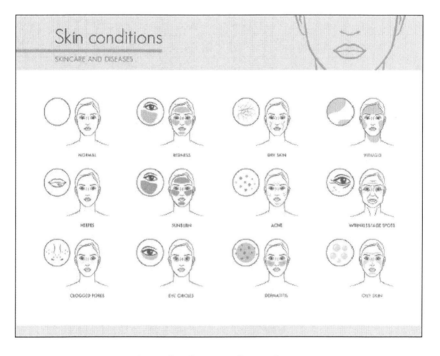

Examples of common skin conditions

Hirsutism, or unwanted hair growth, is a condition characterized by overgrowth of hair in areas of the body where hair is normally minimal or absent. It is also known as male-pattern hair growth when it affects women. This is more of a cosmetic and emotional concern due to the dark, course hair that appears on places on the body where men would normally have hair growth, including the face, chest, and back.

Pruritus is also known simply as itching of the skin, which can be annoying and frustrating, especially when no treatment provides comfort. This condition can occur anywhere on the body and is more common among older adults, as skin tends to become drier with age. Scratching at itchy skin usually makes the condition worse, and skin can become more reddened, rough, and bumpy. Sometimes excessive scratching can cause bleeding of the skin and infections. Itching induced by pruritus can be associated with external temperature changes, parasites, stress, diabetes, nerve damage, inflammation, or allergic reactions to medications.

Psoriasis is a chronic, long-lasting autoimmune skin disease. It is caused by an overactive immune system that produces symptoms such as flaking, inflammation, and thick patches of skin that are red, white, or silver. These symptoms occur due to skin cells dividing themselves too quickly and building up to form these patches of discolored skin. Psoriasis can affect any part of the skin but is usually found on the knees and elbows. The condition can be triggered by stress, infections, smoking, and excessive use of alcohol.

Seborrhea is an inflammatory skin condition that appears on sebaceous-gland rich areas of the skin, including the face, back, and chest. It can also occur in areas where the skin folds and maintains skin-to-skin contact. When it affects the scalp, it is called dandruff. It causes a red and itchy rash, dryness, peeling, flakiness, and white scales.

Systemic sclerosis, also known as scleroderma, is a chronic autoimmune disease that is characterized by an accumulation of connective tissue (diffuse fibrosis), degenerative changes, and vascular problems throughout the skin, joints, and internal organs of the body like the esophagus, lower GI tract, kidneys, lungs, and heart. Symptoms may include hardened, tough or tight skin, discolorations, and/or tight facial tone.

Traditional Therapies for Skin Conditions

While this isn't the place to describe treatments for each skin disorder, there are common therapies recommended for many different types of skin conditions. So this section will be a generalized overview of treatments for skin issues. The first line of defense against skin conditions is generally some kind of medicine like topical lotions and creams, or systemic (oral) pharmaceuticals like steroids or antihistamines to reduce the symptoms of each condition. Some of the most commonly used medications include antibacterials, antifungals, corticosteroids, retinoids, nonsteroidal ointments, salicylic acid, coal tar, and benzoyl peroxide. Other oral and injectable medications include enzyme inhibitors, biologics, immunosuppressants, and antiviral agents.

Common Skin Medications
Antifungals: Tinactin, Lotrimin
Corticosteroids: Prednisone, Hydrocortisone
Retinoids: Ativa, Retin-A, Tazorac
Non-Steroidal Ointments: Voltaren, Solaraze

People may also purchase drugstore remedies and treat themselves with various topical preparations like ointments, creams, lotions, gels, oils, foams, and powders. They can also purchase cleansing products that can keep the areas around the skin problem clean. Other over-the-counter solutions may involve protective, drying, or moisturizing agents, and anti-itch, anti-inflammatory, and anti-infective medications.

Beyond medications, there are plenty lifestyle and everyday practices that can help keep skin healthy and reduce symptoms of some skin conditions. Maintaining a healthy diet is recommended for healthy skin. A diet rich in fruits and vegetables (antioxidants and anti-inflammatories), whole grains, and healthy fats may be best for most people. Yellow and orange fruits and dark-green leafy vegetables are healthy for the skin. Tomatoes, blueberries, brown rice, quinoa, and turkey are skin-friendly foods that may prevent issues with the skin or help maintain it. Some experts believe that getting dark chocolate, cayenne, coconut, garlic, oregano, rosemary, and turmeric in the diet can be very helpful for many skin issues.

In general, if it's good for the body, it's good for the skin. Some people may choose a gluten-free diet because gluten is known to cause inflammation. Being aware of food allergies is critical, and you should always consult with a physician or dermatologist if you experience an unpleasant reaction to something new in your diet. Avoiding certain foods that can cause skin problems may be the best route of prevention.

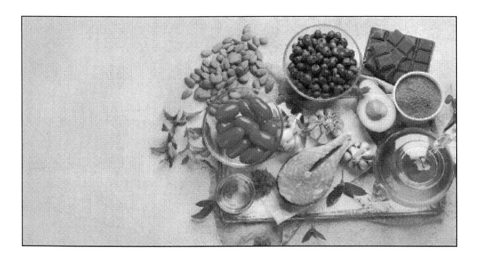

Skin-healthy foods: Salmon, avocados, almonds, dark chocolate, tomatoes, green tea, and blueberries

Research Findings on CBD and Skin Conditions

An important paper was written in 2009 entitled "The Endocannabinoid System of the Skin in Health and Disease: Novel Perspectives and Therapeutic Opportunities." In it, researchers from the United States, Germany, UK, and Hungary stated:

> Recent studies have intriguingly suggested the existence of a functional ECS (endocannabinoid system) in the skin and implicated it in various biological processes…It seems that the main physiological function of the cutaneous ECS is to constitutively control the proper and well-balanced proliferation, differentiation, and survival, as well as immune competence

and/or tolerance, of skin cells. The disruption of this delicate balance might facilitate the development of multiple pathological conditions and diseases of the skin (e.g. acne, seborrhea, allergic dermatitis, itch and pain, psoriasis, hair growth disorders, systemic sclerosis and cancer).[43]

This means that the endocannabinoid system exists within the skin and when it is out of balance, skin conditions can develop. But when it's healthy, it maintains homeostasis of the skin.

The endocannabinoid system can help fight skin allergies; inflammation; pain; itchy, dry skin; acne and seborrhea; psoriasis; dermatitis; systemic sclerosis; and other skin diseases. It may keep skin healthy and prevent many of the effects of aging. Using cannabidiol or CBD can boost the endocannabinoid system's ability to do its job. Ethan Russo believes that when a person experiences chronic endocannabinoid deficiency, he or she may develop all sorts of unhealthy conditions, including skin problems. He also believes that the gut-skin-brain axis is behind many disorders, and when it is properly cared for, this system can keep us healthy and well balanced.

Researchers found that cannabinoid CB2 receptors are involved in wound repair. They state:

> Our previous study showed that cannabinoid CB2 receptors are detected in the epidermis, hair follicles, sebaceous glands, cutaneous muscle layer, and vascular smooth muscle cells in the skin of mice, and are dramatically expressed in neutrophils, macrophages and myofibroblasts during skin wound healing in mice. The primary physiological function of the cutaneous endocannabinoid system is to constitutively control balanced proliferation, differentiation and survival, as well as immune competence and/or tolerance of the skin cells.[44]

The same year, another research team found that cannabinoids may be helpful in treating refractory psoriasis.[45]

A research team in 2014 declared that they provided the first evidence that CBD exerted a unique "trinity of cellular anti-acne actions." This means that CBD controlled the pathologically elevated lipogenesis induced by pro-acne agents, suppressed cell proliferation, and prevented the actions of TLR activation, or pro-acne agents, to elevate pro-inflammatory cytokine levels, which usually result in inflammation.[46] A research paper in 2019 reported that CBD may be effective in treating certain skin diseases like eczema, psoriasis, and atopic and contact dermatitis. The keys to the healing process are CBD's anti-inflammatory properties.[47] Researchers in 2018 conducted an analysis of the current literature on CBD and skin problems in preclinical studies and found that cannabinoids have the potential to treat many skin conditions, including acne, dermatitis, Kaposi's sarcoma, pruritus, psoriasis, skin cancer, and systemic sclerosis.[48]

An earlier study in 2006 reported that due to the anti-inflammatory nature of cannabinoids, they may be a viable treatment in skin conditions like eczema and psoriasis.[49] Another study discovered the immunosuppressant actions of cannabinoids to reduce overactive immune responses causing inflammatory rash.[50] Still another study found that psoriasis, an inflammatory skin disorder, responds to the anti-inflammatory effects of cannabinoids and cannabinoid receptors.[51] Hungarian researchers in 2007 found that hair follicles on the scalp contain endocannabinoids and endocannabinoids receptors, which are both involved in the regulation of hair growth.[52]

Summary

The skin is an amazing organ that provides so many functions that we rarely, if ever, think about. It protects us from environmental invaders, insulates us in the cold, regulates our body temperature in the heat, and constantly regenerates itself throughout our lifetime. It's also one of the most vulnerable organs and can become affected by a number of skin diseases, disorders, and conditions. Some will be mild and easily treated, while others will be chronic, frustrating, and difficult to manage. After viewing the handful of studies examining CBD, the endocannabinoid system and its receptors, and their possible use for such disorders, will CBD become a common, everyday product that most of will use to keep our skin healthy, prevent problems, and manage the symptoms of skin conditions?

Here is one last interesting note on CBD, skin, and diet. Since CBD comes from hemp, it contains many important nutrients, like vitamins A, D, C, E, and B-complex (B_1, B_2, B_3, and B_6). It also provides omega-3 and omega-6 fatty acids, protein, and fiber and is a source of iron, beta carotene, zinc, and potassium. Hemp contains calcium, selenium, phosphorus, manganese, magnesium, flavonoids, terpenes, and terpenoids. These can all be helpful in maintaining healthy and youthful skin.

7

CBD and Addiction, Anxiety, Depression, and Eating Disorders

> *Just when the caterpillar thought the world was ending, he turned into a butterfly.*
>
> —Anonymous proverb

Introduction

This chapter provides a snapshot of research examining the relationship between the endocannabinoid system, cannabinoid receptors, and cannabinoids and their influence on mental health conditions. Because most forms of mental, emotional, or behavioral disorders are treated with psychoactive medications, which may provide relief of symptoms, they are also known for troubling and sometimes dangerous side effects. We will recognize major themes throughout the literature regarding the effectiveness of CBD and its ability to provide neuroprotection and help manage symptoms of depression, anxiety, psychotic disorders, and other mental and emotional conditions. The potential for CBD to effectively manage symptoms of social phobia, post-traumatic stress disorder (PTSD), sleep and appetite disorders, and psychotic features in Parkinson's disease is found in current research. Some experts believe that CBD may also be helpful in treating some forms of substance abuse and addiction.

I must tell you that I have a profound love of psychology, psychiatry, and gerontology and have been a student of each edition of the *Diagnostic and Statistical Manual of Mental Disorders*, published by the American Psychiatric Association, or the *DSM*, including the latest one, the *DSM-5* (the fifth edition). Each edition of the *DSM* is what I have turned to for decades to improve my knowledge of psychiatric illnesses. The *DSM-5* lists over four hundred known forms of mental illness within 947 pages and provides important information about each condition, including signs and symptoms, possible causes, and other related information. I'd like to give you an overview of each psychiatric condition described in traditional terms so that you have a clear picture of what each one is before providing any research-based evidence about the potential effectiveness of CBD.

I should also share with you my background in mental health. Many years ago, I had the great opportunity to work with several geropsychiatrists and provided psychotherapy under their clinical supervision. All of our work was with adult and elderly populations residing in senior care, including skilled nursing facilities, assisted-living, and group homes. I gained an incredible amount of experience working with people diagnosed with almost every psychiatric condition I can think of, from schizophrenia to anxiety and depression, and of course the neurodegenerative diseases like Alzheimer's, Parkinson's, and Huntington's disease. I observed hundreds of psychiatric evaluations and medication changes for several years. As I look back at all of the psychiatric drugs prescribed to countless seniors, I now wonder if CBD would have been safer and effective.

Where there simply isn't enough room in this book to cover every condition in the *DSM-5*, I'd like to concentrate on some of the most common psychological disorders affecting many people, inducing addictions, anxiety, depression, eating disorders, obsessive-compulsive disorder (OCD), post-traumatic stress disorder (PTSD), schizophrenia, sleep disorders, and stress. I have scanned hundreds of research papers, books, websites, and other sources and present to you a summary of findings on the effectiveness of cannabidiol for various mental health conditions. The roles of the endocannabinoid system and cannabinoids will also be reviewed. Some studies go back to the 1970s, and some were published most recently. Since there has been interest in CBD and mental health for decades, why has there not been progress in the development of cannabinoid-derived medications for mental disorders throughout all of these years?

Aging and Mental Health

As a gerontologist, I have studied many aspects of aging, including mental and emotional conditions in later life. While mental issues are common in older adults, they are not inevitable. Older adults who have co-occurring health problems are especially vulnerable to anxiety, depression, sleep disorders, and appetite changes. Older adults may engage in self-medicating behaviors and use, misuse, or abuse prescription medications, over-the-counter remedies, illegal drugs, and alcohol. It is well known that older adults are prescribed the largest amounts of prescription drugs in the United States and are at risk for negative side effects and even death related to their use. Psychotropic medications are usually recommended along with supportive counseling or therapy. A typical problem with medication is the potential for negative and unwanted side effects, which may then lead to noncompliance. If the individual stops taking his or her medication, the effectiveness of the treatment is diminished.

Addiction

Introduction

Substance abuse and addiction are very serious problems in the United States and are responsible for significant physical and mental health problems, loss of income, marital and relationship difficulties, and premature death. It seems like we all know someone who has been affected by alcohol or drug problems. Alcohol abuse alone is associated with the pain and suffering caused by domestic violence, homicide and suicide, overdose, accidents, injuries, loss of driving privileges, and unemployment. Chronic alcoholism is associated with a number of health issues, including cancer, cirrhosis of the liver, pancreatitis, depression, dementia, seizures, and psychosis. Neurochemical changes in both brain physiology and structure can develop with prolonged alcohol abuse, which in turn causes the physical and psychological desire to drink even more, leading to dependence.

The number of lives negatively impacted by addiction is staggering. According to the National Survey on Drug Use and Health, almost twenty million Americans had a substance use disorder in 2017.[1] The same survey reported that 74% of those dealing with substance addiction also had an alcohol use disorder. Around 38% were battling an illegal drug problem, and one out of every eight adults had both an alcohol use disorder and a drug problem at the same time. Experts once referred to an alcohol and drug problem as a dual diagnosis, meaning two different conditions occurring together, but now it's known as a co-occurring disorder. Many Americans who have co-occurring disorders are also suffering from some form of mental illness, which makes the clinical picture more complex and treatment and recovery more challenging. Besides the human tragedy associated with addiction, there's also a high financial price involved. The National Institute on Drug Abuse reported that $300 billion was spent on tobacco abuse, $249 billion on alcohol abuse, $193 billion on addiction to illegal drugs, and $78.5 billion on misuse of prescription opioids.[2]

What about older adults and the elderly? According to the Substance Abuse and Mental Health Services Administration, over one million people over age sixty-five had a substance use disorder in 2017. Around two-thirds of older adults with a substance use disorder develop it before the age of sixty-five. And between 21% and 66% of elderly people who have a substance use disorder also suffer from a co-occurring mental health disorder.[3]

Overview of Addiction

According to the *DSM-5*, substance-related disorders fall into ten different categories based on the type of drug. They include alcohol, caffeine, cannabis, hallucinogens, inhalants, opioids, (sedatives, hypnotics, and anxiolytics), stimulants, tobacco, and other unknown substances. The DSM-5 also differentiates two groups of substance-related disorders: substance *use* disorders and substance-*induced* disorders: "All drugs that are taken in excess have in common direct activation of the brain reward system, which is involved in the reinforcement of behaviors and the production of memories."[4] Addiction, then, is a brain disorder characterized by compulsive engagement in rewarding stimuli, regardless of any negative consequence or outcome. It is a chronic disease typified by motivation, rewarding the brain, and memory. An addicted individual finds relief or reward by using a substance. The National Institute on Drug Abuse defines drug addiction:

> A chronic disease characterized by compulsive, or uncontrollable, drug seeking and use despite harmful consequences and changes in the brain, which can be long lasting. These changes in the brain can lead to harmful behaviors seen in people who use drugs. Drug addiction is also a relapsing disease. Relapse is the return to drug use after an attempt to stop.[5]

In much of the literature on addiction, dopamine (the neurotransmitter that emits signals in the brain's areas regulating pleasure, movement, emotions, and motivation) is mentioned frequently. Dopamine makes us happy. Many forms of addiction occur due to the brain's reward system flooding the circuit with dopamine. Drugs increase dopamine output, causing us to feel good. But drugs also alter the way that dopamine works in the brain. Long-term use of substances that stimulate dopamine become required to produce feelings of happiness or satisfaction because the brain is unable to do this on its own. Another part of the brain is also affected: the hippocampus. This part of the brain is involved in memory, and after the use of drugs or alcohol, it creates memories of the quick rush of good feelings they produce. Then, the amygdala, which is responsible for emotional responses, develops a conditioned response to the substance being used. Just to make this a little more complex, glutamate, the neurotransmitter responsible for learning and memory and found largely in the hippocampus, increases symptoms of craving for substances, like alcohol or painkillers.

Although some of the most widely abused drugs include alcohol, marijuana, cocaine, heroin, fentanyl, ecstasy, methamphetamine, Vicodin, Xanax, and inhalants, people can become addicted to almost any substance. Some can become addicted to over-the-counter medications, and others may become dependent on prescription medications. Opioids are highly addictive and are responsible for tens of thousands of overdoses and deaths. In the short term, opioids are very effective in treating pain and discomfort. They relax the body and can bring great relief. They also have a number of negative side effects, like excessive drowsiness, nausea, confusion, constipation, and slowed breathing, which can cause hypoxia, a condition that results when too little oxygen reaches the brain. Hypoxia can lead to both short- and long-term problems, including brain damage, coma, psychological and neurological problems, or death.

Some adults may misuse or abuse psychostimulants, which are medications generally prescribed to younger people for attention deficit hyperactivity disorder or ADHD. These drugs slow children down, whereas they speed up adults, just like amphetamines. Some commonly prescribed psychostimulants are Ritalin, Concerta, Adderall, Strattera, Vyvanse, and Dexedrine. These drugs stimulate norepinephrine and dopamine and induce feelings of pleasure and euphoria. The side effects, though, are potentially dangerous and deadly. Since norepinephrine regulates heart rate, blood pressure, and breathing, people can experience increased blood pressure and heart rate, decreased breathing, and increased blood sugar. Overuse of these drugs can lead to a dangerously high body temperature, irregular heartbeat, heart failure, and seizures. It can also lead to paranoia, excessive anger, and psychosis.

People who don't use stimulants but prefer a more mellow drug experience may become addicted to central nervous system depressants like sedatives, hypnotics, or tranquilizers. These types of medications can be prescribed to treat anxiety, stress, panic, and sleep disorders. Sedatives include barbiturates and sleep medications like Ambien and Lunesta. Tranquilizers primarily including benzodiazepines such Valium and Xanax, which may be prescribed to treat anxiety. Side effects of these medications include drowsiness, poor concentration, slurred speech, slow movements, memory difficulties, lowered blood pressure, slowed breathing, confusion, and dizziness.

Numerous risk factors are associated with addiction. Genetics and heredity play a role in becoming addicted to a substance. Some experts believe that up to half of all addictions to alcohol, nicotine, or other drugs are based on genetics. If members of your family have experienced addiction, this theoretically puts you at a higher risk for addiction. Some people may have an addictive personality, meaning that if you have a parent who is addicted to alcohol, you might choose not to drink but might become addicted to nicotine and smoking.

The environment has a very powerful influence on us, both as children and as adults. Lack of parental involvement is a risk factor for developing an addiction through experimentation. Abuse or neglect can be associated with addiction as well. Young people may turn to substances to cope with negativity in their environment. The availability of substances has also been shown to be a risk factor for addiction, as is the influence of one's social group.

Having co-occurring disorders such as a mental health problem and a substance abuse issue puts one at a particularly high risk of becoming addicted to a substance. Some people may drink because they are depressed and continue to be depressed because they drink too much. This pattern can become a vicious cycle in which the individual self-medicates to either feel better or to kill the pain. It has been shown that underlying mental and emotional conditions are associated with addiction and that substance abuse is a risk for developing a psychiatric condition. Under these conditions, addiction tends to increase more rapidly, leads to severe consequences, and is more difficult to treat. Recovering from a surgery can lead to one's dependence on pain pills, and an injury can alter one's lifestyle and lead to substance misuse or abuse.

Common Types of Behavioral Addictions

- Gambling
- Sex
- Binge eating
- Internet
- Shopping
- Video games
- Food
- Work
- Exercise

Another risk factor involves the strength or power of the drug that one is consuming. For instance, cocaine, heroin and methamphetamines are more physically addictive than marijuana or alcohol. People who engage in drugs that speed them up usually go through a rough time coming down or withdrawing from the drug. It can be a painful experience in many ways, including physically, emotionally, and psychologically. In order to deal with the pain of withdrawal, people may use harder drugs or increase the dose they are taking. This type of situation is dangerous and can lead to complications including overdose and death.

This book is about the aging process, but it is worth mentioning that the earlier in life an individual experiments with drugs and continues to use them regularly, the higher their risk for addiction. Young adults between the ages of eighteen and twenty-four are most likely to experience coexisting disorders. Using drugs earlier in life can also interfere with brain development, which in turn can make one more prone to developing mental health disorders as one ages.

Another risk factor associated with addiction is the method in which one uses drugs. Certain drugs are more addictive than others, and the way they enter a person's body matters. For instance, drugs that are smoked or injected are likely to be more addictive than those that are swallowed. Smoking the drug gets it directly into the bloodstream and brain, where it takes effect. Swallowing a drug means that it is digested and passes through the liver and other organs, where they are filtered out before taking full effect.

substance-related disorders fall into ten different categories While most addictions can be treated, it's not easy. Addiction is a chronic disease, and most people can't simply stop using a substance for a short while and then be cured. It doesn't work that way. Many individuals will require long-term treatment or care that is repeated over months or years before they can recover completely and return to normal life. In a very simplistic way, addiction treatment needs to help people stop using substances, remain drug free, and return to a productive life.

Treatments range from seeing a counselor who specializes in substance use therapy, to following up with a psychiatrist who evaluates the need for psychotropic medications. An evaluation would provide evidence that there may be co-occurring disorders that require medical or psychological attention, like

Substances Commonly Abused
• Alcohol
• Opioids
• Heroin
• Fentanyl
• Marijuana
• Benzodiazepines
• Cocaine
• Crack
• Crystal meth
• Ecstasy

depression or anxiety. Behavioral therapies can address the person's attitudes and behaviors associated with drug use. It can help to enhance healthy life skills and develop more effective coping mechanisms.

Sometimes the individual requires outpatient behavioral treatment consisting of a variety of programs, including individual and group therapy, cognitive behavioral therapy, family therapy, motivational interviewing, and motivational incentives. If the substance use disorder is severe enough, outpatient treatment may not be effective enough, and the individual may require inpatient or residential treatment. This involves living in therapeutic communities that are highly structured for six to twelve months. Shorter-term residential treatment is another option and focuses mainly on detoxification and intensive therapy. Recovery houses are available and provide short-term, supervised living arrangements for people who have successfully gone through a program and are graduating to a less regimented environment. Here they learn how to transition back into the community and return to their former lives.

Medications may be used as part of the recovery process and can be used from the beginning stages of detoxification through relapse prevention and maintenance. Detoxification itself is not a treatment but is a process the individual goes through while substances wear off completely from the body and brain. Opioids like methadone, Suboxone, and Vivitrol may be used to treat opioid addiction. They work on the same targets of the brain but do not produce the same high and are meant to deal with cravings associated with addiction. Naltrexone may be prescribed for people battling alcohol addiction; it works by blocking opioid receptors associated with the rewarding effects of drinking alcohol and the craving for alcohol. Campral can reduce some symptoms of long-term withdrawal found in people with severe addictions. It may help with symptoms like insomnia, restlessness, anxiety, and dysphoria. Antabuse may be prescribed for people who want to quit drinking and works by making the individual physically ill when he or she consumes alcohol. Compliance with certain treatments may be a problem, but for those who are highly motivated to quit, it can help keep people on the path to recovery.

Research Findings on CBD and Addiction

Researchers from Mount Sinai School of Medicine in the United States and others from Spain found that CBD had an effective impact on heroin self-administration and drug-seeking behavior. They reported that "it specifically attenuated heroin-seeking behavior reinstated by exposure to a conditioned stimulus cue. CBD had a protracted effect with significance evident after 24 hours and even 2 weeks after administration." The authors believe that CBD may be a potential treatment option for people suffering from heroin craving and the risk of relapse.[6]

In 2013, two researchers examining the connection between the endocannabinoid system and cocaine addiction discovered that a dysregulation of the CB1 receptor and related signaling networks induced by cocaine use might be behind brain alterations and neurotoxicity in the brains of cocaine addicts.[7] In 2012, a larger group of researchers found that CBD can be an effective treatment for "cannabis withdrawal syndrome," which may be experienced by heavy users who stop consuming marijuana. Cannabis withdrawal can lead to symptoms including anxiety, insomnia, migraine, appetite loss, restlessness, irritability, and other physical and psychological effects. They indicate that tolerance to cannabis and the resulting withdrawal syndrome may be a product of the desensitization of CB1 receptors by THC. After treating the subject for ten days, the researchers noted the absence of significant withdrawal signs.[8]

Another study in 2013 found that cannabidiol could be useful in treating opioid addiction. They explained that CBD works by interfering with reward mechanisms in the brain that are responsible for the expression of the acute reinforcing properties of opioids.[9] The opioid crisis in the United States has increased significantly since 2013, and alternative treatments are badly needed. An important paper was published in the *Journal of the American Medication Associations* reporting that states initiating medical marijuana programs had an almost 25% lower rate of opioid-related overdoses compared to those with no such program.[10] Leinow and Birnbaum state, "That itself is powerful evidence of the potential for cannabis to treat addiction to pharmaceutical painkillers."[11] A systematic review was written in 2015 and reported that CBD has been shown throughout the literature to have anxiolytic, antipsychotic, antidepressant, and neuroprotective properties. The researchers state, "CBD may have therapeutic properties on opioid, cocaine, and psychostimulant addiction, and some preliminary data suggest that it may be beneficial in cannabis and tobacco addiction in humans."[12] Biologically, cannabidiol is associated with neural circuits included in addiction and drug-seeking behaviors.

Another paper published in 2015 stressed the importance of the endocannabinoid system being the target of drugs for the treatment of addiction:

> Cannabinoid CB1 receptor antagonists/inverse agonists reduce reinstatement in responding to cocaine, alcohol and opiates in rodents. However, compounds acting on the endocannabinoid system may have a broader application in treating drug addiction by ameliorating associated traits and symptoms such as impulsivity and anxiety that perpetuate drug use and interfere with rehabilitation.[13]

Yasmin Hurd and a team of researchers provide a review of both preclinical studies involving animals and human studies on CBD as a therapeutic intervention used for opioid relapse. Common problems associated with opioid withdrawal are recurrent episodes of intense desires to use drugs again, known as "craving." Another problem for many people addicted to heroin or opioid-based medications is going back to using these drugs after a series of treatments. This is known as "relapse." Their team found that CBD may inhibit drug-seeking behavior and has almost no abuse potential. It also has no notable side effects and may be a good treatment for symptoms associated with addiction such as anxiety, depression, insomnia, and pain:

> Currently most medications for opioid abuse directly target the endogenous opioid system. CBD could thus offer a novel line of research medication that indirectly regulate neural systems modulating opioid-related behavior, thus helping to reduce side effects normally associated with current opioid substitution treatment strategies.[14]

Research examining the medical uses of cannabinoids is in its early stages, but results seem promising. Can targeting the endocannabinoid system become an effective treatment for people addicted to opioids and other substances? Another author explains:

> Symptoms of craving are mediated by increasing the transmission of the neurotransmitter glutamate, found in areas of the brain such as the hippocampus (the region in the brain responsible for learning and memory). This may explain why cravings such as anxiety, irritability, sweating and palpitations can occur years into abstinence, when a situation or person stimulates a drug-related memory, creating a greater risk of relapse.[15]

substance-related disorders fall into ten different categories While dopamine has been shown to play a role in addiction, glutamate has more recently received attention as the neurotransmitter that may play a greater role in the development and maintenance of addiction. Glutamate is involved in the reinforcement and habit-development of addiction. It has a strong impact on cravings, relapse, and drug-related memory. Opioid addiction in particular has been associated with the powerful influence of glutamate, and addiction has been called a disorder of both learning and memory.

A paper in 2017 examined the possibility of CBD being an effective treatment for nicotine and cocaine addiction and found that the answer may lie within the endocannabinoid system.[16] The same year a team of researchers from the UK wrote a review article for the *British Journal of Pharmacology*. In it they explain that CBD shows the ability to regulate anxiety, learned fear (phobias), and fear memory (PTSD), and therefore may regulate emotions and emotional memory processing, as well as reduce anxiety, all associated with substance abuse disorders.[17] This can be a very important finding since there are connections between anxiety disorders like PTSD, phobias, and others and the use of substances used to self-medicate unwanted fear and memories. Anxiety and substance abuse also tend to influence one another, and a vicious cycle can emerge.

One year later, a paper described the potential of CBD as a viable treatment for alcoholism. Using rodents, the researcher found that cannabidiol significantly affected the compulsive seeking of alcohol and that the effects lasted up to five months after treatment was terminated. Weiss explains, "CBD reverses neuroplasticity linked to maladaptive learning underlying EtOH craving and relapse, beyond mere transient pharmacological amelioration of vulnerability to relapse," and this "may therefore have major implications for treatment, drug development and understanding of the neural and molecular basis of compulsive EtOH seeking."[18] He also stresses that there is a need for a more effective treatment for alcohol relapse prevention, and CBD may have potential in this area.

More recent research on rodents, CBD, and drug use published in the journal *Neuropsychopharmacology* concluded that CBD affected context-induced and stress-induced drug-seeking behavior in the animals without tolerance, sedation, or interfering with normal behavior. CBD also reduced experimental anxiety among the rodents and prevented high impulsivity in rats with a history of alcohol dependence. The researchers conclude that "the results provide proof of principle supporting potential of CBD in relapse prevention."[19] A press release from a Mount Sinai study in New York found that CBD reduces both the cravings and feelings of anxiety that often accompany people who are addicted to heroin. The study also found that CBD reduced stress, heart rate, and cortisol levels that are brought on by drug cues: "The specific effects of CBD on cue-induced drug craving and anxiety are particularly important in the development of addiction therapeutics because environmental cues are one of the strongest triggers for relapse and continued drug use." Dr. Hurd also states, "Our findings indicate that CBD holds significant promise for treating individuals with heroin use disorder," and "A successful non-opioid medication would add significantly to the existing addiction medication toolbox to help reduce the growing death toll, enormous health care costs, and treatment limitations imposed by stringent government regulations amid this persistent opioid epidemic."[20]

Summary

According to these research findings and so many more that I couldn't squeeze into this book, it appears that CBD is being taking very seriously by researchers and experts in the field of addiction. We all know the terrible news about opioid and heroin addiction and are reminded daily about the number of overdoses and deaths across the nation. The research is telling us that CBD can be effective in treating heroin, opioid, cocaine, morphine, nicotine, and alcohol addictions. It can be useful to help people going through withdrawal, which can be horribly painful for the individual and for their family to watch. If CBD can reduce craving, extinguish fear and memories associated with PTSD and phobia, and help people avoid relapse, isn't it worth continuing this line of research and seeking ways to use it in treating co-occurring addictions?

Anxiety

Introduction

While anxiety disorders can develop at any age, some are more prevalent in older adults, particularly in women. Some level of anxiety and stress are actually good for us. They help us handle certain situations and avoid danger. Anxiety disorders, on the other hand, can cause intense feelings of fear, apprehension, worry, or dread that are considered excessive when compared to the problems or issues being experienced. When anxiety and stress are overwhelming or to the point where they interfere with daily tasks, relationships, and social life, there may a clinically significant anxiety disorder that needs to be addressed. Chronic anxiety can significantly impair one's quality of life.

Ten to twenty percent of the older adult population experience anxiety disorders. Many times, these disorders go unnoticed and undiagnosed. Anxiety is the most common psychiatric disorder for women and the second most common for men, after substance abuse. There are many types of anxiety, including social anxiety disorder, panic disorder, panic attack, agoraphobia, generalized anxiety disorder, substance/medication-induced anxiety disorder, and anxiety disorder due to another medical condition.

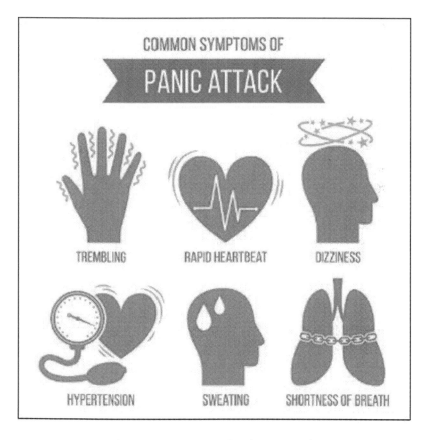

Symptoms most associated with panic attacks

Overview of Anxiety

Anxiety is a general term that consists of several different diagnoses that all share similar features, such as constant fear, apprehension, dread, and associated behavioral disturbances. Anxiety disorders may be diagnosed when these feelings are persistent and excessive. Some anxiety disorders listed in the *DSM-5* include specific phobia, social anxiety disorder or social phobia, panic disorder, generalized anxiety disorder, substance/medication-induced anxiety disorder, and anxiety disorder due to another medical condition. Some of these anxiety disorders have been studied more than others concerning the effectiveness of CBD on the specific disorder.

Despite the specific type of anxiety, many of them share common signs and symptoms, such as panic, unease, fear, sleeping difficulties, dry mouth, dizziness, shortness of breath, tenseness in the muscles, and the inability to stay calm or still. According to the Anxiety and Depression Association of America,[21] anxiety is the most commonly diagnosed disorder in the United States and affects forty million people, or over 18% of the population. There are three million new cases diagnosed annually. People suffering from anxiety disorders are more likely to go to their physician and to be hospitalized. While older adults experience anxiety disorders as much as younger people do, they tend to be diagnosed with generalized anxiety disorder more than younger people. Generalized anxiety disorder is, in fact, the most commonly diagnosed anxiety disorder among older adults. Some anxiety disorders develop after the senior experiences a traumatic event, like an acute illness or a fall, with or without injury.

Although there may be a number of causes or risks factors associated with the development of an anxiety disorder, some are more common than others. Some believe that genetics make certain people more vulnerable to anxiety than others, and under the perfect storm of conflict, stress, and other environmental triggers, symptoms may emerge. An individual's anatomical brain structure may also make one more vulnerable to developing anxiety. The limbic system of the brain is involved in the automatic fear response, emotion, and memory. Anxiety disorders like post-traumatic stress disorder (PTSD) and generalized anxiety disorder may originate within this structure of the brain. An increased volume of gray matter has also been associated with generalized anxiety disorder. Other risk factors or sources of anxiety may be linked to life events and circumstances, such as childhood trauma, abuse or neglect, death of a loved one, divorce, or living in isolation. Growing up with an anxious person may inadvertently teach us to behave in the same manner, making anxiety a learned behavior. And today more than ever, social factors like excessive use of social media can produce symptoms of anxiety. Other factors, like the use of substances, alcohol, and caffeine; poor relationships; and job stress, may all contribute to developing an anxiety disorder.

Traditional Therapies for Anxiety Disorders

There are many ways to effectively treat anxiety disorders. Self-care is usually the first line of treatment and involves interventions including getting exercise, relaxing, managing stress, meditating, eating healthily, stopping smoking, decreasing caffeine intake, and drinking alcohol in moderation. Seeing a mental health specialist may also be helpful. Seeking spiritual help can be effective in reducing anxiety and stress. Trying meditation or prayer may help. Avoiding caffeine and drinking chamomile tea can relieve some symptoms of anxiety. Using aromatherapy and essential oils of lavender, neroli, and chamomile may also be effective.

Self-care is such an important topic concerning anxiety that I'd like to dive into it a bit more. Many times, the most important person who will help you—is you. Think about it: no one knows you better than you do. Therefore, it's important to learn to manage how you think. Are your thoughts mostly happy or negative? Do you think with great confidence or with doubt? Self-care begins with managing your thoughts.

Another important element in self-care is surrounding yourself with positive and healthy people whom you know, love, and trust. They can be helpful resources to turn to when dealing with anxiety and panic. I've heard many times in my career that a strong support group is sometimes better than an experienced psychiatrist. Relationships matter. They can be comforting and supportive during good times and bad.

If your thoughts and relationships are critical for healthy self-care, your body and how you care for it matters as well. Exercise has been found to help many people burn off stress and anxiety. The food you eat can either keep you calm or trigger anxiety and panic. Limiting caffeine is a good start. Reducing or eliminating sugar from your daily diet can also help. Sugar has been found to trigger anxiety and depression.

Finally, at the end of the day, getting the proper amount of sleep can help in reducing symptoms of anxiety and panic. On the other hand, ruminating about problems, overly planning for tomorrow, and stressing over what happened today can all affect one's sleep quality. To get better sleep, start new nighttime habits like putting the cell phone away a couple of hours before bedtime, performing routine hygiene, dimming the lights, reading, listening to relaxing music, and avoiding food or caffeine at least four to five hours before going to bed.

There are also a number of psychiatric medications, such as anxiolytics, antidepressants, and sedatives, which can be effective but come with a number of unwanted side effects. Benzodiazepines are commonly prescribed medications that provide sedation and relaxation and may be helpful in managing symptoms of generalized anxiety disorder, panic disorder, and social anxiety disorder. Brand name benzodiazepines include Xanax, Ativan, Valium, Klonopin, and Librium. They come with side effects including drowsiness, loss of balance, and memory problems, and they can become habit forming. Other common side effects include depression, headaches, confusion, and vison problems, and while these could be dangerous side effects for anyone, older adults run a higher risk of injury.

Buspirone (Buspar) is another medication that might be prescribed by a physician for anxiety disorders. It is used to treat both acute and long-term anxiety disorders. It takes most people several weeks before they begin to feel the effects of this medication. Some side effects include nausea, headaches, dizziness, bizarre dreams, and sleeping problems.

Antidepressants are also widely used to treat anxiety disorders, and many times depression accompanies anxiety. It is believed that half of the people experiencing anxiety also have symptoms of depression. Two of the most commonly prescribed classes of antidepressants are selective serotonin reuptake inhibitors (SSRIs), and serotonin and norepinephrine reuptake inhibitors (SNRIs). SSRIs include brands such as Celexa, Prozac, Zoloft, Paxil, and Lexapro. Examples of SNRIs are Pristiq, Cymbalta, and Effexor XR.

Like other psychiatric medications, these have unwanted aside effects. The most common are nausea, dry mouth, dizziness, headache, and excessive sweating. Other possible side effects include fatigue, constipation, insomnia, changes in sexual function, and loss of appetite. Antidepressants may also cause suicidal thinking or behavior, and the FDA requires that all antidepressants carry the "black box warning."

Another class of antidepressant that may be prescribed are the tricyclics. These are older medications but work just as well as the SSRIs, except they usually cause more unpleasant side effects, so people may choose the SSRIs or SNRIs. Drugs like Anafranil and Tofranil are tricyclics and may cause side effects including drowsiness, lack of energy, dizziness, dry mouth, nausea and vomiting, blurred vision, constipation, and weight gain.

Research Findings on CBD and Anxiety

Cannabinoids have been used for their calming and relaxing effects for thousands of years. There are numerous studies that show promise concerning the use of cannabidiol to reduce feelings of anxiety and stress. In 2010, an article in the *Journal of Psychopharmacology* reported that CBD does have anxiolytic or anti-anxiety effects for generalized social anxiety disorder. The study involved the use of functional neuroimaging to measure regional cerebral blood flow, and when compared to a placebo, CBD was associated with significantly decreased anxiety. The authors conclude that cannabidiol reduces anxiety in social anxiety disorder and is related to its effects on brain activity in both the limbic and paralimbic areas.[22]

A much-referenced study took place in 2010 and involved the effects of cannabidiol on people who had public speaking anxiety. It is well known that public speaking is the most common cause of anxiety and phobia in the United States and is considered a generalized social anxiety disorder. This form of anxiety is very problematic and is associated with impaired social adjustments to everyday aspects of life, increased disability, dysfunction, and a loss of productivity.[23] Based on the work from another study, the authors state: "As this anxiety disorder is often poorly controlled by the currently available drugs (only 30% of the subjects achieve true recovery or remission without residual symptomatology…), there is a clear need to search for novel therapeutic agents."[24]

Years later, a team of researchers boldly say that CBD has therapeutic potential for both nonpsychiatric and psychiatric conditions like anxiety, depression, and psychosis.[25] They bring up the work of others who examined the impact of cannabidiol on certain types of anxiety, including panic attacks, post-traumatic stress disorder (PTSD), and obsessive-compulsive disorder (OCD). Although these studies involved experiments with mice, it is believed that the results can be applied to human subjects. In one such study, CBD decreased defensive behaviors brought on by a predator, proposing a model of panic attacks and PTSD.[26] In another study, CBD was shown to reduce marble-burying behaviors in mice, which means it could be effective in treating OCD.[27] CBD has also been shown to interfere in learning and/or memory of aversive events, which are processes associated with PTSD.[28] The authors conclude by saying that CBD is a safe compound that has a wide range of therapeutic actions in treating anxiety and other psychiatric conditions.

Researchers from Brazil have been interested in the psychological and psychiatric effects of cannabidiol for many years. In a 2012 article, they state, "Future clinical trials involving patients with different anxiety disorders are warranted, especially of panic disorder, obsessive-compulsive disorder, social anxiety disorder, and post-traumatic stress disorders."[29] They remind us that the first study examining the anti-anxiety effects of CBD was back in 1982, when researchers used it to reduce the anxiety-induced effects of THC.[30] They conclude:

> Together, the results from laboratory animals, healthy volunteers, and patients with anxiety disorders support the proposition of CBD as a new drug with anxiolytic properties. Because it has no psychoactive effects and does not affect cognition, has an adequate safety profile, good tolerability, positive results in trials with humans, and a broad spectrum of pharmacological actions, CBD appears to be the cannabinoid that is closer to have its preliminary findings in anxiety translated into clinical practice.

Researchers in 2015 reported that they found preclinical evidence that strongly supports CBD as a treatment for generalized anxiety disorder, panic disorder, social anxiety disorder, obsessive-compulsive disorder, and post-traumatic stress disorder when administered acutely. Human studies also show support of CBD effectively reducing symptoms of anxiety. They also remind us that since the new edition of the *DSM-5* was published in 2013, PTSD and OCD are no longer classified as classic anxiety disorders. Regardless, they both share symptoms of excessive anxiety: "Currently available pharmacological treatments include serotonin reuptake inhibitors, serotonin-norepinephrine reuptake inhibitors, benzodiazepines, monoamine oxidase inhibitors, tricyclic antidepressant drugs, and partial 5-hydroxytryptamine (5-HT) receptor agonists."[31] Anticonvulsants and atypical antipsychotics are also used to treat PTSD. These medications are associated with limited response rates and residual symptoms, particularly in PTSD, and adverse effects may also limit tolerability and adherence.

Another research paper was published in 2016 reporting on the effectiveness of CBD in alleviating anxiety associated with phobias and PTSD. The authors explain that CBD works at reducing learned fear, associated with both phobias and PTSD, in three ways. First, CBD decreases the intensity of fear expression. Next, it disrupts memory associated with traumatic experiences that would provoke anxious reactions. Last, cannabidiol improves *extinction*, or the psychological process by which exposure therapy reduces learned fear. The authors state, "This line of investigation may lead to the development of cannabidiol as a novel therapeutic approach for treating anxiety and trauma-related disorders such as phobias and PTSD in the future."[32] The researchers remind us that these disorders affect up to one in four people in their lifetime and can be very debilitating. Current psychiatric medications are available but are not fully effective in a large proportion of people who take them. Because of the side effects of these medications, people may also be less likely to continue them. Therefore, there is a strong need to find better treatments for anxiety and related emotional disorders.

In a recent article, researchers found that in the majority of test subjects, CBD reduced anxiety scores initially and then remained decreased throughout the duration of the study. Not only did anxiety improve, but it was reported by many subjects that sleep improved as well. This paper is another example of the surge in scientific investigations, using both animals and humans, to test the effectiveness of cannabidiol in treating anxiety and other disorders like epilepsy and schizophrenia. The authors believe that CBD may hold benefits for anxiety and sleep, among other conditions.[33]

Summary

Overall, it appears that cannabidiol (CBD) has gained much scientific evidence as a potentially effective treatment for anxiety, obsessive-compulsive disorder, post-traumatic stress disorder, panic disorder and other conditions. CBD shows an ability to impact a wide range of symptom domains, including anxiety and panic, acts as an anticompulsive, decreases autonomic arousal and learned fear expression, and enhances fear extinction. CBD has reduced experimentally induced anxiety in test subjects and people who experience social anxiety disorder. CBD may be an effective adjunct to counseling and psychotherapy for some people. It has been documented in scientific literature as safe and well tolerated, with very few to no side effects. Can CBD become the basis of a new line of treatment for those suffering from a variety of anxiety disorders?

Depression

Introduction

While depression can develop anytime throughout our lives, we may be more vulnerable as we age due to losses in physical and cognitive abilities, the losses of friends and family, perhaps our homes, and eventually our independence. It makes sense that depressive reactions and conditions would be more probable later in life. Besides the psychosocial causes of depression, the aging brain may change neurochemically and make older adults more susceptible to depressive disorders. One neurotransmitter implicated in depression is serotonin. It appears that low levels of serotonin are associated with many symptoms, including sleep difficulties, excessive worry, depressed mood, cravings for sugars and carbohydrates, obsessive behaviors, and a strong desire for alcoholic beverages in the daytime.

Although many people will experience a bad day, sad mood, or feelings of low energy and lack of motivation, these can be fleeting and not long term. When symptoms like a lack of interest in normal activities, thoughts about death or suicide, sleep or appetite problems, fatigue and difficulty concentrating last for long periods of time, they can be indicative of a depressive disorder. According to the *DSM-5*:

Depressive disorders include disruptive mood dysregulation disorder, major depressive disorder (including major depressive episode), persistent depressive disorder (dysthymia), premenstrual dysphoric disorder, substance/medication-induced depressive disorder, depressive disorder due to another medical condition, or specified depressive disorder, and unspecified depressive disorder.[34]

The *DSM-5* has separated depressive disorders and bipolar and related disorders, which appeared in the same chapter in previous editions. They are now considered two different conditions. Regardless, all of these disorders are characterized by common symptoms like being irritable or sad, feeling empty, experiencing different physical aches and pains, and undergoing changes in cognition that lead to difficulties with concentration and memory.

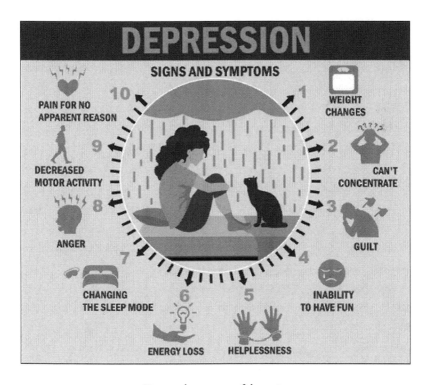

Signs and symptoms of depression

Overview of Depression

Depression is a very serious mental and emotional health condition that affects millions of Americans. The National Institute of Mental Health (NIMH) estimates that 16.2 million adults in the United States have experienced at least one major depressive episode, 1.5% of the US adult population has symptoms of dysthymia annually, 2.8% are affected by bipolar depression each year, and up to 83% of cases are severe, and seasonal affective disorder, or SAD, occurs in around 5% of the population annually. Another form of depression, known as "psychotic depression," is accompanied by hallucinations, delusions, or paranoia and affects around 25% of people hospitalized for depression.[35] It appears that women experience depression more than men do, sometimes twice as much as men.

Symptoms of depression affect both the brain and the body, and people can experience them in different ways. As we age, signs and symptoms may not be as apparent, and we may attribute them to simply growing older or to old age itself. Of course, this is usually not the case, and many older adults suffer from depressive symptoms that may go unnoticed and untreated. Suicide is highest among older white males in the United States, and sometimes symptoms of depression were written off as old age. We should not forget that geriatric suicide is a real problem in the United States. Some experts call it a "silent crisis."

Some classic symptoms of most depressive disorders include persistent sadness, irritability, fatigue, loss of appetite, new aches or pains, thoughts about death or suicide, sleeping problems, anxiety and restlessness, anger, loss of interest in activities, loss of libido or interest in sex, trouble concentrating or making decisions, and obsessing about the past or about bad times in one's life. While there is no single cause of depression, risk factors include brain chemistry (lack of serotonin), hormones, and genetics (family history of depression). Other common risk factors include age, gender, race, and geography; the use of certain prescription medications; and alcohol or drug misuse or abuse. Chronic illnesses such as heart disease, cancer, diabetes, and multiple sclerosis are associated with depression. Experiencing physical or sexual abuse may be linked to the development of depressive disorders. Certain psychiatric conditions like anxiety, borderline personality disorder, and PTSD, along with low self-esteem or poor self-image, may all be directly related to depression.

Having depression itself puts one at risk for developing other physical or emotional problems. It is associated with a higher risk for death and disability and can lead to suicide, substance abuse, and poor outcomes for physical disorders. Depression can significantly impair the ability to function on a daily basis. It can interfere with one's family life, career, and overall quality of living.

Traditional Therapies for Depression

A wide range of home-based, alternative, and clinical treatments exist that may decrease symptoms and make the condition more tolerable. Some researchers have found that certain foods like salmon, eggs, spinach, and chocolate may be involved in increasing low levels of serotonin and dopamine, which are neurotransmitters associated with regulation of mood. Eating foods that contain the essential amino acid tryptophan can help the body produce more serotonin. Reduced serotonin levels are associated with memory problems and low mood. It is also good to get carbohydrates into your diet. Since most of the body's serotonin is made in the gut, carbohydrates are needed to carry tryptophan to the brain to create serotonin. Try to eat foods that provide both tryptophan and carbs at the same time. Researchers in India found that nutmeg has antidepressant effects and state, "The antidepressant-like effect of the extract seems to be mediated by interaction with the adrenergic, dopaminergic, and serotonergic systems."[36]

Although Sant-John's-wort has not been approved by the FDA for the treatment of depression, this plant has been shown to increase serotonin in the body and reduce depressive symptoms. Omega-3 fatty acids may also help improve mood and are found in some fish, Brazil nuts, and chia seeds. Folate, or folic acid, is found in a variety of foods like beans, lentils, and dark leafy greens, and may improve the effectiveness of medications for mood disorders. SAM-e is a naturally occurring compound in the body and can also be bought as a supplement. It helps to regulate hormones and maintain cell membranes, and it may reduce symptoms of depressive disorders.

Dr. Simon Young writes in his paper "How to Increase Serotonin in the Human Brain without Drugs" substance-related disorders fall into ten different categories that serotonin is important in the treatment of depression as well as in susceptibility to both depression and suicide. Because prevention is far better than trying to treat a condition, finding ways to increase the body's serotonin is important. Serotonin is also associated with happiness and overall well-being, which are factors protecting us against mental and physical disorders. He stresses that negative moods are associated with negative outcomes and uses the relationship between hostility and coronary heart disease as an example.

Mood is very important and can influence social behavior, and social support is one of the most studied psychosocial factors associated with health and illness. Poor social support is related to depression, higher levels of stress, dysthymia, and PTSD, as well as increased sickness and death from numerous medical illnesses. As we can see, the relationship between mood and social life can become a vicious cycle. It is therefore important to try natural ways to increase the brain's levels of serotonin. Dr. Young recommends four strategies to boost serotonin, all based on scientific findings. Meditation, exposure to bright light, exercise, and diet have been found to increase levels of serotonin and dopamine and act as natural antidepressants and anti-anxiety agents. Exposure to bright light is effective at increasing serotonin and decreasing depressive symptoms, as evidenced by an interesting study that found that serotonin levels in the human postmortem brain were higher in those who died in the summer than those who died in the winter months.[38]

Some people benefit from seeing a mental health specialist, like a counselor or psychologist. Various types of therapy can be helpful in understanding the disorder and doing things to improve symptoms. Most times, therapy is coupled with psychiatric medication. The reason behind this is that if the depression is biological—meaning that it is due to an imbalance of neurotransmitters like serotonin or dopamine—the medications may be useful in correcting this imbalance. On the other hand, if the depression is cognitive or thought based, talk therapy might help. It's sort of like killing two birds with one stone.

Taking antidepressant medications is another method of managing symptoms of depression. The reuptake inhibitors are some of the most commonly prescribed and include the selective serotonin reuptake inhibitors (SSRIs), serotonin and norepinephrine reuptake inhibitors (SNRIs), and norepinephrine and dopamine reuptake inhibitors (NDRIs). You will recognize names like

Celexa, Paxil, Prozac, and Zoloft. They are from the SSRI group. SNRIs you may recognize include Cymbalta, Effexor, and Pristiq. Wellbutrin is the commonly prescribed NDRI.

Antidepressant medications, like all psychiatric drugs, come with side effects, some of which can be unpleasant and others dangerous and deadly. Here are some of the most common side effects of antidepressants in general: nausea, diarrhea, stomach upset, headaches, dizziness, weakness and fatigue, dry mouth, trouble sleeping, anxiety, and sexual problems like low sex drive. Other side effects include sweating, constipation, and loss of appetite. The more dangerous side effects include low blood pressure when standing up (orthostatic hypotension), high blood pressure, abnormal heart rate or arrhythmia, and suicidal thoughts or actions.

Research Findings on CBD and Depression

Depression appears to be one of the most studied phenomena concerning the effects of cannabinoids and cannabidiol (CBD). A study in 1995 and another in 2002 both found that cannabinoids might have therapeutic value in reducing symptoms of depression and improving mood. substance-related disorders fall into ten different categories Scientists in 2009 found evidence that a deficit in the endocannabinoid system may be related to depression and that the endocannabinoid system regulates depression, anxiety, and emotional and cognitive processes.[41] They also found in preclinical studies that facilitation of endocannabinoid neurotransmission produces both antidepressant and anxiolytic effects. A research paper in the *British Journal of Pharmacology* also found antidepressantlike effects of cannabidiol in mice and proposed that CBD may be mediated by the activation of 5-HT_{1A} receptors. This time the researchers compared CBD to a common psychiatric drug called imipramine, or Tofranil, and found that CBD worked just as well as the antidepressant. A later study found similar results, and the authors wrote that "CBD could represent a novel fast antidepressant drug, via enhancing both serotonergic and glutamate cortical signaling through a 5-HT_{1A} receptor-dependent mechanism."[42]

Another study in 2014 suggested that CBD works as an antidepressant and anti-anxiety agent in animal studies, including the forced swimming test, elevated plus maze, and Vogel conflict test.[43] These are all experiments with mice that are put into certain situations and then observed with and without CBD administration. The researchers believe that CBD can have great potential for treating both depressive symptoms and those of anxiety. Other studies reported similar findings with animals and found that CB1 activity in the hippocampus produced antidepressant effects and modified mood.[44, 45] Leinow and Birnbaum, in their book *CBD: A Patient's Guide to Medicinal Cannabis*, state, "The neural network of the endocannabinoid system works similarly to the way that serotonin, dopamine, and other system do, and, according to some research, cannabinoids have an effect on serotonin levels."[46]

An interesting study took place in China examining the endocannabinoid system and its role in depression, reward, and pain. They indicate that depression and pain co-occur very often, in up to 80% of people, and that these two conditions are associated with impaired quality of life and high mortality. They report, "The most common debilitating disorders affecting society at large are pain and depression, which are the most prevalent among neurological and psychiatric disorders." Pain is experienced subjectively, and no two people go through it the same way. It can be felt physically, emotionally, and mentally. Some people may find relief from the use of certain medications, but in general, pain and depression are difficult to treat, and one set of symptoms exacerbates more symptoms. The paper concludes, "The endocannabinoid system is involved in eliciting potent effects on neurotransmission, neuroendocrine, and inflammatory processes, which are known to be deranged [unbalanced] in depression and chronic pain."[47]

CBD is being examined as a real potential for treatment of depression that is associated with chronic stress, which has been shown to reduce levels of a healthy, functioning endocannabinoid system.[48, 49] Researchers looked at the relationships between deficient CB1-receptor-mediated signaling that results in depressionlike symptoms; activation of CB1-receptor-mediated signals that result in behavioral, endocrine, and other effects similar to those of antidepressants; and conventional antidepressants working through enhanced CB1-receptor mediated signaling. They concluded that reduced endocannabinoid signaling explains most of the measurable behavioral, endocrine, and other changes seen in depression. Poor endocannabinoid signaling is associated with depression, and increasing signaling would be effective in treating mood disorders. They also state that increased endocannabinoid signaling could mimic the effects of conventional antidepressants and help with chronic stress. The bottom line of this study is that "cannabinoid-based antidepressants could be at least as efficacious as conventional therapies."[50]

Researchers in 2018 examined the association between cannabidiol and brain serotonin and norepinephrine levels in mice who were subjected to the forced swimming test and found that CBD induced antidepressantlike effects of the mice in the test.[51] The takeaway of the study is that CBD is shown to interact with naturally occurring brain chemicals or neurotransmitters in our brain. When serotonin, norepinephrine, and cannabidiol all combine to do their work, the outcome is diminished despair and relief of low mood and other depressivelike symptoms. Another study testing CBD on rodents showed that a single dose of CBD induced antidepressantlike effects when mice were subjected to the forced swim test. Similar effects were also seen among rodents undergoing a learned helplessness test. While there are many antidepressant drugs available, they have a significant lag time before a therapeutic response is noticed. Some of these drugs simply don't work well with some people, so there is a need for a new line of antidepressant treatments. The authors concluded that CBD induced fast and sustained antidepressantlike effects and believe that their findings support a promising profile for CBD as a new fast-acting antidepressant medication.[52]

Summary

Depression affects millions of people of all ages and backgrounds. It can become more complicated when diagnosed with other psychiatric or medical conditions. While there are psychiatric medications available, they may come with undesirable side effects, some of which can be very dangerous and life limiting. Not all people respond well to the current medications available. Older adults take more prescription drugs than any other age group in the United States. Can CBD be an effective prevention for mood disorders like depression as we age? Might it become an antidepressant treatment once depression becomes a problem? Can we cut down on the number of prescription and over-the-counter drugs that might produce unwanted side effects? There appear to be many studies indicating its promise as a new and viable antidepressant.

Eating Disorders

Introduction
Some of the most common and complicated psychiatric conditions are eating disorders. According to experts, around twenty million women and ten million men in the United States will experience eating disorders at some time during their lives.[53] Binge-eating disorder is a major problem and is three times more common than both anorexia and bulimia combined. As a matter of fact, binge-eating disorder is more common than breast cancer, schizophrenia, and HIV.[54] Despite popular thought that eating disorders affect mainly women, and in particular, young females, 25% of people with anorexia and bulimia, and 36% with binge-eating disorder, are men. Despite these figures, eating disorders are the third most common chronic disorder among adolescent girls.[55] A sad but probably little-known fact is that anorexia nervosa has the highest mortality rate of any psychiatric disorder, and only roughly one-third of people suffering from this disorder ever receive any treatment. The prevalence of eating disorders is similar for non-Hispanic Whites, Hispanics, African Americans, and Asians in the United States, and only anorexia nervosa is more common in non-Hispanic Whites.

Because this book focuses on the aging process, I address special types of eating disorders among older adults and elderly people. Conditions like geriatric anorexia, Alzheimer's-related cachexia (a "wasting" disorder that leads to extreme weight loss, muscle deterioration, and fat loss), and failure to thrive are examined on their own. I then provide research findings examining the use of CBD and any outcomes reported in the literature.

Overview of Eating Disorders
In order to provide a good overview of eating disorders, I turn to the "Bible" of psychiatric conditions, the *DSM-5*, for a list and description of each eating

disorder. In the chapter entitled "Feeding and Eating Disorders," such disorders are "characterized by a persistent disturbance of eating or eating-related behavior that results in the altered consumption or absorption of food that significantly impairs physical health or psychological functioning."[56] The disorders listed in the *DSM-5* include pica, rumination disorder, avoidant-restrictive food intake disorder, anorexia nervosa, bulimia nervosa, and binge-eating disorder. An interesting note from the American Psychiatric Association is that eating disorders and substance-use disorders have common features, including craving and compulsive use patterns. This relationship may be due to the involvement of the same neural systems involved in regulatory self-control and reward.

Another special note in this chapter is that obesity, while being a national epidemic and serious health concern, is not considered a psychiatric condition. There are numerous factors implicated in the development of obesity, including genetics, physiological, behavioral, and environmental variables, as well as a side effect of certain medications. Despite this, there are strong associations between obesity and several mental disorders, such as binge-eating disorder, depression, bipolar disorder, and schizophrenia.

I'd like to focus on some of the more common eating disorders and then provide some information on those affecting older adults and seniors. Binge-eating disorder is associated with three or more of the following conditions: eating until you feel uncomfortably full, eating large quantities of food when you're not hungry, eating faster than normal, eating by yourself because you feel embarrassed by the amount of food being consumed, and feeling disgusted, depressed, and guilty after you have overeaten. Binge eating is not associated with purging or excessive exercise. If you have three or more of these conditions at least twice a week for more than six months, binge-eating disorder may be a problem.

Bulimia nervosa is an eating disorder characterized by a cyclical pattern of binge eating and then purging to avoid any weight gain. Purging includes self-induced vomiting, the use of laxatives or diuretics, excessive exercise, and fasting. Anorexia nervosa, on the other hand, is expressed as the loss of appetite altogether, along with obsessive fears of becoming overweight or obese. It involves body image disturbances, significant weight loss, refusal to maintain a normal weight, excessive exercise, and the absence of periods in females.

Eating disorders among older adults are particularly dangerous due to frailty, co-occurring illnesses, and many other factors. The nutritional goals for older adults are to maintain or improve their overall health and well-being and to enhance their quality of life. Important, too, is the goal of prevention of an age- or nutrition-related condition before it creates health-related problems. Nutrition is vital for older adults as it influences the aging process itself as well as other physiological systems and functions, body composition, and the onset and management of chronic health conditions. Just as nutrition influences aging, the aging process affects nutritional status. As we age, changes in social status and finances may contribute to decreased access to food, poor food choices, nutrient deficiencies, and overall poor nutritional status. These, in turn, can affect health, independence, mobility, and increased risk of illness. Other factors such as education, social support, gender, and culture can play a role in nutritional status as we age. Older adults who live alone may not be able to afford nutritious diets. Those without higher education may not understand the importance of nutritional supplements. And those who live alone and have few to no support networks may be at a higher risk for nutritional deficiencies and health problems.

Many people don't associate eating disorders with older adults or the elderly and assume they are reserved for younger people, especially young girls. But this isn't the case. Unfortunately, eating disorders go unnoticed and untreated because early warning signs are missed by family, friends, and even health care providers. Some of these early warning signs of an eating disorder include an increased sensitivity to hot or cold foods and fluids, behavioral changes like going to the bathroom right after eating, hair loss, dental problems, gastrointestinal issues, and the desire to eat alone.

Eating disorders that commonly affect older adults are anorexia nervosa and bulimia nervosa. A report indicated that 81% of older adults in a study had anorexia nervosa, and 10% had bulimia nervosa, and that late-onset eating disorders are more common (69%) than early-onset eating disorders.[57] Older adults may refuse meals because they say they're not hungry or are too full, or they feel sick. Some have distorted body image problems, engage in secret eating, have difficulty talking about their emotions, or are experiencing family problems, and this is how they cope. While some older adults may purge, overuse of laxatives is far more common among elderly people. Bulimia nervosa, in particular, may present severe health risks for older adults due to its connection with cardiovascular problems. Besides heart problems, eating disorders can take a serious toll on the health of seniors. The body is aging and is not as resilient as it once was. Eating disorders in later life can do much more damage to the body—and a lot faster.

"Geriatric failure to thrive" is a condition marked by a multifactorial decline that may be caused by chronic co-occurring illnesses and functional impairments. The condition is characterized by weight loss, poor nutrition, decreased appetite, and inactivity. According to experts, four syndromes are common and predictive of undesirable consequences in seniors diagnosed with failure to thrive. They include impaired physical function, malnutrition, depression, and cognitive impairment. Health care providers should conduct evaluations of medication to ensure they are not contributing to the decline. Interventions should target easily treatable causes of failure to thrive with the goals of maintaining or improving overall functional status.[58]

Alzheimer's-related cachexia is a condition characterized by unexplained weight loss and a wasting syndrome among people who have Alzheimer's disease. It is a complicated metabolic process associated with several end-stage organ diseases such as cancer, renal disease, and advanced heart and lung failure, known to occur in persons with advanced dementia. The connection between sarcopenia or the degenerative loss of skeletal muscle, malnutrition, and inactivity may worsen with aging. This can make older adults particularly vulnerable to cachexia, which is also associated with insulin resistance, myolysis (or the destruction of muscle tissue), and systemic inflammation. Cachexia is known to increase morbidity and mortality. An interesting note by the authors of "Cachexia and Advanced Dementia" is that "unintentional weight loss may in fact be a harbinger of AD, appearing before the detectable clinical onset of dementia…patients with AD sometimes exhibit a paradoxical pattern of overeating concomitant with weight loss. This pattern may suggest a hypermetabolic state."[59]

Geriatric anorexia nervosa is the most common eating disorder among adults over age fifty, and the morbidity and mortality are significant. Among deaths related to this disorder, the eating disorder itself or complications related to the eating disorder are to blame.[60] While geriatric anorexia nervosa is highly associated with mood disorders, especially major depression, other factors are involved, including alternations in sense of taste and smell, especially due to medication side effects, cognitive and memory problems, loss, feelings of isolation and loneliness, refusal to eat as a form of control, the environment, and suicidal thoughts. It is a complex and potentially deadly disorder, affecting the older adult's emotional, psychological, and social well-being and quality of life.

Researchers in Japan found that anorexia is not only common in the elderly but one of the major symptoms of depression in elderly people. They also believe that the rates of anorexia and depression will become worse in the future, as they are experiencing a similar growth in their aging population. Older adults diagnosed with an eating disorder may also be prone to develop other illnesses such as osteoporosis, electrolyte imbalance, gastrointestinal problems, changes in hormones, seizures, heart problems, and leukopenia (low white blood cell count). They also discuss "anorexia tardive," which is an eating disorder specific to elderly individuals. It is characterized by a loss of appetite as well as significant weight loss but has more depressive symptoms associated with it than other eating disorders.[61]

Traditional Therapies for Eating Disorders

In this section, I'd like to separate treatments for eating disorders among the general population and then those most associated with older adults. The type of treatment depends on the diagnosis and other co-occurring disorders and symptoms. Most times, treatment involves a combination of psychological therapy, counseling, nutrition education, and the use of certain medications. Perhaps there are other health issues the individual is dealing with alongside the eating disorder. These will need to be addressed too. After an attempt to treat and resolve the eating disorder with no improvement, inpatient programs and hospitalization may be necessary. There are programs that offer intensive outpatient treatment, partial hospitalization, residential treatment, and inpatient care.

Most people start the treatment process by talking with their primary care physician or a mental health professional. This is usually just the beginning, as it generally takes a long time to successfully treat an eating disorder. If the individual requires psychotherapy, it can be very effective in normalizing eating patterns, monitoring eating and mood, switching out unhealthy foods for healthier ones, improving relationships, and developing coping and problem-solving skills. Types of therapy include cognitive behavioral, acceptance and commitment, dialectical behavior, family-based, group cognitive behavioral, and interpersonal psychotherapy. Most treatment centers offer evidence-based treatment, meaning that the particular type of therapy has been used in research studies and was found to be effective.

Antidepressants are the most commonly prescribed medications to treat eating disorders, especially those involving binge eating and purging. Taking antidepressants can be helpful for people diagnosed with bulimia and binge-eating disorder and can help manage symptoms like depression and anxiety. No medication has been approved by the FDA for the treatment of anorexia nervosa. There is some evidence that atypical antipsychotic drugs, like Zyprexa, may lead to slight weight gain. Benzodiazepines may also be recommended to reduce anxiety, although they can be addictive. Birth control pills are commonly prescribed when younger females have lost their monthly period due to their eating disorder and are also used to minimize bone weakness.

Drug treatment for bulimia nervosa include the use of selective serotonin reuptake inhibitors (SSRIs) and are the most researched class of medications for this eating disorder. SSRIs are generally well tolerated by people who use them. Of the SSRIs, Prozac is by far the most studied drug for the treatment of bulimia nervosa and is the only drug specifically approved for adults diagnosed with this disorder. Sometimes the anticonvulsant Topirimate is prescribed off-label for bulimia nervosa. When it comes to binge-eating disorder, three different classes of medications are recommended: SSRIs (antidepressants), antiseizure drugs (for epilepsy and seizure disorders), and Vyvance, an ADHD medication. These drugs may help with the binge-eating behavior associated with binge-eating disorder. They can help manage obsessive thoughts, impulsivity, and depressive symptoms. Vyvanse became the first drug approved by the FDA for treating binge-eating disorder. Wellbutrin should be completely avoided, as it has been associated with seizures in people who have purging bulimia and is not recommended for anyone with an eating disorder.

Lifestyle modifications may help manage symptoms of eating disorders. Activities like yoga and tai chi as well as treatments involving acupuncture and biofeedback can be helpful. Eating a well-balanced, nutrient-dense, and sugar-free diet and taking vitamins C, B-complex, and a multivitamin are recommended. Support from family, friends, and other sources can be comforting.

In terms of treating older adults with eating disorders, there is no one way to approach them all, but they do have enough in common to provide some general information about treatment options. Older adults would most likely start out with a thorough physical examination and assessment of their eating disorder. The examination would take many factors into account, including any socioeconomic problems, swallowing and chewing problems, living alone or in a senior care facility, whether they are bedridden or chair-bound, and a review of other acute or chronic health conditions. Possible interventions include food manipulation, which involves improving food palatability, texture, flavor, and variety as well as any assistance in eating. Another possibility is making environmental changes to improve the dining experience and eliminate social isolation during mealtimes. The use of nutritional supplements, particularly protein supplementation, may be useful in treating geriatric eating disorders.[62]

Research Findings on CBD and Eating Disorders

As I was researching the area of eating disorders and cannabinoids, I was pleasantly surprised to find studies that go back to the early 1990s. One study in 1991 concluded that cannabinoids alleviate symptoms of cancer-induced cachemia (physical wasting, loss of weight, and malnutrition associated with certain diseases). In another article appearing in the *Journal of Pain and Symptom Management* in 1995, researchers reported that dronabinol provided "excellent" results and was safe and effective for anorexia and weight loss associated with AIDS. They also stressed that there were no adverse effects.[63] Another study examined the effectiveness of dronabinol on weight gain in individuals with HIV. This drug is a synthetic form of THC approved by the FDA for the treatment of nausea and vomiting induced by cancer treatments and has been used for many years to increase weight in instances of the "wasting syndrome" characteristic of some people with HIV and Alzheimer's disease. In this study, researchers found that dronabinol increased the weight of seven out of ten individuals with HIV. They also said that the drug improved appetite in people with HIV and cancer.[64]

In 2002, an important study in Madrid using mice found for the first time that peripheral endocannabinoid CB1 receptors have a strong effect on the regulation of eating.[65] Three years later, a study reported that CB1 receptors stimulate appetite and ingestion. They also found strong evidence that the endocannabinoid system plays an important part in energy metabolism and fuel storage in the body.[66] In 2006, a study confirmed the effectiveness of nabilone for cancer-related anorexia symptoms, including pain, anxiety, depression, nausea, night sweats, and insomnia.[67] One year later, researchers in Orlando, Florida, studied the impact of dronabinol on people living with HIV/AIDS experiencing loss of appetite and weight and found that it quickly improved the participants' weight and appetites.[68] Researchers the same year in St. Louis, Missouri, who followed twenty-nine elderly senior care residents experiencing weight loss from a number of conditions, discovered that dronabinol helped them gain an average of nearly eight pounds.[69]

In Ottawa, Canada, a group of researchers wondered if cannabinoids might be effective in managing severe side effects of antiviral therapy used to treat hepatitis C. They already knew that cannabinoid medications were effective in the treatment of nausea caused by chemotherapy and wasting syndrome seen in some people with AIDS. The findings were impressive, as 64% of individuals receiving interferon-ribavirin therapy experienced symptom improvement after receiving cannabinoids.[70]

A 2009 paper published in the *Journal of Psychiatric Research* examined the effects of leptin, ghrelin, and endocannabinoids and found that all three had therapeutic value in treating anorexia nervosa. Leptin, a hormone that regulates energy by reducing hunger, could restore menstrual cycles, decrease motor restlessness, and prevent osteoporosis in chronic patients. Ghrelin, the "hunger hormone" and endocannabinoids, on the other hand, may accelerate nutritional restoration. They also found that both leptin and endocannabinoids improved depressive and anxious symptoms.[71] Two years later, a very intensive article was published in *Frontiers in Behavioral Neuroscience* by a team of researchers headed by Eva Marco. The overall aim of the paper was to study the role of the endocannabinoid system on psychiatric conditions and found there to be connections between defects in endocannabinoid signaling and eating disorders like binge eating, anorexia nervosa, and bulimia nervosa. Much evidence is involved supporting this finding, including the fact that the endocannabinoid system "is strategically located in all the key points involved in food intake and energy expenditure, both at the central and peripheral level," and the endocannabinoid system "influences feeding behavior at the CNS by acting on circuits located in the hypothalamus, the reward system and the brain stem." The team goes on to say that a dysregulation in the endocannabinoid system appears to be an underlying cause of many neuropsychiatric disorders, including eating disorders. Enhancing the signaling within the endocannabinoid system with the use of medications has led to good results in rodents and could be used to treat depression and anxiety. They believe that CBD is a good candidate to modulate the endocannabinoid system and has consistently been shown to have antidepressant and anti-anxiety effects. Its potential as an antipsychotic is also gaining ground in research.[72]

That same year, an international team of researchers from Spain, France, and the United States studied the relationship between the endocannabinoid system, eating disorders, and addiction. In a very detailed report, they conclude that while the causes of eating disorders are still largely unknown, there is an increasing body of evidence of the endocannabinoid system's influence on brain circuits involved in feeding behavior, especially those associated with the reward system. A dysregulation of the endocannabinoid system may lead to eating disorders and many other conditions.[73] Another team of researchers agreed in their work performed in 2012. They indicated that since the endocannabinoid system plays an important role in energy homeostasis, such as in obesity and eating disorders, cannabinoids can be safe and effective tools in managing disorders like cachexia caused by various diseases. Eventually, cannabinoids may become a new treatment approach for diseases of endocannabinoid dysregulation, imbalanced body homeostasis, and energy expenditure.[74]

Two important studies in 2014 examined the effectiveness of cannabinoid-based treatments for eating disorders. An Italian team echoed the findings of previous studies and reported that there does seem to be a link between a defective endocannabinoid system and eating disorders, including obesity. They also call for the clinical development of a drug that could modify the endocannabinoid system in the treatment of such disorders.[75] The other study examined the effectiveness of dronabinol for severe anorexia nervosa and found that it did indeed lead to a small but significant weight gain in anorexic nervosa patients.[76] An article published in a 2015 issue of *Cosmopolitan* reported that cannabinoids helped anorexic mice return to their normal, healthy weight.[77] In another paper published the same year in *The American Journal of Clinical Nutrition* it was found that "endocannabinoids and endocannabinoid-related compounds are involved in food-related reward and suggest a dysregulation of the physiology in anorexia nervosa." The research team was specifically looking at hedonic eating, or the consumption of food simply for pleasure and not for energy. They conclude that "a dysregulation of peripheral endocannabinoid signaling in both underweight and recently weight-restored patients with AN [anorexia nervosa] who undergo hedonic eating, thereby suggesting an alteration of the biochemical mechanism implicated in food-related reward."[78]

A year later, more research papers were published, all reporting similar themes and findings. Natasha Devon, in her article "Obesity is an Eating Disorder just like Anorexia and it's Time we Started Treating it that Way," stresses that many diseases of either extreme weight loss or gain, including obesity and binge eating, have comparable biological and psychological features. Remember, that obesity is not officially an eating disorder according to the American Psychiatric Association and is not listed in the *DSM-5* as such. Her argument is that there is plenty of evidence showing a clear link between defects within the endocannabinoid system and eating disorders.[79] Another study examined the relationship between CBD and "brown fat," or brown adipose tissue, which is the type of fat cell that burns calories to produce heat rather than stores them. This type of fat is activated when the body is exposed to cold and produces heat to help maintain body temperature. Exercise may stimulate the hormones responsible for activating brown fat, and it could play a role in weight loss. This study suggests that CBD may induce brown fat, which could be key in prevention of obesity.[80] Another article published in 2016 by an Italian team of researchers looking specifically at anorexia in old age called for the use of simple interventions like nutritional supplements and diet modification. While they do not examine CBD as a potential method of treatment, it has been established in the literature that CBD might work to improve appetite and help older adults with eating disorders.[81]

Lastly, another Italian team examined the relationship between endocannabinoids and eating disorders. They conclude:

> The endocannabinoid system plays an important role in the control of eating behavior by acting via central (brain) and peripheral (gut, liver, muscle and fat) mechanisms. The CB1 receptor is believed to be responsible for most of the central and peripheral effects of cannabinoids on the eating behavior. While some studies have clearly demonstrated that dysregulation of cannabinoid physiology can have detrimental effects on eating behavior, conversely, optimizing endocannabinoid tone appears to have beneficial effects on eating behavior regulation.

They also believe that the endocannabinoid system may be a target for the development of drugs to treat eating disorders.[82]

Summary

As I began doing research for this section of the book, I was concerned about finding much in the scientific literature on cannabidiol and eating disorders, but I was wrong. Many researchers from around the world are interested in the effects of CBD as well as dysregulation of the endocannabinoid system in relation to the treatment of eating disorders. Younger people may experience symptoms of anorexia, bulimia, and binge eating, and older adults may develop geriatric anorexia, Alzheimer's-related eating disorders, and failure to thrive. Anorexia has the highest mortality rate of any psychiatric disorder, and the other eating disorders can present great difficulties, diminished quality of life, and early mortality. While there are traditional means to treat symptoms of the disorders, such as lifestyle changes, nutritional education, therapy, and hospitalization, psychotropic medications are often prescribed and have both unwanted and sometimes life-threatening side effects. Much evidence from these studies indicate that the endocannabinoid system plays a role in eating, weight gain, and weight loss. They also show that CBD may increase appetite in those who need to gain weight and regulate eating behaviors for those who may binge eat. The endocannabinoid system also plays an important role in energy homeostasis. Can CBD become a viable treatment for eating disorders in the near future?

8

CBD and Obsessive-Compulsive Disorder, Post-Traumatic Stress Disorder, Schizophrenia, and Late-Onset Schizophrenia

Not until we are lost, do we begin to understand ourselves.
—Henry David Thoreau

Obsessive-Compulsive Disorder

Introduction
A mental health condition known as obsessive-compulsive disorder, or OCD, has gained more attention over the past couple decades and is now considered more common than once believed. OCD affects both men and women equally, people of all ages, races, ethnicities, and cultural backgrounds. It is usually identified by parents or teachers of school-aged children between eight and twelve, and then again between the late teen years and early adulthood. It has also been known to be diagnosed after the age of thirty-five. According to the Anxiety and Depression Association of America, 1.2% of adults are affected by OCD within the past year, and it currently affects one in forty adults and one in one hundred

children in the United States.¹ The International OCD Foundation sites that roughly the number of people living in Houston, Texas—between two to three million—represents how many people in the United States are currently diagnosed with obsessive-compulsive disorder.² It is also estimated that over 80% of people diagnosed with OCD experience moderate to serious impairment in many areas of life. Suicidal thoughts occur in about 50% of people with OCD, and suicidal attempts are reported in about 25% of people with OCD. Males tend to have an earlier onset and are more likely to have comorbid tic disorders. Females experience more obsessive-compulsive thoughts about cleaning, and men have more regarding taboo and forbidden topics.

Overview of Obsessive-Compulsive Disorder

While obsessive-compulsive disorder used to be considered an anxiety disorder in other editions of the *DSM*, it now has its own chapter and is no longer considered an anxiety disorder. The latest edition of the *DSM-5* includes the following disorders in the chapter entitled "Obsessive-Compulsive and Related Disorders": obsessive-compulsive disorder (OCD), body dysmorphic disorder, hoarding disorder, trichotillomania (hair-pulling disorder), excoriation (skin-picking) disorder, substance/medication-induced obsessive-compulsive and related disorder, obsessive-compulsive and related disorder due to another medical condition, and other specified obsessive-compulsive and related disorder and unspecified obsessive-compulsive and related disorder (e.g., body-focused repetitive behavior disorder, obsessional jealousy).

The obsessions involved in the disorder are uncontrollable and recurring thoughts, urges or mental images that cause anxiety and can include fixations on things like dirt, germs, or contamination; unwanted or taboo thoughts about sex, harm, or religion; aggressive thoughts toward others; and having things in perfect order or symmetrical. Some individuals may have repeated mental images of themselves hurting someone else. Compulsions, on the other hand, are repetitive behaviors that an individual with OCD feels the urge to do in response to the obsessions. The goal of compulsions is to neutralize or eliminate the obsessions. Common compulsions include handwashing, excessive cleaning, checking and rechecking, ordering and arranging things in a very particular and precise manner, and compulsive counting.

Some individuals with OCD will experience a tic disorder. Tics are defined as sudden, brief, and repetitive movements. These include eye blinking, facial grimacing, shoulder shrugging, and head and shoulder jerking movements. There are also vocal tics, which include repetitive throat clearing, grunting sounds, and sniffing. OCD can be diagnosed with other disorders, such as anxiety, major depression, eating disorders, psychotic disorders, and obsessive-compulsive personality disorder.

There are some risk factors associated with obsessive-compulsive disorder, including genetics (especially if the first-degree relative developed OCD as a child or teen), brain structure and functioning (particularly differences in the frontal cortex and subcortical structures of the brain), and the environment. Individuals who experienced child abuse, sexual assault, or trauma as children run a higher risk of developing OCD. The *DSM-5* also lists being "temperamental" as a risk and prognostic factor, and defines it as "greater internalizing symptoms, higher negative emotionality, and behavior inhibition in childhood."[3]

Traditional Therapies for Obsessive-Compulsive Disorder

People with OCD have many options when it comes to treatment and symptom management. They can begin by modifying things about their lifestyle and trying several home remedies. It's important to note that people taking medications for OCD should remain compliant about their medications and take them as prescribed. Even when symptoms seem to be managed and the person is feeling better, they should remain on the medication. Paying attention to triggers and warning signs can help reduce symptoms as well. Before taking any supplements or drugstore medications, always make sure to speak with your physician.

Individuals can also learn as much as they can about their condition, join a support group, and find healthy coping mechanisms like exercise, healthy eating, and recreational activities to deal with triggers and behavioral reactions. Stress management techniques may help and include meditation and prayer, massage, yoga, tai chi, deep breathing, and visualization. The point is to try whatever is necessary to not let OCD impair one's health, well-being, and quality of life.

Beyond self-care, treatments such as cognitive behavioral therapy (a form of treatment that helps people cope with and change problematic thoughts, behaviors, and emotions), and exposure and response prevention (purposely confronting situations that induce distress and working through it until the anxiety is diminished) have been shown to be helpful for many people diagnosed with OCD. A note on exposure and response prevention: it is exactly what it sounds like. An individual is exposed to something that triggers their anxiety a little at a time. The individual then learns how to respond to them instead of using repetitive behaviors. Group therapy, teletherapy (video conferencing), and acceptance and commitment therapy may be useful for some people. Medications can also be prescribed for OCD and associated conditions. The most common include antidepressants like Anafranil, Prozac, Luvox, Paxil, and Zoloft. If these don't work well, antipsychotics may be prescribed, like Risperdal, particularly for people who have both OCD and tics.

More intensive options for OCD include outpatient and intensive inpatient treatment programs. Perhaps a day program or partial hospitalization are better for some people. If very close supervision and around-the-clock care is required, residential treatment and inpatient programs are available. Some people may benefit from other treatments if they do not respond well to therapy and medications. Clinical trials may be one route. Deep brain stimulation or electroconvulsive therapy (ECT) might also help manage the disorder.

Research Findings on CBD and Obsessive-Compulsive Disorder

An early study in 2004 by a team of Brazilian scientists found that cannabidiol significantly decreased anxiety and increased "mental sedation." It had anxiolytic (anti-anxiety) effects mediated by action on the limbic and paralimbic systems of the brain. These two areas are responsible for the regulation of emotion, arousal, stimulation, memory, learning, and motivation.[4] Six years later, another Brazilian team performed an interesting study using mice that mimicked the effects of obsessive-compulsive disorder by participating in marble-burying behavior, which can be seen as an obsessive-compulsive behavior in rodents. The team gave the mice CBD, Paxil (an antidepressant), and Valium (a benzodiazepine). CBD decreased the behavior compared to Paxil and Valium, and even more compelling, the effect of CBD was still seen seven days later, whereas the effects of Valium disappeared. Both CBD and Paxil decreased the marble-burying behavior through "distinct pharmacological mechanisms."[5]

In February 2012, a paper was published in the journal *Psychopharmacology*, examining how certain drugs move throughout the body, namely CBD, CBDV, THCV, and CBG. They reported that CBD inhibited obsessive-compulsive behaviors in rats and mice.[6] Another paper in 2012 stated that cannabidiol is indeed an anxiolytic drug and can be effective not only for obsessive-compulsive disorder, but also for panic disorder, social anxiety disorder, and post-traumatic stress disorder. This, too, was from a group of researchers in Brazil.[7]

Yet another research group from Brazil, led by Mirella Nardo from the Department of Pharmacology, University of São Paulo, did something very interesting to mice in their study. They were interested in examining what CBD could do when they gave meta-chloro-phenyl-piperazine (mCPP), also known as the street drug "ecstasy," to mice, knowing that the drug would induce obsessive-compulsive behaviors. This study involved the marble-burying test and, after administration of CBD, found that it had anticompulsive effects on the mice, and they significantly reduced the behavior in which they buried marbles.[8]

A chapter entitled "Cannabinoids and Obsessive-Compulsive Disorder" appeared in the textbook *Cannabinoids in Neurologic and Mental Disorders* in 2015. In it, Plinio C. Casarotto and his team provide an extensive overview of OCD, its genetic components, brain structures that are involved—specifically the cortico-striato-thalamo-cortical (CSTC) circuit—neurochemical changes associated with CBD, the role the endocannabinoid systems plays in OCD, and the effects of drugs on this system. The team concludes that while the number of studies examining CBD and OCD is rather small, there appears to be a dysfunction of the CSTC circuit in OCD. They explain:

Cannabinoid receptors are significantly expressed in most parts of this circuitry and can modulate the release of key neurotransmitters related to this disorder, including glutamate, dopamine, GABA, and serotonin. Together, these pieces of evidence indicate that the endocannabinoid system could be an important target for new therapeutic approaches in OCD. Additional studies are clearly needed to investigate the role of these neurotransmitters in this disorder.[9]

Summary

Despite there being only a small number of studies, there does appear to be some evidence that CBD can help people diagnosed with obsessive-compulsive disorder. CBD seems to interact positively with parts of the brain that regulate emotions and arousal. It has also been shown to act together with major neurotransmitters that also help to regulate mood, specifically anxiety and depression. Ecstasy-induced mice appear to calm down their marble-burying behaviors, which scientists believe is a reliable model of human OCD. CBD may be as effective as Paxil and more effective than Valium in treating symptoms of the disorder in animal studies. Considering its ability to reduce anxiety in animals and humans, it is hoped that more research will be conducted specifically on the effectiveness of CBD for OCD.

Post-Traumatic Stress Disorder (PTSD)

Introduction

According to the US Department of Veteran Affairs, post-traumatic stress disorder can happen to anyone, and while not everyone who experiences a trauma will have PTSD, many will. Around seven or eight out of every one hundred people, or 7–8% of the US population, will have PTSD at some point during their lives. Around eight million adults have PTSD in any given year. Ten out of every one hundred women, or 10%, develop PTSD at some point in their lives, compared to four out of every one hundred, or 4% of men. These numbers are higher for veterans of war. Between 11% and 20%

of military personnel who served in Operations Iraqi Freedom and Enduring Freedom have PTSD in any given year. Among those who served in the Gulf War or Desert Storm, 12% have PTSD in any given year, and the highest percentage of veterans experiencing PTSD were in the Vietnam War; among them, 30% had PTSD in their lifetimes.[10] PTSD has a history prior to these wars, and soldiers in World Wars I and II were diagnosed with conditions that physicians were calling "battle fatigue" or "shell shock." The condition wasn't called PTSD until the Vietnam War, when thousands of soldiers came home experiencing symptoms of depression, anxiety, guilt, insomnia, flashbacks, and the inability to be close to loved ones. In 1980, the *DSM-3* added PTSD as an official mental disorder.

Rates of PTSD are also higher among first responders, including emergency medical services (EMS) personnel, firefighters, and police officers. It is estimated that around 30% of first responders develop emotional and behavioral conditions, including depression and PTSD, compared to 20% in the general population.[11] According to a study in 2016, firefighters have a higher rate of suicidal thinking and attempts than the general population.[12] And among police officers, between 125 and 300 commit suicide every year.[13] A research team from West Virginia and New York examined PTSD among police officers and the associations with frequency, recency, and types of traumatic events. They found that "the frequency of several traumatic events was associated with higher PTSD scores in women, while the recency of seeing victims of assault was associated with higher PTSD scores in men."[14]

Overview of Post-Traumatic Stress Disorder (PTSD)

Whereas prior editions of the *DSM* housed post-traumatic stress disorder in the chapter on anxiety disorders, it is now found in the *DSM-5* chapter on trauma and stressor-related disorders. According to the *DSM-5*, "Trauma- and stressor-related disorders include disorders in which exposure to a traumatic or stressful event is listed explicitly as a diagnostic criterion. These include reactive attachment disorder, disinhibited social engagement disorder, posttraumatic stress disorder (PTSD), acute stress disorder, and adjustment disorders."[15]

Post-traumatic stress disorder is defined as a chronic and debilitating psychiatric condition that can develop after experiencing a traumatic, shocking, dangerous, or intensely stressful event. It affects the mind and body and is related to the brain's "extinction process," which reduces the impact of traumatic memories. It is important to note that not everyone who experiences such an event will experience PTSD, and not everyone with PTSD has gone through these types of events. Some individuals may rely on substances like alcohol and drugs to cope with their problems associated with PTSD.

For those who do develop PTSD, symptoms usually start to appear within three months after the event but can emerge years later. In order for a psychiatrist or psychologist to diagnose an individual with PTSD, symptoms must last more than one month and be severe enough to interfere with many aspects of the person's life, work, and relationships. The course of the illness varies. Some people will recover within months, others will experience symptoms for years, and there are people who will have PTSD for the rest of their lives.

The four groups of symptoms that are most common with PTSD are reexperiencing, avoidance, arousal and reactivity, and cognition and mood. To be diagnosed, the individual must have all of the following for at least one month: at least one reexperiencing symptom, at least one avoidance symptom, at least two arousal and reactivity symptoms, and at least two cognition and mood symptoms. Reexperiencing symptoms include flashbacks, bad dreams and nightmares, and recurring frightening thoughts. These types of symptoms can truly impair an individual's quality of daily living. Avoidance symptoms involve staying away from places, objects, or events that are reminders of the trauma the individual experienced. For example, if the person had a bad car crash on a particular street, he or she may avoid driving down that street. Other symptoms include avoiding thoughts or feelings related to the traumatic event. Arousal and reactivity symptoms include being easily startled, feeling tense or on the edge, having difficulty sleeping, and experiencing outbursts of anger or rage. A loud noise may cause great distress to someone who experienced a terrible event in a war, for instance. Cognition and mood symptoms consist of trouble remembering key features of the traumatic event, negative thoughts about oneself or the world in general, distorted feelings like self-blame and guilt, and a loss in interests and activities that one used to enjoy. These symptoms can make an individual feel very alone, isolated, and detached from friends, family and other people.

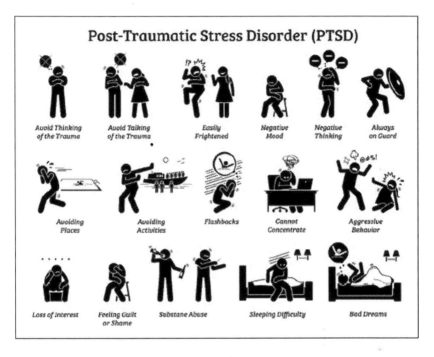

Symptoms of PTSD

PTSD can develop at any age, in any person. People who have experienced horrible events like physical or sexual assaults, severe medical issues, being abused, living through natural or man-made disasters, or being in serious accidents are at a higher risk for developing PTSD. Other risk factors include seeing other people being hurt or traumatized, witnessing a murder, seeing a dead body, experiencing childhood trauma, having little to no social support after the event, dealing with stress brought on by the loss of a loved one, going through a divorce, or losing one's job. A major risk factor is having a history of either mental illness or substance abuse, or both. PTSD most often develops from a sudden and devastating trauma that happens with no warning and was not expected.

Physiological changes take place in the limbic system, and particularly, the amygdala, which is responsible for processing fear in persons who have PTSD.

Changes are also being detected using neuroimaging research in the medial prefrontal cortex, involved in decision-making, and the hippocampus, which forms long-term memories. When PTSD is activated in a person, the hippocampus reduces in size, neuronal integrity, and functional integrity. The medial prefrontal cortex also appears to lose volume and becomes hyporesponsive during PTSD episodes. There is also heightened responsivity of the amygdala during these episodes.[16] This information will become more important as you read about the research findings on CBD and PTSD.

Traditional Therapies for Post-Traumatic Stress Disorder (PTSD)

The most common treatments for post-traumatic stress disorder involve psychotherapy, medications or both at the same time, which is the preferred model of care. Every person is different, and some will respond to one treatment better than others will. The most commonly prescribed medications are SSRI and SNRI antidepressants like Prozac, Paxil, Zoloft, and Effexor. Paxil and Zoloft are the only two that are FDA approved specifically for PTSD. Other medications include antipsychotic drugs, beta-blockers, and benzodiazepines, like Valium, Xanax, and Ativan. Sleeping pills may also be recommended if the person is experiencing insomnia.

Therapy for PTSD has three main goals: alleviating or managing symptoms, improvement of coping skills, and rebuilding confidence and self-esteem. Various forms of cognitive behavioral therapy can be helpful in changing one's thought patterns that produce anxiety and fear and take away from the quality of life. Individual or group therapy may be recommended depending on the individual and types of symptoms he or she is experiencing. The general course of therapy is usually up to twelve weeks and can involve cognitive processing therapy, prolonged exposure therapy, eye movement desensitization and reprocessing, and stress inoculation therapy. All of these therapies are meant to help people learn how to react to events in their lives that may trigger their PTSD symptoms. People can learn more about trauma and its effects; learn how to change one's lifestyle and eat, sleep, and live better; learn stress management and relaxation skills; and learn how to manage anger, guilt, and shame.

Research Findings on CBD and Post-Traumatic Stress Disorder (PTSD)

In 2008, researchers from Virginia were interested in studying the effects of the endocannabinoid system on learning and forgetting both pleasant and unpleasant experiences. They discovered that the endocannabinoid system did indeed play an important role in the extinction of avoidance-motivated behaviors and is of little significance for "appetitively motivated behaviors," or activities that increase the likelihood of satisfying a specific need, like finding food when you're hungry.[17] One year later, several papers were published on cannabidiol and post-traumatic stress disorder. In one paper, a Canadian research team examined the effects of nabilone on PTSD symptoms and found that 72% of the patients in their study experienced either the cessation of nightmares or a significant reduction in nightmare intensity. Some patients also reported other improvements in sleep time, quality of sleep, night sweats, and a reduction in daytime flashbacks.[18] Another study in Israel discovered that the amygdala (the fear-processing part of the limbic system) contains a large number of CB1 receptors. When researchers injected a synthetic cannabinoid into the amygdala of rats, the cannabinoid lowered anxiety responses, especially extinction learning. The synthetic cannabinoid also supported inhibitory avoidance (learning and memory processing) and extinction, which are the goals of psychotherapy. In plain English, the cannabinoid reduced stress.[19] Jose Crippa and his team from Brazil provided a review of some advances in the development of both the experimental and clinical use of CBD in neuropsychiatry. They reported that CBD does show potential in treating many disorders, including epilepsy, substance abuse, social phobias, schizophrenia, depression, bipolar disorder, sleep disorders, Parkinson's disease, and post-traumatic stress disorder. They call CBD a "useful and promising molecule" that may help people who have these and many other conditions. They also remind us that this type of research is not new and actually goes back to the 1970s and call for more controlled clinical studies with larger groups of participants.[20]

An important paper was published in 2013 examining the reductions in endocannabinoid levels in people with PTSD following the 9/11 attacks on the World Trade Centers in New York. The research team reported that they had evidence of a reduction in circulating endocannabinoid levels in people with PTSD after being exposed to the traumatic event. They believe their data supports the hypothesis that deficient endocannabinoid signaling may be a part of the glucocorticoid dysregulation that is associated with post-traumatic stress disorder.[21] A couple of years later, researchers found that the endocannabinoid system plays a critical role in the brain's fear circuitry. Whereas targeting fear memories through the endocannabinoid system produced mixed results, activation of cannabinoid receptors accelerated the extinction of fear memories. They admit that further work is needed to find out if the use of cannabinoids would truly help people with PTSD.[22]

Another Israeli research team added a new spin to the research on cannabinoids and PTSD. It was reported that there is enough evidence from studies in both animals and humans that the endocannabinoid system plays an important role in the control of emotions. On the other hand,

> there is increased prevalence of cannabis use in post-traumatic stress disorder (PTSD) patients and *vice-versa*. Clinical studies suggest that PTSD patients may cope with their symptoms by using cannabis. This treatment-seeking strategy may explain the high prevalence of cannabis use among individuals with PTSD. Preliminary studies in humans also suggest that treatment with cannabinoids may decrease PTSD symptoms including sleep problems, frequency of nightmares, and hyperarousal.[23]

Another paper was published the same year by researchers in Brazil and the UK examining cannabidiol's regulation of learned fear, which is characteristic in post-traumatic stress disorder and phobias. While exposure therapy may be effective temporarily and the use of medications come with risks or may be ineffective altogether, cannabidiol may be effective in reducing the fear associated with PTSD. The authors state:

> The evidence indicates that cannabidiol reduces learned fear in different ways: (1) cannabidiol decreases fear expression acutely, (2) cannabidiol disrupts memory reconsolidation, leading to sustained

fear attenuation upon memory retrieval, and (3) cannabidiol enhances extinction, the psychological process by which exposure therapy inhibits learned fear.

They also believe that future research should be conducted to shed light on the neural circuit, psychological, cellular, and molecular systems underlying the regulation of fear memory processing and cannabidiol. The team also stated that CBD might be an improvement over other commonly prescribed drugs like benzodiazepines and antidepressants because of its favorable side effects profile. CBD can also be an added treatment for those receiving therapy because combining the two may lead to better outcomes.[24]

A year later, an article was published in *Current Opinion in Psychology* proclaiming the success of CBD in its antidepressant and anxiolytic effects. The researchers point out that there is a growing interest in finding a treatment to help people with trauma-related disorders. They conclude that neurobiological research indicates cannabinoids as possible pharmacological treatments for PTSD.[25] In 2017, another team from the UK and Brazil published a paper in the *British Journal of Pharmacology*. In it, they examined cannabidiol as a possible treatment for both anxiety-related disorders and substance abuse disorders. They found that CBD reduces fear memory expression and an enduring reduction in learned fear expression like those found in PTSD and phobias. They conclude by saying, "This makes CBD a potential candidate for testing as a pharmacological adjunct to psychological therapies or behavioral interventions used in treating PTSD and phobias."[26]

In 2018, two Brazilian researchers provided a great overview of scientific work that had been done on CBD and PTSD. They point specifically to one element of PTSD—inappropriate retention of adverse memories—as a set of symptoms that can be managed with cannabidiol and believe that pharmacological intervention of the endocannabinoid system holds promise as a therapeutic treatment for PTSD and other trauma- and stress-related disorders. In their article, they also provide a thorough history of the advances in research on the use of CBD for PTSD. Bench research, or that conducted with mice or rats, has been going on since 2008 and human studies since 2012. That's a lot of good years of investigation into the effectiveness of cannabidiol for post-traumatic stress disorder, and the results are fairly consistent and positive. Work with rodents yielded decreases of the total extinction of fear-based memories, and research with human subjects produced diminished PTSD symptoms.[27]

A recent study by a research team in Colorado provided the very first case study examining the clinical benefits of cannabidiol for patients diagnosed with PTSD. Eleven patients receiving treatment in an outpatient psychiatric clinic were given CBD by a mental health professional over the course of eight weeks. They also received routine therapy and received psychotropic medications at the same time. The researchers found that 91% of patients, or ten out of eleven, experienced a decrease in PTSD symptom severity. CBD was well tolerated; no one had to stop taking it due to any unpleasant side effects. They concluded by stating:

> Administration of oral CBD in addition to routine psychiatric care was associated with PTSD symptom reduction in adults with PTSD. CBD also appeared to offer relief in a subset of patients who reported frequent nightmares as a symptom of their PTSD. Additional clinical investigation including double-blind, placebo-controlled trials, would be necessary to further substantiate the response to CBD that was observed in this study.[28]

Summary

With research spanning from the 1970s through today, it seems that CBD has produced some good results in treating symptoms of post-traumatic stress disorder using both animal and human subjects. It is also apparent that the endocannabinoid system plays a significant role in this disorder and that by targeting it, researchers may develop a CBD-drug treatment to help people manage their symptoms of PTSD. Can CBD become an adjunct treatment alongside psychotropic medications and therapy to help people with PTSD, or will it be effective on its own? More time and research will hopefully answer this and many other questions regarding its full therapeutic potential.

Schizophrenia

Introduction

Sometimes referred to as the "Holy Grail" of psychiatry, schizophrenia is one of the most mysterious and disabling mental disorders affecting millions of people in the United States and around the world. Being the Holy Grail means that psychiatry is endlessly in search of the truth about schizophrenia, and perhaps the only way to find it is to go where no one else has. Dr. Eugene Blueler, a Swiss psychiatrist, is credited for first using the term "schizophrenia," which he derived from two Greek words: *schizo*, meaning "to split," and *phren*, which means "mind" or "brain." Dr. Bleuler also was the first to create two categories of symptoms—positive and negative. Briefly, positive symptoms of schizophrenia mean the presence of abnormal functions such as highly exaggerated thoughts or behaviors that are not based in realty. These include hallucinations, delusions, confused thoughts and disorganized speech, trouble concentrating, and movement disorders. Negative symptoms, meaning the absence of or lack of functioning in thoughts and behaviors, include lack of pleasure or motivation, little to no eye contact or affect (emotion), inappropriate emotional expressions, poor hygiene, trouble with speech, difficulty with or inability to carry out activities of daily living, and poor follow-through on projects or activities or initiating them.

According to the Schizophrenia and Related Disorders Alliance of America (SARDAA), schizophrenia is found in 1.1% of the world's population (21 million), and 3.5 million people in the United States, and it is one of the leading causes of disability.[29] Almost 75% of people with the disorder are diagnosed between the ages of sixteen to twenty-five years of age. But as we will see later in this section, schizophrenia can develop much later in life, after age sixty, and is known as "late-life schizophrenia." Some cases are believed to have genetic roots. Around 25% of people with schizophrenia will recover completely, another 50% will improve over the course of ten years or so, and the remaining 25% will never recover. Schizophrenia is a very costly disorder, with estimates between $32 and $65 billion annually. Between 33% and 50% of homeless people have schizophrenia, and half of them will receive no treatment.

The World Health Organization indicates that people with schizophrenia are two to three times more likely to die early compared to the general population. This is due to many preventable diseases, including cardiovascular disease, stroke, diabetes, and infections. Some will also die from accidents and suicide. Schizophrenia is more common in males than females, and symptoms begin earlier in men.[30]

Overview of Schizophrenia

Official information about schizophrenia can be found in the *DSM-5*, published by the American Psychiatric Association. The chapter is called "Schizophrenia Spectrum and Other Psychotic Disorders." Key features of psychotic disorders include delusions, which are fixed beliefs not grounded in reality, with various themes such as being harmed by others (the most common delusion), that others are talking about the individual, that one possesses great wealth or special abilities, that others are in love with him or her, that something catastrophic is going to take place, or that something is wrong with one's health. Delusional content can also be considered bizarre, such as the belief that one's internal organs have been removed and replaced with someone else's without any surgical scars, that one is under police surveillance, that one's thoughts have been removed or inserted by an alien force, or that one's actions are being controlled by an outside force.

Hallucinations include distorted perceptionlike experiences of any of the senses, but auditory hallucinations are the most common in schizophrenia and other psychotic disorders. Auditory hallucinations are experienced as either familiar or unfamiliar voices and are distinct from one's own thoughts. Disorganized thinking and speech are characterized by switching from one topic to another, answering questions with unrelated responses, and at times, severely disorganized speech that is almost incomprehensible. Grossly disorganized or abnormal motor behavior, including catatonia (diminished reactivity to one's environment), involves symptoms ranging from childlike "silliness" to unpredictable aggression. Catatonic features include resisting instructions, maintaining rigid or bizarre postures, being mute, having purposeless or excessive physical movement, grimacing, staring at others, and repeating other people's speech. As noted earlier, negative symptoms are also key features of psychotic disorders.

To be diagnosed with schizophrenia, an individual must exhibit two or more of the following for at least one month: delusions, hallucinations, disorganized speech, grossly disorganized or catatonic behavior, and negative symptoms. Levels of functioning must also be significantly lower in major life areas like work and personal relationships. There must be continuous signs of disturbance for at least six months. Other disorders must have been ruled out, like schizoaffective disorder and bipolar disorder with psychotic features, and the disorder cannot be explained by substance abuse.[31]

Traditional Therapies for Schizophrenia

Some of my earliest work in mental health was providing psychotherapy to mentally ill people living in group settings. Under the supervision of psychiatrists, my team and I assisted with psychiatric evaluations, provided various forms of therapy to clients, educated the staff, and maintained clinical records and therapy notes. That was quite a while ago, when Haldol was the number one drug being prescribed to people with schizophrenia and other psychotic disorders. A lot has changed in the treatment of people with these disorders, and while there have been improvements, much is still unknown about them. I'm still not sure if moving people from group settings to community clinics was the best thing for them. Many went from larger psychiatric institutions to nursing homes, which were ill prepared to provide appropriate care or treatment. Others became homeless. Regardless of my opinion, here is a rundown of the current state of treatment for people diagnosed with schizophrenia.

The individual will start out with a complete physical examination, go through a myriad of tests and screenings, and have a psychiatric evaluation. The traditional model of care involves both medications and therapy together, and in severe cases, hospitalization may be required for a period of time. Most people will receive lifelong treatment due to the chronic nature of schizophrenia. The goal of treatment is to reduce and manage symptoms using the lowest possible doses of medication. Some individuals will respond well to one medication; others will require multiple medications. One of the greatest problems with psychiatric drugs are the side effects they produce. Many people will simply stop taking their medications if the side effects are too unpleasant. There are many injectable forms of antipsychotic medications now to help with compliance.

Drugs prescribed for schizophrenia and other psychotic disorders are classified as first- and second-generation antipsychotic medications. First-generation drugs have more and potentially severe side effects like tardive dyskinesia, a movement disorder that can last a lifetime in some individuals. Thorazine, Prolixin, Haldol, and Trilaphon are some examples. These medications can be effective and are less expensive than second-generation drugs, which are newer, have fewer side effects, and are generally more tolerable. They include Abilify, Clozaril, Latuda, Zyprexa, Invega, Geodon, Risperdal, and Seroquel.

Mental health professionals can provide ongoing therapy, counseling, and support for individuals with schizophrenia. Partial hospitalization, full hospitalization, and other programs may also be effective in managing symptoms and improving life skills. Electroconvulsive therapy (ECT) may be effective for people with treatment-resistant forms of schizophrenia as well as for those who have a combination of the disorder and depression. Everyday treatments include joining support groups, learning to cope with symptoms, developing healthier lifestyles, learning more about the disorder, getting support and services from the community, and engaging in stress management techniques.

Research Findings on CBD and Schizophrenia

I have to admit that I was shocked to find a study on cannabinoids being used to treat schizophrenia in 1997. In the journal *Pharmacology, Biochemistry and Behavior* is an article indicating that the endocannabinoid system—and in particular the endocannabinoid *anandamide* (the "bliss" or "happy" molecule)—may play an important role in the treatment of schizophrenia. Anandamide is responsible for memory and motivation, control of movements, and higher thought processes. It also plays a role in pain, appetite, and fertility. In terms of schizophrenia, this endocannabinoid can help restore cognitive balance and regulate perceptual processes.[32] Another early study in California reported that anandamide levels of untreated schizophrenics were eight times higher than those of healthy individuals. This level of anandamide is not present in schizophrenics taking newer antipsychotic drugs like Risperdal, Zyprexa, and Seroquel. These were all FDA approved to treat symptoms of schizophrenia between 1993 and 1997. It was theorized that anandamide increases in people with acute schizophrenia as a way for the body to compensate for the disorder.[33]

Years later, in 2008, a researcher from Germany reported that there appeared to be a complicated interaction between the dopaminergic and endocannabinoid receptor system. Dopamine has been the focus of discussion for decades as one cause of schizophrenia. The "dopamine hypothesis" supports the idea that an overabundance of dopamine is behind the disorder. The author concludes that CBD improves symptoms of schizophrenia.[34] Another study that year reported that the endocannabinoid system may play a large part in the development of schizophrenia. They described an increased density of CB1 receptor binding and increased levels of anandamide (the molecule responsible for mood, pain, and cognition) in cerebrospinal fluid. They propose a cannabinoid hypothesis alongside the traditional dopamine hypothesis of schizophrenia since there exists an interesting relationship between the two. They conclude that cannabidiol or CBD may one day be beneficial in the treatment of psychosis.[35]

In 2010, an article appearing in *Pharmaceuticals* suggested that "a disturbance of the cannabinoid system could contribute to the general understanding of the biological bases of schizophrenia and it may also be involved in its associated comorbidities." Written by a research team in Montreal, the article explains that anandamide binds to CB1 and CB2 receptors naturally, but in the case of schizophrenia, this process is broken down, and there is a disruption in the endocannabinoid system. They also state that "there seems to be an association between schizophrenia and polymorphisms of the CB1 receptor gene." CB1 receptors have been found in greater quantities in several parts of the brain associated with schizophrenia, such as the prefrontal cortex, hippocampus, and basal ganglia. The team also found that anandamide levels run higher in the cerebrospinal fluid and in the serum of people diagnosed with schizophrenia. The team clearly saw a connection between the endocannabinoid system and schizophrenia.[36] Researchers from Brazil and Italy that same year provided an intensive review of current literature on CBD and schizophrenia and found that CBD emerged as possessing the most consistent antipsychotic properties in dopamine- and glutamate-based models of schizophrenia.[37] One year later, a paper was published stating that many recent studies have found that cannabinoids improve several areas of schizophrenia, including neuropsychological performance, reduction in negative symptoms, and general antipsychotic effects. The Australian authors admit that the neurochemical effects of cannabinoids are complex but found that they do appear to have a "restorative" effect on neurotransmitter dysfunction in schizophrenia.[38]

In many scientific communities around the world, interest in cannabidiol and other cannabinoids in the treatment of schizophrenia was growing, and as a result, numerous studies were conducted examining the relationship between the two. Brazilian researchers provided an in-depth, systematic review of the literature available through the year 2012 on the endocannabinoid system and its role in schizophrenia. They found links between changes within the endocannabinoid system and the development of symptoms of schizophrenia and proposed a cannabinoid hypothesis of schizophrenia. They stressed that this is important not only for theoretical reasons, but for practical and therapeutic purposes:

> The current pharmacological therapy of schizophrenia is limited to the antagonism of dopamine receptors, which presents limited efficacy and significant side effects. Thus, alternative pharmacological strategies must be pursued; one approach involves the characterization of other neurotransmitter systems affected in this disorder.

For instance, they continue, glutamate may play a significant role in schizophrenia and there have been attempts to target and enhance this neurotransmitter to manage symptoms of schizophrenia.[39] Another team of researchers agreed with these findings and wrote:

> Data reported so far clearly indicate the presence of a dysregulation in the endocannabinoid system (both in terms of cannabinoid receptors and endocannabinoid ligands) in animal models of psychosis as well as in schizophrenic patients. Based on these observations, the pharmacological

modulation of the endocannabinoid system has been taken into account as a new therapeutic possibility for psychotic disorders.[40]

Another team of researchers in 2012, motivated by the search for safe and effective medications to treat schizophrenia, discovered that CBD enhances anandamide signaling and helps to manage symptoms of the disorder at the same time. Technically, "biochemical studies indicate that cannabidiol may enhance endogenous anandamide signaling indirectly, by inhibiting the intracellular degradation of anandamide catalyzed by the enzyme fatty acid amide hydrolase (FAAH)." They also believed that psychosis is derived from a state of hyperactivity of the endocannabinoid system and that certain elements of this system can play a protective role in schizophrenia. The researchers conclude by stating that "cannabidiol exerts clinically relevant antipsychotic effects that are associated with marked tolerance and safety, when compared to current medications."[41] This was quite a discovery because it spells out that high levels of anandamide are not the problem when it comes to the disorder, but rather are the result of the brain's attempts to solve it and reduce stress. The bottom line appears to be that CBD prevents the deactivation of anandamide, which in turn reduces symptoms of schizophrenia. This could lead to a new targeted treatment for schizophrenia.

One report from 2012 is important to note here. In it, Antonio Waldo Zuardi and his research team from Brazil remind us that cannabidiol was once thought in the scientific community to have no important pharmacological effects or activity and was always in second place compared to research on THC. Most studies focused on the medicinal properties of THC and ignored CBD. But now the research team states:

> CBD appears to have a pharmacological profile similar to that of atypical antipsychotic drugs as seen using behavioral and neurochemical techniques in animal models. Additionally, CBD prevented experimental human psychosis and was effective in open case reports in patients with schizophrenia with a remarkable safety profile. Moreover, fMRI [functional MRI] results strongly suggest that the antipsychotic effects of CBD in relation to the psychotomimetic

effects of THC involve the striatum and temporal cortex that have been traditionally associated with psychosis.[42]

Again, these researchers stress that CBD may have real potential as a treatment for psychosis in general and in schizophrenia in particular. CBD may become a safer alternative to psychiatric drugs or an add-on treatment.

In an issue of *Schizophrenia Bulletin,* Kirkpatrick and Miller make an interesting connection between schizophrenia and inflammation. They maintain that an association between the two have been found before in various studies and remind us that chronic inflammation plays a key role in a number of diseases and disorders, including Alzheimer's disease, diabetes, cardiovascular and cerebrovascular diseases, and some cancers. Studies have shown that individuals with schizophrenia have increased blood concentration of inflammatory cytokines, which are essential molecules that regulate inflammation and play an important role in the immune system. There are other abnormalities in schizophrenia associated with inflammation including oxidative stress, increased autoantibodies, circulating lymphocytes, and CRP. Autoantibodies work against a person's own proteins, lymphocytes produce antibodies and are an important source of cytokines, CRP is produced in the liver as a result of inflammation, and oxidative stress may be a factor in the decreased levels of blood and central nervous system membranes of polyunsaturated fatty acids seen in schizophrenia.[43]

A significant amount of work was done in 2015, examining the effects of CBD on schizophrenia and the role of the endocannabinoid in this disorder. A medical textbook, *Cannabinoids in Neurologic and Mental Disease,* was published that year by an international group of researchers. They provided scientific findings on neuroinflammation, Alzheimer's disease, Parkinson's disease, Huntington's disease, ALS, epilepsy, schizophrenia, bipolar disorder, Tourette's syndrome, PTSD, addiction, appetite disorders, and OCD. In terms of schizophrenia, Rohleder and Leweke state that "a neurobiological role of the ECS involving the disruption of endogenous cannabinoid signaling and functioning in schizophrenia…[has] been suggested." They believe that while the dopamine hypothesis has played an important role in science for decades, the endocannabinoid system must be taken seriously as a part of the pathophysiology of schizophrenia.[44]

A review paper published in the *Annals of Clinical Psychiatry* by Brazilian researchers in 2015 sheds light on the mechanisms behind cannabidiol and how it helps with symptoms of schizophrenia. They point out that CBD has various neuroprotective effects, just like many other scientists have. They state that CBD has been shown to help with sleep, convulsions, and hormones and is a neuroprotective substance. All of these effects support the educated guess that CBD could have anti-anxiety and antipsychotic effects. They agree that CBD has a strong impact on oxidative stress and inflammation, which have both been found in schizophrenia.[45] The same year, another team from the Department of Psychiatry, New York University Langone Medical Center, reported that CBD is a very well-tolerated substance and produces few psychoactive effects on its own. It is helpful in counteracting the negative effects of THC like psychosis, anxiety, and euphoria. CBD actually diminishes the memory impairment caused by THC. They conclude, "The evidence for an association between cannabis use and schizophrenia is compelling…whether CBD might present a general alternative or augmentative therapeutic strategy for patients with schizophrenia will require much additional research."[46]

Another report came from Germany supporting the role of inflammation in schizophrenia. Muller and his team report that high levels of cytokines and other pro-inflammatory substances have been found in the blood and cerebrospinal fluid of people with schizophrenia. They present a "vulnerability-stress-inflammation" model of schizophrenia and believe that long-lasting and chronic stress increases pro-inflammatory outcomes among people who are genetically vulnerable to developing schizophrenia. This is another fascinating way of looking at schizophrenia and how CBD may contribute to alleviating symptoms of the disorder.[47]

One study in 2016, examining the means by which CBD produces antipsychotic effects, found a neurobiological basis for its effectiveness. In the report, the researchers identified that CBD triggers molecular signaling pathways that are associated with the effects of many antipsychotic medications. One of the benefits of these results is that CBD is safe and tolerable and has nowhere near the potentially negative, unwanted, and dangerous side effects that these medications carry.[48] In a 2017 supplement to the journal *European Psychiatry*, two researchers report that CBD may have promising therapeutic benefits for the treatment of schizophrenia-induced psychosis.[49] In another study in Brazil in 2017, researchers proposed that the endocannabinoid and endovanilloid systems are dysfunctional in schizophrenia. The signaling across mesocorticolimbic circuits might be disrupted and thereby contribute to psychotic symptoms.[50]

Several researchers stated in another study in 2018 that CBD not only has antipsychotic properties, but also is effective and safe for people with schizophrenia.[51] This study was very important, because it was the first placebo-controlled trial of CBD with schizophrenic individuals. After six weeks of treatment with CBD and antipsychotic drugs, significant progress was observed. Illness severity decreased, cognitive performance improved, and overall functioning was increased. The team also informed the scientific community that CBD does not appear to be dependent on dopamine receptor antagonism, which means that CBD might represent an entirely new class of treatment for people diagnosed with schizophrenia.

The last article reviewed for this chapter is from the publication *Current Psychiatry*. Dr. Joseph M. Pierre from the University of California, Los Angeles, asks the question: Is CBD for schizophrenia a real possibility or just wishful thinking? He provides an outline of studies reaching back into the mid-1990s through today and makes several conclusions. First, CBD may be a limited benefit as an add-on treatment for people who have already responded well to their antipsychotic medications. On the other hand, it may not work so well for those who are treatment resistant and do not respond so well to the drugs. Second, he states that "CBD might be effective as standalone therapy as an alternative to antipsychotics that is better tolerated." In summary, CBD may work for some people with schizophrenia but not for everyone with schizophrenia.[52]

Late-Onset Schizophrenia: A Special Age-Related Disorder

Overview
This book is about aging well and how we might accomplish this by incorporating cannabidiol (CBD) into our daily routines. I therefore felt compelled to add this section on later-life schizophrenia. While schizophrenia will develop

earlier in life, experts estimate that at least 20% to 29% of people have an onset of the disorder between the ages of forty and sixty. There is debate whether early- and late-onset schizophrenia are the same thing or whether they are truly distinct and separate disorders. That debate will continue. The *DSM-5* doesn't have an official diagnosis for late-onset schizophrenia. The book simply states, "Late-onset cases can meet the diagnostic criteria for schizophrenia, but it is not yet clear whether this is the same condition as schizophrenia diagnosed prior to mid-life."[53]

An article published in 2014 by researchers from the University of California–San Diego provide some distinguishing characteristics between early- and late-onset schizophrenia. Many older adults who develop late-onset schizophrenia have successful occupational and marital histories compared to those with early-onset schizophrenia. Inflammation appears to play a role in late-onset schizophrenia but not early-onset schizophrenia. Maglione and her team reported, "A number of studies have found associations between inflammatory conditions, such as autoimmune diseases and infections, and schizophrenia. Given that aging is associated with an overall increase in inflammation, [it] could play a role in the pathophysiology of LOS [late-onset schizophrenia]." Another difference between the two forms of the disorder is that atypical antipsychotic medications may be helpful in the short term but are neither safe nor effective when used over long periods of time for middle-aged and older adults. Older adults also show more positive symptoms of the illness (delusions and hallucinations) and tend to respond to lower doses of antipsychotic medications. One last differentiating factor is more older women are diagnosed with late-onset schizophrenia compared to earlier-onset schizophrenia.[54]

Chen and her team add to the risk factors involved in later-onset schizophrenia. They report:

> Older age of onset was associated with weaker family history of schizophrenia, lower rates of substance use, better early psychosocial functioning and higher educational achievement. Female preponderance and comorbid physical health problems were particularly notable in the late onset cohort. Later life schizophrenia

also showed a relatively greater association with psychosocial factors proximal to psychosis onset, such as unemployment.[55]

A year prior to this article, a team of researchers reviewed issues surrounding another type of age-related schizophrenia called *very-late-onset schizophrenialike psychosis*, or VLOSP for short. Some of the defining features include cognitive deficits and problems, neurodegenerative changes like those observed in Alzheimer's disease and other dementialike disorders, a generalized atrophy of the brain, and increased ventricle-to-brain ratio. A subgroup of individuals with VLOSP will develop dementia, and the associated cognitive deterioration will be characterized by deficits in working memory, language, psychomotor speed, and executive functioning (e.g., self-control, multitasking).[56]

An older but very enlightening article was published in 2002 in *Current Psychiatry*. In it, the authors point out that very-late-onset schizophrenia goes widely undiagnosed for a number of reasons but mainly due to the social isolation of these older individuals: "Their symptoms of paranoia and reluctance by family members to intervene also can prevent them from receiving treatment that could control psychotic symptoms and improve their quality of life." Some risk factors involved in elderly people developing very-late-onset schizophrenia include sensory deficits, personality disorders prior to the onset of schizophrenic symptoms, social isolation, neuropsychological abnormalities, and being female. People with this form of the disorder respond to one-half the antipsychotic dosage required for younger people with schizophrenia. Older people are more susceptible to negative side effects of antipsychotics, even at lower doses. They are at a higher risk for extrapyramidal side effects, including Parkinsonism, akathisia (a movement disorder that makes it difficult for a person to be still), urinary retention, constipation, delirium, blurred vision, and exacerbation of glaucoma. Other negative side effects include cardiovascular problems, falls, injury, and tardive dyskinesia (a very unpleasant movement disorder characterized by jerky or stiff movements of the body and face that cannot be controlled). Atypical or newer antipsychotic drugs are preferred for individuals diagnosed with late-onset and very-late-onset schizophrenia.[57]

Summary

According to research that spans decades, there appears to be a connection between the endocannabinoid system, CBD, and other endocannabinoids like anandamide and schizophrenia. This disorder remains one of the most elusive for doctors and scientists alike. As stated in the beginning of this section, it is the Holy Grail of psychiatric illnesses. Despite this, many researchers have spent years of their careers in search of better ways to manage symptoms and improve the quality of the lives of people who live with this illness. The current practice of prescribing antipsychotic drugs comes with both benefits and potentially dangerous side effects. It is well known that when patients experience unwanted and unpleasant side effects, the likelihood that they will stop using their medications is rather high. What kinds of outcomes does this produce? Surely, not positive ones. CBD, on the other hand, appears to produce fairly consistent and positive results. It is safer than many prescribed drugs and is well tolerated. Although more research needs to be conducted on this topic, for now it is hoped that people living with schizophrenia can find some relief, better manage their symptoms, and maximize their quality of life by using CBD.

9

CBD and Sleep Disorders

A well-spent day brings happy sleep.

—Leonardo da Vinci

Introduction

Insomnia is such an epidemic in the United States that between roughly fifty and seventy million Americans suffer nightly from disordered sleep. Sleep disorders are usually associated with chronic stress, depression, anxiety, and pain. As we age, we may become more susceptible to difficulties achieving good, restful sleep. Some older adults experience excessive daytime sleepiness and then find it difficult to sleep throughout the night. Prescription medications may carry negative side effects that interfere with sleep. Neurodegenerative disorders, such as Parkinson's, Huntington's or Alzheimer's diseases, can also trigger disruptions in the normal sleep cycle. Sundowning is a classic example of disruption of circadian rhythm patterns due to dementia associated with Alzheimer's disease. According to the Cleveland Clinic, females are 1.3 times more likely to report insomnia than males, insomnia is more common in men than women over the age of sixty-five, and older adults are 1.5 times more likely to complain about insomnia than younger people.[1]

According to the American Sleep Association, there are a significant number of problems associated with sleep disorders. Roughly 48% of people in the United States report snoring, almost 38% unintentionally fall asleep during the day, and 4.7% report nodding off or falling to sleep while they are driving. Drowsy driving has its consequences. Around 1,550 people die, and another 40,000 are hurt annually due to drowsy driving. Around 30% of adults report short-term sleep problems, and 10% have chronic, long-lasting insomnia. Here are some more staggering statistics: twenty-five million adults in the United States have obstructive sleep apnea (9% to 21% of women and 24% to 31% of men). Roughly 37% of those twenty to thirty-nine years old and 40% of those forty to fifty-nine years old report short sleep duration. One last frightening statistic: One hundred thousand deaths occur in hospitals every year due to medical errors caused by sleep deprivation among health care professionals. The bottom line is that sleep disorders are a huge problem in the United States and around the world.[2]

Overview of Sleep Disorders

In general, a sleep disorder is defined by changes in an individual's sleep patterns that negatively impact physical and mental health. The *DSM-5* outlines ten different sleep disorders. They include insomnia, hypersomnolence disorder, narcolepsy, breathing-related sleep disorders, nonrapid eye movement sleep arousal disorders, nightmare disorder, rapid eye movement (REM) sleep behavior disorder, restless leg syndrome, and substance/medication-induced sleep disorder: "Individuals with these disorders typically present with sleep-wake complaints of dissatisfaction regarding the quality, timing and amount of sleep. Resulting daytime distress and impairments are core features shared by all of these sleep-wake disorders."[3] Many times, sleep disorders are accompanied by mental and emotional problems like depression, anxiety, and cognitive issues. Chronic sleep disturbances are risk factors for developing mental illness and substance use disorders. Sleep disorders can also be early signs or symptoms of underlying mental or emotional disorders. Getting medical or psychiatric attention early is recommended before the sleep disorder becomes a full-blown psychiatric problem.

INSOMNIA CHECKLIST	SLEEP APNEA CHECKLIST
☐ DIFFICULTY FALLING ASLEEP ☐ WAKING UP THROUGHOUT THE NIGHT ☐ WAKING UP TOO EARLY IN THE MORNING ☐ DAYTIME FATIGUE ☐ IRRITABILITY ☐ DEPRESSION/ANXIETY ☐ DIFFICULTY PAYING ATTENTION ☐ INCREASED ERRORS ☐ ACCIDENTS ☐ POOR FOCUS ☐ IMPAIRED MEMORY	☐ INTERRUPTED BREATHING ☐ LOUD SNORING ☐ GASPING FOR AIR WHILE ASLEEP ☐ INSOMNIA ☐ MORNING HEADACHES ☐ DECREASED SEX DRIVE ☐ TOOTH GRINDING ☐ IRRITABILITY ☐ EXHAUSTION ☐ DIFFICULTY PAYING ATTENTION ☐ INCREASED BLOOD PRESSURE ☐ DEPRESSION ☐ OBESITY

The two most common sleep disorders affecting millions of people are insomnia and sleep apnea. Insomnia involves the difficulty with or inability to fall or stay asleep, and it is estimated that one in four people in the United States have the disorder. Many people will experience insomnia for a short period of time for various reasons like experiencing stress, changing jobs, or having a baby. It can interfere with physical, mental, and emotional well-being and performance. Insomnia can bring about a number of related problems, like anxiety, depression, fatigue, hallucinations, and diminished immunity—all of which, if left untreated, can lead to cardiovascular and other serious conditions like sleep apnea. There are two types of insomnia: primary and secondary. Primary insomnia involves sleep problems not associated with or caused by another physical or mental health problem. Secondary insomnia is caused by another condition like depression, pain due to arthritis or cancer, or the use of drugs or alcohol. Some symptoms of insomnia include difficulty falling asleep, waking in the middle of the night, having trouble getting back to sleep, early waking, feeling tired upon waking, irritability, and memory and concentration problems.

Sleep apnea, on the other hand, is a potentially dangerous disorder in which breathing repeatedly starts and stops throughout the night. Three types of sleep apnea include obstructive sleep apnea, central sleep apnea, and complex sleep apnea syndrome. Obstructive sleep apnea is the most common form of the disorder and occurs when throat muscles relax. Central sleep apnea occurs when the brain doesn't send the proper signals to the muscles that control breathing. Complex sleep apnea syndrome is also called "treatment-emergent central sleep apnea" and occurs when an individual has both obstructive and central sleep apnea. Symptoms of sleep apnea include snoring loudly, gasping for air while asleep, having episodes of not breathing while asleep, waking up with a dry mouth or throat, and having headaches in the morning. Other symptoms like experiencing difficulty staying asleep, excessive sleepiness throughout the day, difficulty paying attention, and an irritable mood can also occur when left untreated.

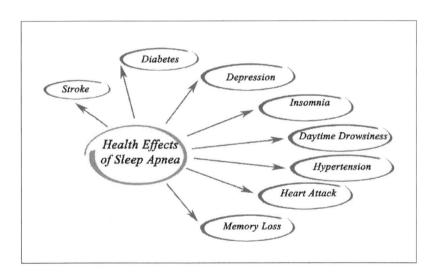

Health conditions associated with sleep apnea

Traditional Therapies for Sleep Disorders

Before considering sleep medications, it may be best to begin with natural remedies for sleeping problems. Getting some exercise into your daily or weekly routine can help, and many experts report that people who exercise regularly sleep better than those who don't. They also recommend working out in the morning because it can help regulate the secretion of hormones that help manage blood pressure, which can lead to better-quality sleep.

Getting natural sunlight has been shown to produce beneficial effects concerning sleep. Our bodies need sunlight to figure out what time of day or night it is and then to produce energizing hormones or those that will bring about relaxation, like melatonin. The hypothalamus, which is responsible for regulating energy levels and sleep, has the ability to sense light and then communicates with our body to produce more or less melatonin. During the day, we feel energized because our bodies are not producing melatonin, and at night, we get sleepy because of the increased production of this hormone.

Engaging in stress management can help with sleep difficulties because stress is one of the reasons for so many sleepless nights. Millions of Americans report that they feel tired, sluggish, or fatigued due to stress. Some stress management methods involve keeping a journal of recurrent thoughts or situations that bring about stress. Learning and performing yoga and engaging in guided imagery and progressive muscle relaxation may also condition the mind and body to manage symptoms of stress and induce sleep. Sometimes simply getting to bed earlier can be effective in promoting better-quality sleep. Also, try to avoid taking naps during the daytime, as they can interfere with sleep at night.

Experts believe that our diet can either enhance sleep or disrupt it. Eating foods rich in tryptophan, like turkey, cheese, and almonds can make you feel relaxed, sleepy, and happy. Salmon provides good levels of omega-3 fatty acid DHA, as does other fish, including tuna, mackerel, and sardines. Whole-grain crackers have healthy carbohydrates, which cause the blood sugar levels to spike and then drop, causing drowsiness. Tart cherry juice or cherries are some of the only edible sources of melatonin and may help with sleep issues. Bananas are rich in carbohydrates and tryptophan as well as potassium and magnesium, which can promote muscle relaxation and a good night's sleep. Try to avoid any foods or beverages high in sugar or caffeine, like dark chocolate, coffee, tea, and soft drinks. Caffeine stays in the system for up to six hours, so if you go to bed any sooner than 11:00 p.m., it may keep you awake. Spicy foods will do the same thing. They increase metabolism, raise body temperature, and can interfere with sleep. Eating any fatty, greasy foods will make the digestive system go into overtime and will most likely cause stomach distress and ruin sleep. Consuming large meals can have the same unwanted results.

Other simple lifestyle changes can be made to increase quality of sleep. For instance, get off your cell phone, tablet, or computer an hour or two before going to bed, because they act like electronic caffeine and increase activity in the brain. Instead, try reading a book for a while before bedtime. Taking a relaxing shower at night instead of the morning may send a message to your nervous system that it is time to slow down, which can induce sleepiness. Using lavender products like candles, mists, and sprays can fill the room with aromatherapy that signals to the brain that it's time to relax. An hour before bed, turning the temperature down can be helpful because it is more difficult to sleep when you are too warm. Turn down anything that makes noise or throws off light. You spend more time in bed than anywhere else, so choosing comfortable bedding and a good mattress are smart investments in creating an environment for relaxation and sleep.

If these simple changes don't work, it may be time to consult your doctor about sleeping pills, including either prescription medication or over-the-counter (OTC) medications. These are also known as sedatives and hypnotics, and there are plenty of them available. The most commonly prescribed medications for sleep are benzodiazepines. Generally speaking, physicians will prescribe the lowest possible dose and monitor for effectiveness with sleep. Commonly used sleeping pills include Ambien, Lunesta, Restoril, Sonata, Desyrel, and other OTCs like antihistamines, melatonin, and herbal remedies. A major problem with these types of drugs is their potential for misuse, abuse, or addiction. Sleeping medications can have some serious and dangerous side effects. Oversleeping, drowsiness while driving or working, allergic reactions, and facial swelling may occur. Side effects tend to be worse when mixing sleep medications with alcohol or other substances. Older adults and people with sleep apnea may experience worse side effects due to age and health conditions. Long-term use of these medications can lead to memory difficulties, mental and behavioral disorders, learning problems, and increased insomnia.

Research Findings on CBD and Sleep Disorders

Searching the literature did not yield a large volume of research studies on sleep and cannabidiol, although there are several to summarize. In 2008 researchers stated that CBD might hold therapeutic promise for people with a condition called "somnolence," or excessive daytime sleepiness, which is associated with poor sleep quality at night.[4] They conclude that cannabidiol is more of a wake-inducing agent than a nighttime remedy for sleep. Using it in the daytime may increase alertness and energy, which may contribute to better sleep quality. Another study in 2008 discovered the importance of the CB1 receptor in the regulation of sleep. Eric Murillo-Rodriguez agreed with the findings of the first study and reported that "to treat somnolence, the development of drugs aimed to block the CB1 receptors…might be considered as new candidates in the near future as therapeutic options."[5]

A few years later, a paper provided information concerning the use of acute systemic administration of CBD on the sleep-wake cycle of rats. When rats were given 10 mg and 40 mg of CBD, sleep significantly increased. Researchers also found that REM sleep latency increased when rats were given 40 mg of CBD. They concluded that CBD appears to increase total sleep time.[6] Another study the same year examined the effects of the drug dronabinol specifically for obstructive sleep apnea. Researchers in the United States found that the synthetic cannabinoid drug dronabinol was safe and well-tolerated in people who were diagnosed with OSA. This finding is important because "poor tolerance and long-term adherence to Continuous Positive Airway Pressure (CPAP) treatment in OSA make discovery of such therapeutic alternatives clinically relevant and important."[7]

In 2017, American researchers provided a review of the current literature on cannabis and cannabinoids and their effects on sleep. They found that CBD could have a therapeutic potential for the treatment of insomnia. Newer studies show that synthetic cannabinoids such as dronabinol and nabilone may provide short-term benefits for sleep apnea due to their effects on apneas associated with serotonin mediation. They state, "CBD may hold promise for REM sleep behavior disorder and excessive daytime sleepiness, while nabilone may reduce nightmares associated with PTSD and improve sleep among patients with chronic pain."[8]

The following year yielded a little more attention and research on cannabidiol, dronabinol, and the role of acetylcholine in sleep quality. Researchers from Brazil and the United States led the way. The Brazilian team looked at the relationship between CBD and sleep in a new and different way. Instead of asking whether CBD helps with sleep, they posed the question, "Does cannabidiol interfere with sleep?" They reported that few studies examined the possible interference of CBD with the sleep-wake cycle and found that it, in fact, did not induce any significant effect on sleep in healthy volunteers in their study. While CBD may help with sleep regulation and REM sleep behavior disorder in people diagnosed with Parkinson's disease, it does not have any negative effects on the quality of sleep among people with no serious physical or mental health conditions.[9]

An American team of researchers from Chicago examined the effects of dronabinol (a drug already used to treat nausea and vomiting induced by chemotherapy) on obstructive sleep apnea. They conclude that their "findings support the therapeutic potential of cannabinoids in people with OSA." They found positive results, like improved self-reported sleepiness and greater treatment satisfaction, among subjects in their study.[10] This is another important study because sleep apnea can be a severe disorder within itself and can lead to greater health and emotional complications. Untreated sleep apnea can lead to cardiovascular problems. There is a great need for new and effective treatments for this and other sleep disorders.

The same year, a team from Brazil examined how injections of CBD could enhance levels of acetylcholine in rat brains. Acetylcholine is a brain chemical that is responsible for quite a few body and brain functions, including muscle contraction, regulation of pain, REM sleep functions, mental arousal, attention, motivation, and memory. It was discovered that CBD increases acetylcholine levels in a brain region related to wake control. This study was the first of its kind to demonstrate the effects of acetylcholine levels in CBD-treated rats and suggests that the part of the brain, the basal forebrain, could be a site of action for CBD to promote wakefulness modulation.[11]

Research in 2019 examined the effectiveness of cannabidiol for anxiety and sleep. The research team from Colorado pointed out the need for more studies due to the "explosion" of interest among people looking to use CBD for a number of physical and emotional health conditions. There is evidence of the physiological and neurological benefits of CBD for anxiety disorders. Their work supports many findings that CBD is safe and is better tolerated than commonly prescribed psychiatric drugs for both anxiety and sleep disorders.[12]

Summary

While there is not an abundance of research articles or books on sleep and CBD, it appears that the scientific community is leaning toward a favorable view of CBD as a potentially effective treatment for sleep disorders. It has been shown to decrease anxiety, which can help with quality of sleep. CBD has also been shown to be a powerful anti-inflammatory and pain reliever. Perhaps people suffering from pain-related conditions can benefit from its effects for sleep. Some studies demonstrate a usefulness for it during the day for alertness and energy, which in turn may improve quality of sleep throughout the night. CBD has shown to help people with Parkinson's-induced REM behavior disorder. The synthetic forms of cannabinoid-based drugs dronabinol and nabilone have produced fairly good results for many conditions, including sleep disturbance. With scant findings, it is necessary to continue research in this area and hopefully find solid evidence that cannabidiol, synthetic cannabinoids, and the endocannabinoid system with all of its components can lead to real therapeutic help for people struggling with sleep problems.

10

CBD and Neurodegenerative Disorders

If I tell you the truth, you don't have to remember anything.
—Mark Twain

Introduction

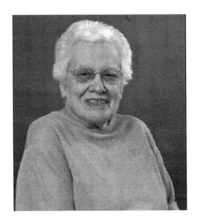

I could not wait to get to this chapter, and for many reasons. My mother passed away in the same skilled nursing center where she worked as a nursing assistant for almost thirty years. She provided care on the same unit of the facility the entire time and delivered person-centered care decades before anyone heard those words. I saw my mom slipping away years before she needed assisted living and then skilled care. Ten years before she moved into a beautiful and caring assisted-living community, her memory was failing; she was falling and had left the stove on several times. I kept her home with our family for over fifteen years until it was absolutely time (*whatever that means*) for her to move into the assisted-living community located only seven minutes from our home. This made it convenient for almost-daily visits. I witnessed the confusion, anger, bitterness, rejection, and sadness she experienced. Once the cognitive decline accelerated, the staff recommended she be moved into the skilled facility up the hill. She actually did better there for a year or so. Her dementia was worsening, and eventually the social worker recommended the memory care unit. I disagreed at least twice and then gave in upon the third request, and again, Mom did better in the smaller, more relaxed atmosphere of the specialized living area. This is where she died another year later, after a massive stroke induced a nine-day coma. She died surrounded by most of her family, friends, and some of the staff who had worked with her before she retired at the age of eighty. She was almost ninety-two when she passed peacefully.

I offer this story because neurodegenerative disorders mean something very special to me. Besides cancer, millions of people will die from conditions like Alzheimer's, Parkinson's, Huntington's, ALS, and multiple sclerosis. These are difficult diseases for the person, their family and friends, and of course, their caregivers. These diseases are characterized by stage after stage of loss and the well-known *long goodbye*. There are no cures. While current treatments may ease some of the symptoms, we need better solutions and hopefully, one day, prevention of these terrible disorders.

It might sound complicated, but simply stated, neurodegenerative diseases are the main causes of neurocognitive disorders. Diseases such as Alzheimer's, Parkinson's, Huntington's, and multiple sclerosis contribute to a group of conditions that eventually lead to impaired mental functioning. This includes memory problems, changes in behaviors, difficulty with language, and trouble performing activities associated with daily living. We used to call such conditions "organic brain syndrome," but the preferred term "neurocognitive disorder" is now the most commonly used terminology. Although neurocognitive disorders are generally considered age related, they can also affect people at younger ages. Neurodegenerative diseases cause the brain and nerves to deteriorate over time, leading to a gradual loss in neurological functioning. These disorders can also develop due to brain trauma or substance use.

Symptoms of each disorder will be somewhat different, but in general they include memory loss, confusion, and anxiety. Some people will also experience other psychiatric conditions like depression, psychosis, and hallucinations. Other symptoms may include headaches, inability to concentrate, short-term memory loss, trouble with routine tasks like driving, loss of balance or ability to walk, and changes in vision. Some risk factors for developing either neurodegenerative or neurocognitive disorders include lifestyle and daily living habits (poor diet, lack of exercise, smoking, excessive alcohol or substance use) and exposure to toxins. Other more common risk factors include advanced age, cardiovascular diseases, and diabetes. These disorders can be diagnosed with the use of CT scans, MRIs, PET scans, and EEGs.

Alzheimer's Disease

Introduction
Many experts agree that Alzheimer's is one of the most important diseases of the twenty-first century. According to the Alzheimer's Association, 5.8 million Americans are currently living with Alzheimer's, and by 2050 that number will balloon to well over 14 million. It is the sixth leading cause of death among all Americans and the fifth leading cause among people sixty-five years and older. One out of every three American dies of Alzheimer's disease. To put this in perspective, Alzheimer's kills more people than breast and prostate cancer combined. Between 2000 and 2017, deaths due to heart disease decreased by 9%, but deaths associated with Alzheimer's increased by 145%. Every sixty-five seconds, someone in the United States is developing this disease, which is quite a staggering fact. It has been estimated that one out of every ten people sixty-five years and older will develop Alzheimer's, and around two-thirds of

them will be women.[1] With all that said, you likely either know someone diagnosed with this crippling disease or an individual who has already passed away from it. Alzheimer's is a slow and agonizing process for everyone around and one that perhaps can be helped with CBD.

Overview of Alzheimer's Disease

In 1907, a German psychiatrist by the name of Alois Alzheimer was the first to describe symptoms of what he then called "presenile dementia." Another German psychiatrist, Emil Kraepelen, later named the condition Alzheimer's disease. Upon examining postmortem brains of his patients, Alois Alzheimer observed neuritic plaques (extracellular deposits of amyloid beta in the gray area of the brain) and neurofibrillary tangles, which are today still considered some of the hallmarks of Alzheimer's disease. Neuritic plaques are formed by the extracellular buildup of amyloid beta, which is a leftover fragment of a larger protein. As amyloid beta clusters together, the fragments have toxic effects on brain cells and disrupt communication between cells. These clusters then form larger deposits called amyloid plaques. Tangles are another hallmark of Alzheimer's disease. These are formed by a protein called tau, which plays an important role in the brain cell's health and functioning. In Alzheimer's, tau detaches and forms neurofibrillary tangles. These changes then result in sustained activation of the immune response.

Fagan and Campbell define Alzheimer's as "a complex age-related neurodegenerative disease characterized by the progressive loss of memory and cognitive function." Symptoms of the disease include memory loss, confusion, difficulty completing difficult tasks, problems with abstract thinking, speech problems, disorientation regarding time and physical space, and changes in mood. Some individuals will experience anxiety and depression during the early and mid-stages of the disease. Agitation, aggression, combativeness, loss of inhibition, apathy, rigidity and/or tremors, and slowness of movement are all well-known symptoms of Alzheimer's disease. Deterioration takes place over the course of years, leading to death within three to nine years proceeding a diagnosis.[2]

Alzheimer's is the most common cause of dementia, which is a medical condition characterized by a decline in thinking and other mental abilities that are severe enough to interfere with daily activities. Behavioral and social skills also deteriorate and disrupt the individual's ability to live and function independently. Memory deteriorates to the point at which the individual gets lost in a familiar place. One's thinking and reasoning fade away; even people who were once accountants may no longer recognize numbers. Judgment and decision-making also disappear, and determining what to wear becomes a difficult or impossible task. Changes take place in one's personality and behavior, many times causing distress for the individual, his or her family, and caregivers. Some common changes include wandering, changes in sleep habits, distrust and paranoia, delusions, social withdrawal, and irritability.

Signs and Symptoms of Alzheimer's Disease

- ✓ Memory Loss
- ✓ Confusion and Disorientation
- ✓ Problems Completing Difficult Tasks
- ✓ Difficulties with Abstract Thinking
- ✓ Speech Difficulties
- ✓ Mood Changes, Anxiety, and Depression
- ✓ Aggression and Combativeness
- ✓ Loss of Inhibition
- ✓ Movement Problems

Beyond these changes, many medical complications are associated with Alzheimer's disease, including dehydration and malnutrition, urinary tract infections, depression, immobility, falls and fall-related injuries, and pneumonia. Constipation, diarrhea, and incontinence are common problems among older adults with Alzheimer's. Oral and dental problems are common as well. Ultimately, the cause of death will be a combination of the disease and dehydration, skin ulcers, and pneumonia. Most individuals will require skilled nursing care throughout the final stages of the disease.

There are several risk factors associated with the development of Alzheimer's disease. Among them, age is by far the greatest known risk, and while the disease is not a part of normal aging, as you grow older, the likelihood of developing Alzheimer's disease increases. Experts believe that one's family history and genetics are also risk factors, especially when one of your parents or siblings has the disease. A specific genetic factor is a form of the apolipoprotein E gene (APOE). Although a variation of this gene, APOE e4, is associated with a higher risk of Alzheimer's, not everyone with this gene will develop the disease. While men and women share an equal risk for developing Alzheimer's, there are more women who have it, mainly due to the greater longevity of women.

Another interesting risk factor is mild cognitive impairment, or MCI for short. This is a condition that occurs between the cognitive decline of normal aging and the development of a serious form of dementia. People with MCI have an increased risk of developing Alzheimer's, especially if the main symptom is memory loss. More attention is focusing on head trauma, particularly associated with sports, as a risk factor for developing the disorder. Other risk factors include poor sleep patterns, lack of exercise, obesity, smoking or being exposed to secondhand smoke, high blood pressure, high cholesterol, and poorly controlled type 2 diabetes.

Traditional Therapies for Alzheimer's Disease
While there is no real way to prevent the condition, modification in a number of lifestyle areas may help reduce its risk. Some studies report that lifelong learning and being mentally and socially engaged may help reduce the risk of Alzheimer's. By making healthy changes in your diet, exercise, and habits, you can not only reduce risk of Alzheimer's but also the risk of heart disease and other cardiovascular problems. An important fact to remember is *what's healthy for the heart is healthy for the brain*, and vice versa. Healthy changes can lower your risk of developing other diseases that are associated with Alzheimer's, like diabetes.

Your diet is incredibly important. Hippocrates in 400 BC preached that "food is medicine," and he was absolutely correct. We simply are what we eat. That being said, whether it's the Mediterranean or ketogenic diet, smart and healthy eating is an essential method of preventing disease and disorders that may be associated with Alzheimer's.

> **Reducing Risk of Alzheimer's Disease through a Healthy Diet**
>
> Eat lots of fresh leafy greens and nonstarchy vegetables like eggplant, tomatoes, cauliflower, and artichokes.
>
> Cook with olive and coconut oil.
>
> Get beans, legumes, nuts and seeds, and herbs and spices in your daily diet.
>
> Whole grains, wild-caught fish, pasture-raised poultry, eggs, and cheese are recommended.
>
> Eat red meat once a week, drink lots of water (not tap water), and some coffee and tea, preferably green or white tea, and drink red wine daily.
>
> Try to stay away from processed foods, excessive alcohol, sugar, and refined grains and foods packaged in aluminum (its's a neurotoxin).

These may help to reduce inflammation, support brain circulation, memory, and communication between brain cells, and prevent the formation of plaques and tangles in the brain.

We are learning more and more about the importance of the gut, gut health, and the microbiome. Some experts are now calling the gut our second brain because of its influence over our brain and brain-related diseases. Researchers are describing what is called the "brain-gut-microbiome axis" and how the three are interrelated and mutually influential in health and disease. Exercise—aerobic exercise, in particular—is important and has brain-protecting qualities. Maintaining a healthy weight and not smoking are also beneficial. Getting adequate amounts of sleep is important because poor sleep may cause or exacerbate the development of dementia. Engaging in productive and somewhat complex work can help maintain cognitive abilities.

When possible, try to avoid taking anticholinergic drugs because they may be a risk factor in developing Alzheimer's disease. These drugs are prescribed by physicians for a number of conditions like depression, allergies, gastrointestinal disorders, Parkinson's disease, psychiatric disorders, COPD, insomnia, motion sickness, asthma, and overactive bladder. Anticholinergic drugs help to contract and relax muscles and work by blocking acetylcholine, a brain chemical responsible for muscle contraction, activation of pain responses, and regulation of endocrine and REM sleep functions. The list of anticholinergic drugs is quite long, but a few examples include Elavil, Flexeril, Tylenol, Tylenol PM and Advil PM, Benadryl, Sinequan, and Mellaril. While there might be some risk involved with these drugs, it certainly doesn't mean that everyone will be affected in the same way. Other drugs that have a lesser anticholinergic effect include Xanax, Zyrtec, Lasix, IMODIUM, and Zantac. It should be noted that in April of 2020, the FDA requested that Zantac be made unavailable to the public due to the presence of a contaminant known as N-Nitrosodimethylamine, or NDMA. It is believed that this substance may cause certain types of cancer.

Above and beyond changes in lifestyle, the use of medications is standard in the treatment of Alzheimer's disease. Currently there are five FDA-approved medications for the disorder. Three of them (Aricept, Razadyne, and Exelon) are from the drug class called "cholinesterase inhibitors." Among them, only Aricept has been approved for all stages of Alzheimer's. Razadyne has been approved for mild to moderate Alzheimer's, and Exelon for moderate to severe Alzheimer's disease. They work by increasing levels of acetylcholine and may be effective in treating symptoms related to memory, thinking, judgment, language, and other cognitive processes. Alzheimer's disease either manages or destroys cells that produce and use acetylcholine, in turn reducing the amount available to carry messages. By maintaining acetylcholine levels, these drugs may help make up for the loss of functioning brain cells. Although cholinesterase inhibitors are usually well tolerated, they do come with side effects, including nausea, vomiting, loss of appetite, and increased frequency of bowel movement.

Namenda is another FDA-approved drug for moderate to severe Alzheimer's and is prescribed to improve memory, attention, reason, the ability to perform simple tasks, and language. It is the first drug to work with

NMDA receptors by regulating glutamate. When glutamate attaches to other cells, it passes calcium into the cells, carrying electrical or chemical signaling, which is important for learning and memory. It may help people with Alzheimer's to carry out daily activities and improve mental functioning. Side effects of Namenda include dizziness, headache, confusion, and constipation.

The last drug, Namzaric, is a combination of Aricept and Namenda and was approved by the FDA for the treatment of moderate to severe Alzheimer's. This drug unfortunately carries more serious side effects than the others. People with asthma or lung diseases may experience worsening of lung problems. Seizures, nausea, vomiting, and difficulty urinating may occur. Namzaric has caused increased stomach acid in people, which increases the risk for ulcers and bleeding. When it is taken with NSAIDs like Advil or aspirin, the risk increases even more. Some people have experienced slowed heartbeat and fainting, especially among people who have a coexisting heart condition. Namzaric has also caused muscle problems in people who have received anesthesia.

Research Findings on CBD and Alzheimer's Disease

CBD is a neuroprotective, antioxidant, and anti-inflammatory agent, which may make it an effective treatment for Alzheimer's disease. Leinow and Birnam state in their book *CBD: A Patient's Guide to Medicinal Cannabis* state that "new science shows that the disease is strongly connected to the endocannabinoid system, and, with the re-immergence of CBD medicine, it is likely that cannabinoid-based treatments will become more standard."[3] They point out that cannabinoids have the ability to protect against the destruction of neural circuits in a number of ways. They neutralize free radicals, reduce inflammation, clear out beta amyloid, improve the function of mitochondria, and remove cellular waste.

One of the earliest articles I found was in the *Journal of Neurochemistry* in 2004. In it, researchers were examining the neuroprotective effects of cannabidiol on beta-amyloid-induced toxicity. Not only did they find that CBD had neuroprotective effects, but it also exhibited antioxidative and antiapoptotic effects against beta-amyloid peptide toxicity, which causes oxidative stress and inflammation in the brain. Apoptosis is programmed cell death, and oxidative stress is an imbalance between reactive oxygen species (ROS) production and the body's inability to detoxify or repair damage caused by beta amyloid.[4]

Four years later a paper was published examining a much broader subject: the role of the endocannabinoid system in Alzheimer's disease. Authors Bisogno and Di Marzo state:

> The available data indicate that endocannabinoids are likely to play in this disorder a role similar to that suggested in other neurodegenerative diseases, that is, to represent an endogenous adaptive response aimed at counteracting both the neurochemical and inflammatory consequences of B-amyloid-induced tau protein hyperactivity, possibly the most important underlying cause of AD.

They add that another attractive feature of CBD for Alzheimer's is its antioxidant actions. Cannabinoids, they believe, might one day become a treatment for this disorder.[5]

The year 2009 yielded a little more research into the use of CBD for Alzheimer's disease. The authors write:

> There is increasing evidence that the cannabinoid system may regulate neurodegenerative processes such as excessive glutamate production, oxidative stress and neuroinflammation. Neurodegeneration is a feature common in various types of dementia and this has led to interest in whether cannabinoids may be clinically useful in the treatment of people with dementia. Recent studies have also shown that cannabinoids may have more specific effects in interrupting the pathological process in Alzheimer's disease.[6]

Another paper published the same year focused on inflammation as the basis of most neurodegenerative disorders and stated that scientists are still searching for treatments to handle the problems caused by it. They admit that neuroprotective and anti-inflammatory strategies would be desirable and believe that CBD may be a promising agent for neurodegenerative diseases like Alzheimer's, Parkinson's, Huntington's, and multiple sclerosis.[7]

Shortly thereafter, in 2010, two scholars from Switzerland provided a review of animal and human studies examining cannabinoids and Alzheimer's, Huntington's, Parkinson's, and vascular dementia. They found an involvement of the endocannabinoid system in the neurotransmission, neuropathology, and neurobiology of these disorders and point to several sources of evidence for therapeutic potential in neurodegenerative diseases. CB1 and CB2 agonists, for instance, "may interrupt excitotoxicity and reduce inflammation in AD brains, modulators of endocannabinoid signaling may reduce hyperactivity in HD, while CB1 agonists could reduce dyskinesia in PD." They propose that CBD may even be able to slow down the cognitive decline associated with Alzheimer's disease as well as manage behavioral symptoms in both Alzheimer's and Huntington's diseases.[8]

In 2011, a large research team from Brazil demonstrated that CBD may account for a significant reduction of amyloid beta-induced neuronal cell death by searching for and reducing reactive oxygen species and by exerting anti-inflammatory properties.[9] That same year, a paper was published in the journal *Drugs & Aging*, stressing the potential for CBD to be an effective treatment specifically for the behavioral and psychological symptoms of dementia. They also examine other phytochemicals (plant-based substances) such as curcumin, ginseng, sage, and resveratrol (found in wine) and find them to have therapeutic possibilities for the treatment of dementia-related problems.[10] In 2012, four scientific investigators reviewed the potential of the endocannabinoid system as a primary target for Alzheimer's treatment. They wrote, "Based on the complex pathology of AD, a preventative, multimodal drug approach targeting a combination of pathological AD symptoms appears ideal. Importantly, cannabinoids show anti-inflammatory, neuroprotective and antioxidant properties and have immunosuppressive effects."[11] Three researchers in 2013 specifically examined the evidence that endocannabinoids such as anandamide and 2-AG play in Alzheimer's disease and the potential for "beneficial therapeutic manipulation of the EC signaling system."[12] A paper in 2014 pointed out the activation of both CB1 and CB2 receptors by either natural or synthetic cannabidiol has positive effects in Alzheimer's experimental models by reducing the harmful amyloid beta peptide action and tau phosphorylation and by promoting the brain's natural repair systems. Cannabinoids show the ability to counteract many harmful processes induced by Alzheimer's disease.[13]

One of the arguments about monotherapy, or using one drug, for Alzheimer's is that the disease is multifaceted and is linked to numerous mechanisms in the brain, in the gut, and elsewhere throughout the body. How can one pill target all of these areas and make a real difference? Researchers in 2015 stated, "The ideal treatment for AD should be able to modulate the disease through multiple mechanisms rather than targeting a single dysregulated pathway." They point to the endocannabinoid system, as many researchers do, as a prime target to treat the disease. Cannabinoids and endocannabinoids both appear to have the ability to modify multiple processes in Alzheimer's disease.[14]

Researcher Celina Liu and her team in Toronto, Canada, found that cannabinoids can be effective in the treatment of certain neuropsychiatric symptoms of Alzheimer's disease, like agitation and aggression. These are typically treated with various psychiatric medications including benzodiazepines, antidepressants, antipsychotic drugs, and others, with each one carrying negative and potentially dangerous side effects. She and her colleagues agree that "the limited efficacy and high-risk profiles of current pharmacotherapies for the management of agitation and aggression in AD have driven the search for safer pharmacological alternatives." They provided a review of the literature and found that six studies showed "significant" benefits from dronabinol and nabilone, which are synthetic cannabinoids, on agitation and aggression."[15]

Then, in 2016, a massive overview of natural phytochemicals in the treatment and *prevention* of dementia was published. The Italian team of academics reviewed studies on Alzheimer's disease, vascular disease, dementia with Lewy bodies, and frontotemporal dementia:

> Currently approved pharmacological treatments for most forms of dementia seem to act only on symptoms without having profound disease-modifying effects. Thus, alternative strategies capable of

preventing the progressive loss of specific neuronal populations are urgently required...We believe that natural phytochemicals may present a promising source of alternative medicine, at least in association with therapies approved to date for dementia.[16]

In 2016, Shelef and his research team from Israel examined the safety and efficacy of medical cannabis oil on behavioral and psychological symptoms of dementia. While this study did not look into CBD specifically, the researchers found that adding medical cannabis oil to prescribed antipsychotic medications, like Risperdal, decreased delusions, agitation, aggression, irritability, apathy, and sleep problems in patients suffering moderate to severe dementia. They conclude by stating, "There is no FDA-approved treatment for [behavioral, psychological symptoms of dementia], but antipsychotic drugs are frequently prescribed off-label yielding only modest improvements and associated with increased mortality."[17]

Another paper published the same year reported that amyloid proteotoxicity (adverse effects of damaged or misfolded proteins found in Alzheimer's) initiates an inflammatory reaction that is blocked by cannabinoids. They state:

> Nerve cell death from the accumulation of aggregated or amyloid-like proteins is a common theme in most age-dependent neurodegenerative diseases. However, there are no drugs that significantly inhibit cell death associated with Alzheimer's disease (AD), Parkinson's or Huntington's diseases. This could be because most interest has been in the late manifestations of the disease, not in the initial changes in cell metabolism that ultimately lead to nerve cell death.

They speculate that the accumulation of clusters of damaged protein in the brain occurs throughout the life course and promotes age-related cognitive changes and might also be behind the initiation of many age-related disorders.[18]

An article in 2017 provided preclinical evidence using mice in labs that CBD can produce beneficial effects for people diagnosed with Alzheimer's and Parkinson's diseases and multiple sclerosis. It showed neuroprotection through its antioxidant qualities and anti-inflammatory effects as well as its ability to alter a large number of targets, like receptors, all of which are involved in the development of neurodegenerative disorders.[19] The same year, a review by Austrian researchers yielded some interesting evidence that CBD may become a multifunctional treatment option for people diagnosed with Alzheimer's disease. In rats, CBD was shown to reverse and prevent the development of cognitive problems. They also believe that the combination of CBD and THC might have greater therapeutic benefits than either of them alone. Being that current drugs for Alzheimer's have limited benefits, CBD seems to be a prime candidate for a new treatment strategy for the disease.[20]

Summary

Alzheimer's disease is a progressive, incurable, neurodegenerative disease that has a very heavy impact on quality of life. It is also a very expensive disorder and takes its toll on both informal and professional caregivers. Alzheimer's is the most common cause of dementia in older adults and progresses from early signs and symptoms to eventual death. Lifestyle changes and the use of prescription medication may help, but most experts agree that there is no prevention for Alzheimer's and the medications are not overly effective. Some medications may actually increase the risk for developing dementia.

Amyloid plaques, neurofibrillary tangles, and inflammation appear to be the hallmarks of this disease. CBD has been shown throughout multiple research reports to have valuable biological and symptom benefits. It has a neuroprotective quality as well as antioxidant and anti-apoptotic effects against amyloid beta peptide toxicity. Many researchers believe that the endocannabinoid system itself is a target for the development of therapeutic agents to help manage symptoms of Alzheimer's and other neurodegenerative diseases like Parkinson's, Huntington's, and multiple sclerosis.

CBD has shown to work in a variety of ways, in multiple systems and channels throughout the body and brain, and appears to hold promise among many experts in their respective fields. If we were to stand back and look at the bigger picture, many diseases and disorders may be the result of a dysfunctional endocannabinoid system. Why or how it becomes dysfunctional is still a mystery, but by feeding our system cannabidiol, we are providing the system with a much-needed boost. It is comforting to know that in the near future, we may not have to rely on so many psychiatric drugs but instead use a substance that is natural. Our bodies prefer natural things and in general reject those that are artificial or synthetic. Could it be that a plant that has been used as medicine for thousands of years, by almost every culture on the planet, is about to make a massive comeback and bring quality of life to people diagnosed with Alzheimer's, neurodegenerative disorders, and many other diseases?

Amyotrophic Lateral Sclerosis (ALS)

I am probably the most selfish man you will ever meet in your life. No one gets the satisfaction or the joy that I get out of seeing kids realize there is hope.

—Jerry Lewis

Introduction

I grew up watching Jerry Lewis movies, especially those costarring Dean Martin. He was always a funny guy to me. I also began watching the Jerry Lewis MDA (Muscular Dystrophy Association) Labor Day Telethon annually with my parents. This is where I saw his serious side and his passion to help young people diagnosed with muscular dystrophy. It wasn't until years later that I realized that MDA was responsible for conducting research in other areas, including another dreadful disease—amyotrophic lateral sclerosis.

The first time I heard about this disease was absolutely shocking. I learned that the first signs and symptoms begin almost unnoticeably and then advance to mild weakness in the hands or feet, accompanied by no to little pain. Within a year or so, ALS advances to severe muscle weakness, serious problems with chewing or swallowing, deterioration of language, and difficulty breathing. Most people do not experience any mental decline characterized by other neurodegenerative diseases, so they are completely aware of their rapidly worsening condition. Movement of limbs, eyes, or tongue becomes impossible as they are overtaken by complete paralysis. The person is trapped inside a failing body. Individuals with ALS eventually die due to respiratory difficulties, as it becomes almost impossible to breathe, because they can no longer get enough oxygen from their lungs into their blood. The one blessing about Lou Gehrig's disease is that many people will die in their sleep.

Amyotrophic lateral sclerosis, or ALS, also goes by the name Lou Gehrig's disease after the famous New York Yankee. It also known as Charcot's disease, after the French neurologist who coined the term "amyotrophic lateral sclerosis." Many people have probably never heard of the disease or, like me, knew very little about it. When Steven Hawking, the famous theoretical physicist, died in 2018, the world started to pay more attention to the disorder. Ice bucket challenges then spread across the internet, and people began money-raising campaigns to support research and promote awareness.

Every day, fifteen people are newly diagnosed with ALS, or around fifty-six hundred annually. Currently, there are around thirty thousand people living with ALS in the United States, and each year, two out of every one hundred thousand people will die from it. To put this into a little more perspective, every ninety minutes, one person is diagnosed with the disease, while another dies from it. The life expectancy after diagnosis is the shortest among all neurodegenerative disorders. Most people will die within two to five years. Despite this, improved medical care has helped many people live more productive lives for a little bit longer.

Overview of Amyotrophic Lateral Sclerosis (ALS)

Amyotrophic lateral sclerosis is a fatal neurodegenerative disease caused by the selective and progressive injury and death of motor neurons located in the spinal cord, brain stem, and motor cortex. When cells in these regions die, the individual loses voluntary muscle control and movement, making chewing, speaking, and walking difficult to impossible. Once the nerve dies, it can no longer send signals to muscles, which causes them to twitch, spasm, become progressively weak, and eventually waste away. Once the disease begins, it almost always progresses, shortening the life span dramatically, leading to an early death. Despite this, progression is not always a straight line, meaning that periods of arrest have been seen in people in which there is little to no loss of function for a few weeks or months.

It is not clear what causes the disease, but we do know that there are two forms it. Sporadic ALS represents almost 90% of cases and has no clear etiology or origin. Familial ALS, which is genetic, represents 5% to 10% of cases. It appears that both athletes and people who have served in the military have a higher risk of developing ALS, and the US Department of Affairs has recognized ALS as a service-connected disease. Two groups of military personnel have shown a higher incidence of ALS—those who served in Guam in the late 1950s and more recently, those serving in the Gulf War. This has led to research trying to find a connection between environmental factors such as exposure to nerve toxins as potential causes of the disease.

ALS appears to be somewhat related to age, as most people who are diagnosed are between the ages of forty and seventy. The average age at onset is fifty-five, and some people in their twenties and thirties have been diagnosed in far fewer numbers. Although ALS is more common in men, with advanced age, the incidence equals out between men and women. Symptoms of ALS include progressive weakening of muscles, slurred speech, abnormal fatigue in the arms and legs, and uncontrollable periods of laughing or crying, called the pseudobulbar affect.

Traditional Therapies for Amyotrophic Lateral Sclerosis (ALS)

ALS is difficult to diagnosis early because it mimics many other neurodegenerative disorders. Physicians will run a series of tests, including an electromyogram (EMG), which evaluates electrical activity in muscles; an MRI to check the brain and spinal cord; a nerve conduction study, which evaluates the nerve's ability to send impulses to the muscles; blood and urine tests; a spinal tap to analyze spinal fluid; and possibly a muscle biopsy, in which a small portion of the muscle is removed and sent to a lab to be tested.

Because breathing issues will develop during the progression of the disease, breathing tests will be performed regularly, and the individual may eventually need mechanical ventilation for assistance with breathing. Physical therapy can address issues like walking, mobility, and pain, as well as any braces or equipment needs. Occupational therapy can work toward continued independence, regardless of how much muscle weakness the individual experiences. OT can help with bathing, grooming, eating, and dressing. Speech therapy can help the individual with different means of communication and ensure that their needs are being expressed and understood. A dietician may be involved to provide help with meals and foods that are easier to swallow. Because the decline in independence is so severe, the individual is likely to experience anxiety or depression. A psychologist, psychiatrist, or other mental health professional can provide emotional support for both the person diagnosed with AL and the family.

The symptoms of ALS can be very devastating and accompanied by intense emotions like fear, guilt, and anger. It's a very difficult disease to adjust to, and living with ALS can take its toll on everyone involved. There will be grieving, sadness, and at times, despair. With this being said, it would be more helpful for everyone to remain as positive as possible and focus on quality of life. ALS will take away many things, including one's psychical independence, but like Steven Hawking, one's mental capacities will be largely intact and can be used to take part in having a social life, speaking to others about the disease, joining or speaking at support groups, and doing other positive activities.

Outside of working closely with a medical team and adjusting socially and psychologically to the disease, the use of medications might provide relief of certain symptoms and even prolong life for a while. One medication that has been FDA approved specifically for ALS since 1995 is Rilutek (riluzole). It is an antiglutamate oral treatment that has been shown in clinical studies to slow the progression of the disease and increase survival by one year or more. It gives people with ALS more time to sustain higher functioning and have greater muscle control and movement. The drug Radicava (edaravone) is another treatment option for people with ALS, and it, too, slows the decline of physical function. It works by protecting nerve cells and helps to remove free radicals in the body. Radicava is an intravenous drug, which means it is given as an IV with a needle inserted into a vein. The treatment lasts about an hour. Both drugs come with side effects, including nausea and fatigue, and elevated enzyme levels might occur with Rilutek. Radicava can cause more severe side effects like allergic reactions—some being life threatening. Other side effects may include hives; swelling of the lips, tongue, or face; fainting; breathing problems; wheezing; trouble swallowing; dizziness; itching; and asthma attacks. It has been reported that the most common side effects are bruising, trouble walking, and headaches. A new oral suspension or liquid form of Riluzole was approved by the FDA in 2018. It can be a better way to administer the drug for people who have trouble swallowing and taking tablets. With this advancement, more accurate dosing and greater compliance to taking medications might be achieved. This drug, too, comes with side effects including hypoethesia (partial or reduced sensitivity to stimuli), asthenia (lack of energy and strength), nausea, hypertension, abdominal pain, and reduced lung function.

One last medication worth mentioning is Sativex, which is an oral mucosal spray containing cannabis extracts. It helps with spasticity in individuals diagnosed with motor neuron diseases, including amyotrophic lateral sclerosis. The drug is a combination of equal parts THC and CBD and has shown significant improvements on certain tests and scales. Since there is no cure for the disease, Sativex may be able to provide a new treatment that will manage symptoms and improve quality of life. This drug can be especially effective for those who do not respond to other treatments for spasticity and pain. Some adverse side effects of Sativex include nausea, dizziness, asthenia, and confusion.

Research Findings on CBD and Amyotrophic Lateral Sclerosis (ALS)

Before getting into specific studies, it is comforting to know that much of what has been found by researchers striving to find a better way to treat people with ALS has been mainly positive. CBD has been found to ease pain due to its analgesic properties. It has helped to reduce muscle tension and induce relaxation. It acts as a bronchodilator, opening airways so that people with ALS can breathe easier. It has shown the ability to slow down or stop the overproduction of saliva, which is seen in many people with ALS. It stimulates appetite, enhances diet, and induces sleep. All of these are wonderful effects of cannabidiol and even better, with minimal to no side effects.

Beginning in 2007, researchers in Little Rock, Arkansas, studied the effects of the CB2 receptor on ALS using mice and found that cannabinoids produced anti-inflammatory actions through the CB1 and CB2 receptors, and delayed the progression of neuroinflammation. More importantly, they add that the survival rate of the mice in the study increased by 56%.[21] One year later, another team of researchers studying the endocannabinoid system and its potential impact on ALS found that CB1 and CB2 exert different effects on the disorder. They found that CB1 receptors slow down the release of glutamate, which reduces calcium release. CB2, on the other hand, may influence inflammation. Cannabinoid agents may exert antioxidant actions, target multiple neurotoxic pathways, and become a valuable treatment for ALS.[22]

Several years later, researchers revisited the ability of the naturally occurring endocannabinoid system to help reduce symptoms of ALS in a review article. Pryce and Baker remind us that studies have shown that cannabinoids have reduced or alleviated limb spasticity and neurodegeneration. They state, "Cannabinoids have efficacy, not only in symptom relief but also as neuroprotective agents which may slow disease progression and thus delay the onset of symptoms."[23] Will cannabinoid therapeutics become a disease-modifying or symptom control agent for slowing this devastating disease? The same year, researchers from Spain made the following remarks concerning endocannabinoids and amyotrophic lateral sclerosis:

> Cannabinoid-based medicines may serve as novel therapy, able to delay/arrest neurodegeneration in ALS, due to their capacity to normalize glutamate homeostasis, to reduce oxidative injury, and/or to attenuate local inflammatory events, and possibly also due to their capacity to activate cellular responses…addressed to control the toxicity of protein aggregates.[24]

In 2016, a large research team concluded that CBD has been demonstrated to be a potent anti-inflammatory and neuroprotective agent in neurological preclinical models.[25] Another paper in 2016 published by Italian researchers asked the question, "Can cannabinoids be a potential therapeutic tool in amyotrophic lateral sclerosis?" They point to studies using mice in which CBD produced positive results, like anti-inflammatory, antioxidant, and neuroprotective qualities. Studies using animals showed the ability of CBD to delay disease progression while prolonging survival. They then turn to the evidence in human studies and start by stating that the endocannabinoid system clearly plays an important role in the development of ALS. Cannabis has been shown to relieve ALS symptoms such as pain, depression, appetite loss, and excessive drooling. It also improved one of the main problems with ALS: spasticity. While there is not enough research on CBD and ALS, they believe "there is valid rationale to propose the use of cannabinoid compounds in the pharmaceutical management of ALS patients. Cannabinoids indeed are able to delay ALS progression and prolong survival."[26]

The following year, in 2017, Gerhard Nahler, a researcher from Austria, presented a case study involving one patient who, while taking Riluzole, experienced progressive deterioration. The patient then decided to take cannabidiol twice a day alongside Riluzole and, after several weeks, increased the dose. Incredibly, "Within 6 weeks, the impaired function of the right hand and foot reversed almost completely, and dysphagia partially. Improvement was maintained for 10 weeks, when again a slow progression of dysarthria and dysphagia was observed…However, symptoms of the limbs (weakness, fasciculation, atrophy) worsened much less." What does this mean? Possibly, the combination of ALS medications and CBD together can improve symptoms and bring some functioning back for the individual dealing with multiple symptoms. Nahler also states, "These mechanisms of CBD are interesting as they fit many of the current hypothetical requirements for a successful drug for motor neuron disease. Further on, CBD seems to be well tolerated and safe in humans, even at high doses and with chronic use and can easily be combined with existing treatment regimens."[27]

In 2019, a research team from Italy tested the effectiveness of nabiximols (Sativex) for motor neuron diseases, including amyotrophic lateral sclerosis. The participants were between the ages of eighteen and eighty and were taking other antispasticity medications along with Sativex. They reported, "In this proof-of-concept trial, nabiximols has a positive effect on spasticity symptoms in patients with motor neuron disease and had an acceptable safety and tolerability profile."[28] Another review paper that year was published in the *Journal of Neurochemistry* summarizing results of experiments using cannabinoids for ALS symptoms in mice. Researchers specifically examined survival time and disease progression. They found an increase in survival time, and eight out of nine studies they scanned revealed significant improvements in motor function. Weight loss was improved in four out of five studies. They conclude, "This review provides some evidence for the efficacy of cannabinoids in prolonging survival time in an ALS mouse model. A delay in disease progression is also suggested following cannabidiol treatment though it was not possible to consolidate the results from reviewed studies."[29]

Summary

If you have not heard a lot about ALS or know much about it, you now have a glimpse into the devastation it causes the individual who is diagnosed with it, as well as their family, friends, and caregivers who provide support and medical treatment. ALS is a disease that attacks nerve cells in the brain and spinal cord that control voluntary motor movement. The disease progresses quickly and ruthlessly, limiting the individual's life expectancy from two to five years after diagnosis. Currently, two medications approved by the FDA may provide some relief of symptoms and add a few more weeks of life. There is no cure or known prevention. Studies have shown that cannabinoids may become a new treatment by itself or as an add-on with other medications for ALS.

Parkinson's Disease

> *Parkinson's patients are the experts on what we have. We have a responsibility as patients to share our experience—what works for us. What we respond to, what we can contribute to research.*
>
> —Michael J. Fox

Introduction

It's only right to begin this chapter by paying tribute to Michael J. Fox and the incredible work that has been done through his foundation, the Michael J. Fox Foundation for Parkinson's Research. Michael was diagnosed with an early-onset form of the disease in 1991 when he was twenty-nine years old, and he only went public with his condition years later, in 1998. He then went on to launch his foundation in 2000 and has raised over $900 million dedicated to finding a cure for this devastating disease.

Parkinson's disease is a neurodegenerative disorder characterized by movement symptoms including tremors, rigidity, slowness of movement, and impaired balance. Neurons in the part of the brain called the substantia nigra malfunction and eventually die. Some of these neurons are responsible for producing dopamine, an important neurotransmitter responsible for muscle movement and coordination. Parkinson's disease is progressive, meaning that symptoms will only get worse over time, until the individual in unable to control his or her own movements. The progression is slow, and only after 70% to 80% of the nerve cells have been lost do symptoms appear, making it a challenging disease to diagnose and treat.

Parkinson's disease is the second most common neurodegenerative and age-related disorder, second to Alzheimer's disease. Around one million people in the United States and between seven and ten million people worldwide have Parkinson's.[30] It affects more people than multiple sclerosis (MS), muscular dystrophy (MD), and amyotrophic lateral sclerosis (ALS) combined. Around sixty thousand Americans are diagnosed with Parkinson's disease annually, and many people go undetected and undiagnosed.

The rate of newly diagnosed cases of the disease increases with age. Around 4% of people are diagnosed before their fifties, and men are roughly 1.5 times more likely to have Parkinson's than women. The disease is a very costly one, with direct and indirect costs estimated at $25 billion annually. Medication costs around $2,500 per year, and surgery can run as high as $100,000 per individual.

Overview of Parkinson's Disease

The cause of Parkinson's disease is still unknown, and while there is no cure, medications, therapy, supplements, and lifestyle changes may help to manage symptoms. While the disease itself is not fatal, many complications can be very serious and life threatening. Symptoms will vary from person to person due to the diversity of the disease. In general, most people affected will experience tremors, bradykinesia (or slowness of movement), limb rigidity, and gait and balance problems.

While Parkinson's may be thought of mainly as a movement disorder, it does have nonmotor symptoms as well, including apathy, depression, loss of sense of smell, constipation, sleep behavior disorders, and cognitive impairment. Lewy bodies found in substantia nigra neurons are associated with cognitive loss.

Various stages of the disease have been identified, and each one is characterized by patterns of progression. Stage one is characterized by mild symptoms with little or no interruption in activities of daily living. Tremor and other movement symptoms occur on only one side of the body. During stage two, symptoms such as tremors and rigidity become worse and affect both sides of the body. Daily tasks become more difficult and take more time, and problems with walking and posture become more evident. Stage three is also known as the midstage. Falls may become problematic, and activities of daily living like dressing and bathing become more difficult to accomplish. The two hallmarks of this stage are loss of balance and slowness of movements. As symptoms become more severe and limiting, the individual is entering the fourth stage of Parkinson's disease. While it is possible to stand on one's own, the individual may need a walker to get around. Living alone may be too dangerous at this stage, and help with almost all activities is necessary. The fifth and final stage is the most advanced and debilitating and is characterized by severe stiffness in the legs, making it impossible to stand or walk on one's own. The individual may be bedridden at this point or require a wheelchair to move around. Psychiatric symptoms like hallucinations and delusions can occur, and the individual will eventually require around-the-clock care.

An interesting theory known as Braak's Hypothesis indicates that perhaps the earliest signs and symptoms of the disease begin in the enteric nervous system, which houses the medulla and olfactory bulb (which controls the sense of smell). Parkinson's only advances as far as the substantia nigra and cortex over an extended period of time. Among the nonmotor symptoms involved, loss of sense of smell (or hyposmia), constipation, and sleep disorders may develop years before the motor symptoms appear. Research is therefore looking into these nonmotor symptoms in order to detect Parkinson's as early as possible and try to stop it before it progresses.

5 Stages of Parkinson's Disease

STAGE 1
MILD SYMPTOMS THAT DO NOT INTERFERE WITH DAILY LIVING

SOME TREMOR AND OTHER MOVEMENT SYMPTOMS ON ONE SIDE OF THE BODY

CHANGES IN POSTURE, WALKING, AND FACIAL EXPRESSIONS

STAGE 2
SYMPTOMS WORSEN, AND DAILY TASKS BECOME MORE CHALLENGING

TREMORS AND RIGIDITY BECOME WORSE AND AFFECT BOTH SIDES OF THE BODY

STAGE 3
MIDSTAGE, AT WHICH SLOWNESS AND LOSS OF BALANCE BECOME AN ISSUE

ACTIVITIES OF DAILY LIVING (EATING, DRESSING) ARE IMPAIRED

FALLS ARE COMMON

STAGE 4
SEVERE STAGE, AT WHICH MOVEMENT IS VERY LIMITED

DEVICES LIKE WALKERS AND CANES MAY BE NECESSARY

INDIVIDUAL CAN NO LONGER LIVE ALONE AND REQUIRES HELP WITH DAILY ACTIVITIES

STAGE 5
INABILITY TO WALK, MAY BE RESTRICTED TO WHEELCHAIR OR BED

HALLUCINATIONS AND DELUSIONS ARE COMMON

Parkinson's disease exhibits both motor and nonmotor symptoms, as mentioned earlier. Parkinson's is known as a movement disorder due to its hallmark and most obvious symptoms, such as tremors, slowness, and stiffening of movements. To be diagnosed with the disease, three movement symptoms must be present: bradykinesia, tremor, and rigidity. Postural instability is another symptom and occurs later in the disease. Other movement symptoms include drooling, cramping, dyskinesia (involuntary writhing movements), freezing (being stuck in place), micrographia (small handwriting), shuffling gait, festination (short, rapid steps), and soft speech, or hypophonia. These movement symptoms are caused by impairment in dopamine which is primarily responsible for controlling movement, ability to feel pleasure and pain, and emotional responses. As Parkinson's gets worse, more dopamine neurotransmitters die until the point in which the brain no longer produces dopamine in any significant amount. The result is severe impairment of movement as well as many other symptoms.

Non-Motor Symptoms	Motor Symptoms
✓ LOSS OF SMELL ✓ CONSTIPTAION ✓ REM SLEEP BEHAVIOR DISORDER ✓ DEPRESSION ✓ WEIGHT LOSS ✓ URINARY PROBLEMS ✓ VISION PROBLEMS ✓ SEXUAL DIFFICULTIES ✓ PAIN ✓ LOSS OF TASTE	✓ BRADYKINESIA (SLOWNESS OF MOVEMENT) ✓ TREMOR AND CRAMPING ✓ STIFFNESS OF MOVEMENT ✓ POSTURAL INSTABILITY ✓ DYSKINESIA (IMPAIRED OR ABNORMAL VOLUNTARY MOVEMENT) ✓ DROOLING ✓ MICROGRAPHIA (SMALL HANDWRITING) ✓ HYDROPHONIA (SOFT SPEECH)

Besides the motor symptoms of Parkinson's disease, several nonmotor or nonmovement symptoms can develop. The most common are loss of smell, constipation, REM sleep behavior disorder, and depression. These symptoms can occur years before the individual is diagnosed with Parkinson's disease. Other nonmotor symptoms include weight loss, urinary problems, vision difficulties, sexual problems, pain, loss of sense of taste, anxiety, vivid dreams, restless leg syndrome, light-headedness, fatigue, increase in dandruff, excessive sweating, early satiety (feeling full after eating very little), and cognitive problems in memory, language, planning, and attention.

Traditional Therapies for Parkinson's Disease

There are no specific tests to diagnose Parkinson's disease. Most likely, a neurologist will diagnose the disease after reviewing the person's medical history, reviewing signs and symptoms, and performing neurological and physical examinations. Lab tests, including blood tests, can be used to rule out other causes of reported and observed symptoms. A specific SPECT scan (single-photon emission computerized tomography) known as a dopamine transporter (DAT) scan may be suggested by the physician. Other imaging tests including an MRI, CT ultrasound of the brain, and PET scans may be helpful in obtaining a clear diagnosis of Parkinson's disease.

While Parkinson's cannot be cured, there are medications that may help manage symptoms and improve daily living. Most medications are prescribed to help with motor movements and manage walking and tremors. Because people with Parkinson's have low levels of dopamine, these types of medications essentially increase or substitute for dopamine. An unfortunate side effect of the medications is that they become less and less effective over time. Levodopa is the most widely prescribed and effective Parkinson's medication that passes into the brain and is converted to dopamine. Lodosyn is a dopamine-promoting medication that protects levodopa from converting too quickly outside the brain allowing it to enter the brain and provide its therapeutic work. Some side effects of levodopa may include nausea or light-headedness. Dyskinesia, or involuntary movements, may develop when higher doses of the drug are consumed.

Other medications, known as dopamine agonists, work not by converting into dopamine, but by mimicking dopamine effects in the brain. These types of drugs include Mirapex, Requip, and Neupro, which is a patch. Apokyn is a short-acting shot that is used for quick relief of symptoms. The side effects of these drugs are close to those of levodopa, but can also include hallucinations, fatigue, and compulsive behaviors such as hypersexuality, eating, and gambling.

Another class of medications are known as MAO B inhibitors and include Eldepryl, Azilect, and Xadago. These medications help to prevent the breakdown of brain dopamine by inhibiting the brain enzyme monoamine oxidase B, or MAO B. Nausea or insomnia are common side effects. Other medications like COMP inhibitors (Comtan), anticholinergics (Cogentin), and amantadine, for early-stage Parkinson's may be prescribed. Side effects generally include gastrointestinal issues, cognitive problems, and difficulty with movement.

When individuals do not respond well to medications and have advanced Parkinson's disease, deep brain stimulation may be an alternative treatment. Deep brain stimulation involves surgeons inserting electrodes into specific areas of the brain. This may help to improve effectiveness of medications, minimize or delay involuntary movements, reduce tremor and rigidity, or improve slowing of movements. There are some risks involved with deep brain stimulation, including infections, stroke, or brain hemorrhage.

Besides medication and deep brain stimulation, many lifestyle changes can be made to enhance one's quality of life and better manage symptoms. Maintaining a diet rich in fiber and fluids can help prevent constipation. Getting adequate amounts of antioxidants in the diet is also recommended. Omega-3 fatty acids, creatine, Coenzyme Q10, calcium, vitamin D, ginger, folic acid (vitamin B_9), vitamin B_{12}, green tea, and milk thistle can also be added to the individual's diet. Exercising as much as possible can increase muscle strength, balance, and flexibility. Getting some physical activity may also reduce feelings of depression or anxiety. Working with a physical or occupational therapist might be beneficial for maintaining an exercise program and enhancing one's activities of daily living. As the disease progresses, falls become a serious concern, and fall prevention should be addressed. Any supportive treatment like massage, yoga, tai chi, stress management, prayer, and meditation may also help with the management of symptoms.

Research Findings on CBD and Parkinson's Disease

A study in 2007 found that CBD exerted antioxidant properties and reduced oxidative stress leading to neuroprotection in a rat model of Parkinson's disease. The researchers stated, "Our results indicate that those cannabinoids having antioxidant cannabinoid receptor-independent properties provide neuroprotection against the progressive degeneration of nigrostratial dopaminergic neurons occurring in PD." They also believe that the activation of the CB2 receptor may contribute to the potential of cannabinoids in Parkinson's disease.[31]

The very next year, another article published in the *Journal of Psychopharmacology* demonstrated how CBD could be useful for people with Parkinson's disease who experienced psychiatric symptoms, like hallucinations. Psychosis in Parkinson's is challenging to treat, and there is a need for a new and more effective pharmacological intervention. This study examined for the first time the efficacy, tolerability, and safety of CBD for Parkinson's with psychotic symptoms. Their conclusion: There were no adverse effects, and CBD was effective, safe, and well tolerated for decreasing psychotic symptoms associated with Parkinson's disease.[32] In another study published in 2008, researchers stated, "In the past 45 years, it has been possible to demonstrate that CBD has a wide range of pharmacological effects, many of which being of great therapeutic interest, but still waiting to be confirmed by clinical trials."[33] Properties such as anti-inflammatory, antioxidative, and neuroprotective effects might benefit a number of disorders, including Parkinson's disease, Alzheimer's disease, cerebral ischemia, diabetes, rheumatoid arthritis, and other inflammatory diseases, as well as nausea and cancer.

A few years later, Brazilian researchers examined the effects of cannabidiol on cognitive impairment associated with neurodegenerative disorders, like Parkinson's disease. They found that CBD had "memory-rescuing effects" in an animal model and stated that "a single acute injection of cannabidiol at the highest dose was able to recover memory in iron-treated rats. Chronic cannabidiol improved recognition memory in iron-treated rats." They suggest that CBD may be potentially effective in treating cognitive decline associated with neurodegenerative disorders.[34]

Another Brazilian study one year later found that CBD reversed L-dopa-induced psychotic symptoms and improved motor function in Parkinson's patients. In their study, mice received acute pretreatment with CBD; it had anticataleptic effects, such as muscular rigidity and pain. They concluded that CBD may be effective in the treatment of movement disorders like Parkinson's disease.[35]

In 2014, researchers performed an exploratory double-blind trial, treating patients with Parkinson's with CBD. The motivation for their study was that to date, no neuroprotective treatment for Parkinson's had been available, but the endocannabinoid system was emerging as a promising possibility. Three groups of subjects were each treated with a placebo, 75 mg per day of CBD, or 300 mg of CBD per day. They found some improvement in quality-of-life measures among the placebo group and the group receiving 300 mg per day. They concluded that CBD may be helpful in treating Parkinson's, with the added benefit of no psychiatric side effects.[36] As noted earlier, one of the nonmotor symptoms of Parkinson's is REM sleep behavior disorder. REM sleep behavior disorder is characterized by the loss of muscle relaxation during REM sleep, nightmares, and behaviorally acting out during these nightmares. Researchers examining Parkinson's disease found that CBD was able to control symptoms of this disorder.[37]

A research team in 2015 found that cannabidiol might be able to treat neurodegenerative diseases like Parkinson's, not only due to its neuroprotective properties (anti-inflammatory and antioxidant effects), but also to its ability to protect against MPP$^+$, a neurotoxin that is relevant to the disease.[38] A year later, another study found more evidence that CBD has neuroprotective effects—but this time, specifically for neuropsychiatric disorders. The research team believes that CBD could have therapeutic effects over a broad range of neuropsychiatric disorders, which would include the nonmotor symptoms of Parkinson's (e.g., hallucinations). CBD may reduce the damage associated with neurodegeneration and have positive effects on psychosis, anxiety, and depression associated with neurodegenerative disorders. They also found CBD facilitates the growth and development of neurons and strengthens synapses between brain cells.[39]

A fascinating study from a team of Italian researchers in 2017 found that the endocannabinoid system "is highly represented in the basal ganglia and has been found altered in several movement disorders, including Parkinson's disease (PD)."[40] They also state, "A number of preclinical studies in different experimental Parkinson's disease (PD) models demonstrated that modulating the cannabinoid system may be useful to treat some motor symptoms." Another study the same year took a broader stance on the use of CBD for neurological disorders. The team examined the potential role of CBD in Parkinson's, Alzheimer's, multiple sclerosis, Huntington's disease, amyotrophic lateral sclerosis (ALS), and cerebral ischemia (stroke). They concluded that preclinical evidence shows that CBD can produce beneficial effects for these disorders.[41] The same year, another team of researchers from Italy examined cannabinoid involvement in neurodegenerative disorders and found that it exerts neuroprotective effects for mental and motor dysfunction in these diseases.[42] These effects may limit neurological damage, alleviate certain symptoms, attempt to delay or arrest the progression of the diseases, and possibly repair damaged neural structures. The study also supports earlier research reporting that the cannabinoid signaling system is abundant in the basal ganglia and that "the cannabinoid system is impaired in different neurological disorders that directly or indirectly affect the basal ganglia, which supports the idea of developing novel pharmacotherapies with compounds that selectively target specific elements of the cannabinoid system." They also report that CBD may induce neuroprotection and reduce psychotic symptoms associated with the disease.

In 2018, a review article published in *Surgical Neurology International* showed how researchers from Pittsburgh concluded that phytocannabinoids have "neurological uses that include adjunctive treatment for malignant brain tumors, Parkinson's disease, Alzheimer's disease, multiple sclerosis, neuropathic pain, and the childhood seizure disorders Lennox-Gastaut and Dravet syndromes."[43] They found evidence of CBD's anti-anxiety, antidepressant, neuroprotective, anti-inflammatory, and immunomodulatory benefits as well as reducing vascular changes and neuroinflammation. CBD was found to help with psychotic symptoms. Overall, they discovered that CBD is safe, and some of the most commonly reported side effects were fatigue, diarrhea, and changes in either appetite or weight. CBD was shown to not alter heart rate, blood pressure, or body temperature. They concluded by saying, "CBD is of particular interest due to its wide-ranging capabilities and lack of side effects in a variety of neurological conditions and diseases."

Another study the same year was driven by the question "Can CBD become a promising strategy in treating or preventing movement disorders?" Here is what the research team from Brazil found after reviewing both preclinical and clinical studies. CBD reduced the frequency of events related to REM sleep behavior disorder, reduced anxiety, depression, and psychosis, ultimately improving quality of life. In terms of safety, CBD did not alter heart rate, blood pressure, glycemia, or prolactin levels. CBD did not induce tolerance or impair cognitive abilities.[44]

Summary

Parkinson's disease is the second most common neurodegenerative disorder after Alzheimer's disease. It affects one million people in the United States and millions of others around the world. There is no cure, and medications may help to manage symptoms for some people, some of the time. CBD has been shown in numerous studies to have many positive benefits for neurodegenerative disorders like Parkinson's disease. We have reviewed its neuroprotective, antioxidant, anti-inflammatory, anti-anxiety, antidepressant, and antipsychotic qualities. It also appears to be safe and well tolerated and has few to no side effects. Can CBD one day become a real medical treatment for Parkinson's and other neurodegenerative diseases? More clinical research is needed before such claims can be made.

Huntington's Disease

Introduction

Huntington's disease is a rare and devastating inherited neurodegenerative disorder of the central nervous system. It is characterized by three major sets of symptoms, including involuntary movements, psychological and behavioral disturbances, and dementia. It is caused mainly by a faulty gene (the huntingtin gene) that causes toxic proteins to build and cause damage in the brain, which leads to neurological symptoms. The disease has been known for a long time, dating back to 1872, when George Huntington provided a full description in his first paper entitled "On Chorea." The disease became known as "Huntington's Chorea" for many decades, based on the unwanted movements observed in multiple patients. It was later changed to Huntington's disease after the medical community developed a greater understanding of the disease's multiple symptoms. Huntington's was no longer just a movement or motor disorder. It was far more complicated than that.

Currently, around thirty thousand people in the United States have the disease, and another 150,000 are at risk. While most people develop signs and symptoms of Huntington's disease in their thirties or forties, it can occur earlier and later in life. If the disease develops before the individual is twenty years old, the disorder is called Juvenile Huntington's disease and is characterized by different symptoms and a faster progression.

Overview of Huntington's Disease

Huntington's disease is diagnosed through a neurological examination involving observation and testing of motor, sensory, and psychiatric symptoms. A neurologist assesses one's memory, language abilities, mental functioning, and reasoning. A psychiatrist evaluates mood, behaviors, coping skills, distorted thinking, and quality of judgment. CRIs or CT scans may be ordered to obtain brain structure images.

Many times, mood and behavioral symptoms will precede problems in motor movements, although symptoms vary by individual. Some symptoms will be more prominent than others. By the time physical movement problems develop, the disease has already progressed. The three hallmark sets of symptoms are movement, cognitive and psychiatric disorders. Movement disorders include chorea (involuntary jerking and writhing movements), dystonia (muscle rigidity and contracture), slow or abnormal eye movements, impaired ability to walk, maintain posture or balance, and speech and swallowing difficulties. The movement problems are particularly difficult to live with and can interfere greatly with work, activities of daily living and quality of life.

Cognitive disorder in Huntington's can involve several difficulties in being able to organize, prioritize or remain on task, act impulsively, inability to learn new information, slowness of thoughts, being inflexible in thought or behavior, and lacking an awareness of one's own behaviors. Psychiatric symptoms occur both as a reaction to the disease and to altered brain functioning. It is common for people with Huntington's disease to experience sadness, apathy, irritability, or withdrawal. Some will become very depressed and think about or attempt suicide. Other will feel tired and lack energy. Some co-occurring psychiatric disorders may accompany the disease, such as obsessive-compulsive disorder (OCD), manic behaviors, and bipolar depression. These conditions make the clinical picture complex and present more challenges for the individual, family, and healthcare professionals providing care and treatment.

Huntington's disease is caused by an inherited defect in one gene, known as the huntingtin gene. Huntington's is called an "autosomal dominant disorder" because the person affected only needs one copy of the defective gene to develop the disease. A parent carrying the gene can pass either a healthy gene or the defective gene onto the child. Among parents diagnosed with HD, every child in the family carries a 50% chance of inheriting the gene that will cause the disorder.

The disease progressively becomes worse over time, and death usually occurs within ten to thirty years after symptoms develop. Functional abilities decline, clinical depression may lead to thoughts of suicide, and later in the disease progression, the individual will need assistance with all activities of daily living and care. The disease will render the individual almost helpless and unable to speak, chew, or swallow. The individual will most likely be confined to his or her bed. Death will be caused by pneumonia, infection, injuries, falls, or complications associated with the inability to swallow. It is by far one of the cruelest neurodegenerative disorders or diseases of any kind.

Traditional Therapies for Huntington's Disease
While there is no cure for Huntington's disease, medication and other interventions may help to manage symptoms and promote quality of life. Medications

for the movement disorders involved in the disease include Xenazine, which was approved by the FDA specifically to suppress the chorea symptoms, such as writhing and involuntary jerking. It comes with a serious side effect of triggering or worsening depression, as well as other psychiatric conditions. Antipsychotic drugs like Haldol are prescribed to suppress movements, but they, too, may make the disease worse by causing more involuntary movements and muscle rigidity. Risperdal and Seroquel may be prescribed, and while they have fewer side effects, they can also worsen symptoms. Other medications—including amantadine, Klonopin, and Kepra—may be prescribed, but they carry side effects including nausea, mood swings, cognitive impairment, and fatigue.

Psychiatric medication may help manage symptoms associated with the disease, like depression, bipolar disorder, and agitation. Antidepressants such as Celexa, Lexapro, Prozac, and Zoloft may be prescribed for depression and can include several negative side effects, with nausea, diarrhea, drowsiness, and low blood pressure as some of the most commonly experienced. Antipsychotic drugs may help with violent outbursts, agitation, and other psychotic or mood symptoms. This class of medication may cause the unwanted side effect of additional movement problems. Bipolar symptoms may be managed through the use of anticonvulsants like Tegretol and Lamictal.

A psychologist or therapist can provide various types of therapy and help the individual work through emotional and behavioral issues. Some goals of therapy include managing behavioral problems, developing effective coping mechanisms and strategies, communicating effectively with others, and keeping realistic expectations as the disease progresses. A speech therapist, physical therapist, or occupational therapist may also be part of an interdisciplinary team that helps the individual with disease-associated difficulties.

Besides the care team, the individual and family can do many things to more effectively handle the disease. People with Huntington's disease are known to struggle with maintaining a healthy body weight, so getting more calories into one's diet would be helpful. Since chewing and swallowing foods become progressively more difficult, using specific utensils designed for people with these difficulties can also help. The use of nutritional supplements may assist in maintaining a healthier weight.

Remaining socially active may improve mood. Being aware of and avoiding anything that causes stress or anxiety might alleviate anger, agitation, aggression, or depression. Keeping the home environment as calm and pleasant as possible can improve the person's mood. Creating and sticking to a routine can help the person manage his or her day and remain as independent as possible for as long as possible. When it comes to managing Huntington's disease, simple is best. Breaking down activities of daily living (e.g., dressing, toileting, cooking) into small steps can make such activities more doable and pleasant. Establishing priorities and organizing activities can also help the individual get things done while experiencing greater confidence and improved self-esteem. Outside the home, a support group may provide a place to talk with others going through the same problems and learn better ways to cope. Just seeing that he or she is not alone with this disease may bring some relief and comfort.

Some things that may need to be addressed are preparing to move into a skilled nursing facility and planning for end-of-life care. These are difficult things to discuss and can be frightening and depressing for everyone involved. There may come a point when the individual can no longer function at home and requires around-the-clock care and supervision. The family, too, will be unable to deliver this level and intensity of care, and finding a care facility will be necessary. Talking about palliative care and hospice is important, and understanding that end-of-life care will involve pain management, comfort measures, support, and education might bring a sense of ease to the individual and family. Finally, having a living will and advance directives in place can make the decision-making process easier for everyone involved.

Research Findings on CBD and Huntington's Disease

I'm beginning this section referencing a research article entitled "Pharmacological Management of Huntington's Disease: An Evidence-Based Review" to stress a point made by its authors, who reviewed 218 publications on medications prescribed for Huntington's disease between 1965 and 2006. They found that Haldol and Prolixin were mainly used to treat chorea, while Zyprexa was used, although not as much. All three drugs were considered "possibly useful" for the treatment of chorea. There was less evidence for using L-Dopa and Mirapex for rigidity, Elavil and Remeron for depression, Risperdal for psychosis, and Zyprexa, Haldol, and busprirone (BuSpar, which has been discontinued in the United States) for behavioral symptoms associated with Huntington's disease. According to the authors and in their own words: "There is poor evidence in the management of HD today."[45] The only medication to be FDA approved for Huntington's is Xenazine, but it has potentially dangerous side effects. That being said, let's review what research has examined over the past few decades regarding the use of CBD for Huntington's disease.

Much to my surprise, a study in 1986 was published and provided the results of CBD used to treat three people who did not respond to medications for Huntington's disease. After one week, there was between 5% to 15% improvement in both subjective and objective tests. After two weeks, improvement increased to 20% and 40% and remained stable for two more weeks. The only side effect was mild and transient hypotension.[46] Another early study in 1991 reported that CBD was only as effective as a placebo when administered to fifteen patients with Huntington's.[47] In 1994, two researchers said, "Selective neuronal vulnerability is a key feature of the neuropathology of Huntington's disease."[48] Specifically, they discovered a greater loss of cannabinoid receptors on striatal nerve receptors, which are clusters of neurons in the subcortical basal ganglia of the forebrain. Since the striatum is critical for motor movement, action planning, motivation and reward perception, it makes sense that Huntington's would be associated with symptoms like both motor disturbances and depression. It is well known that atrophy of the striatum is involved in Huntington's and other movement disorders.

Curtis and Rickards, in their paper "Nabilone Could Treat Chorea and Irritability in Huntington's Disease," reported that cannabinoids might have a neuroprotective property that could delay the onset of Huntington's symptoms or prevent the death of striatal neurons.[49] Micale and his team wrote in 2007 that there exists a possible neuroprotective role of endocannabinoids and their regulating action on neurotransmitter systems affected in several neurodegenerative disorders like Alzheimer's, Huntington's, and multiple sclerosis.

Imbalance in the endocannabinoid system may be present in these diseases: "In HD, a reduced EC signaling, given both the loss of cannabinoid CB1 receptors and decrease of ECs in the brain structures involved in movement control as basal ganglia, has been well documented in preclinical and clinical studies."[50]

In 2011, a research team reported on a downregulation (reduction in cellular response related to a decrease in the number of CB1 receptors) in the basal ganglia, which play an important role in the control of movement. They suggest that pharmaceutical activation of CB1 receptors in people with early-stage Huntington's might change or slow the progression of the disease. They use evidence from other studies that show when CB1 receptors are activated, it promotes neuronal survival and anti-inflammatory results. They also cite evidence that when the brain is injured, it overproduces endocannabinoids in an effort to protect and heal itself.[51] Another study in 2011 demonstrated how Sativex, a cannabis-based medicine, provided neuroprotection in rat models of Huntington's disease.[52]

One year later, an international research team asked, "Can cannabidiol be effective in treating neurodegenerative diseases?" and found many sources of support that it indeed could. Published in the prestigious *British Journal of Clinical Pharmacology*, they report that CBD has shown neuroprotective effects in experiments with rodents. CBD was found to be effective in human studies as well when the target symptom was chorea, the movement symptom involved in Huntington's disease. They call CBD "an unusually interesting molecule" in that "its actions are channeled through several biochemical mechanisms and yet it causes essentially no undesirable side effects and its toxicity is negligible." It is a powerful antioxidant, anti-inflammatory, and neuroprotective agent, and it lowers anxiety: "CBD has tremendous potential as a new medicine…Because the mechanisms that underlie its anti-inflammatory effects are different from those of prescribed drugs, it could well prove to be of considerable benefit to a large number of patients, who for various reasons are not sufficiently helped by existing drug."[53] Another paper in 2012 agreed that CBD could become a new medicine for Huntington's disease.[54] Later in 2015, researchers found that before motor symptoms begin, levels of CB1 receptors decrease in the basal ganglia, which are strongly associated with chorea and cognitive problems.[55]

Summary

The disease that began as Huntington's Chorea many decades later became simply Huntington's disease. While it has been known about for a long time, most clinicians thought that it was only a disorder of movement. They discovered later that it wasn't and actually involved behavioral, cognitive, and psychiatric problems. The disease is incurable, and most experts agree that there are few medications that can make a real difference in the lives of people living with the disorder. Most medications only help to manage some of the symptoms. After reviewing the research available, CBD seems to be a candidate in the treatment of many neurodegenerative disorders, including Huntington's disease.

Multiple Sclerosis

Introduction

Multiple sclerosis, or MS for short, is a chronic and progressive inflammatory demyelinating disease of the central nervous system that affects the ways that nerves work. It affects roughly four hundred thousand people in the United States and 2.3 million around the world. While symptoms vary among people diagnosed with MS, pain, muscle spasticity, inflammation, fatigue, and depression are most common. These symptoms and others can lead to reduced activity, impaired functional ability, and a decline in quality of life. Despite advances in treatments, there is still no way to prevent or cure MS.

Multiple sclerosis is usually diagnosed between the ages of twenty and forty with the average age being thirty-two. In some cases, children have been diagnosed at earlier ages. The disorder is more common in woman than men, and the ratio between the two is three to four women to one man. It is possible for symptoms to be invisible, making these numbers somewhat questionable.

Risk Factors for Multiple Sclerosis
✓ WHILE NOT A GENETIC DISEASE, HAVING IMMEDIATE FAMILY MEMBERS INCREASES RISK ✓ LIVING IN NORTHERN REGIONS AROUND THE WORLD ✓ INCREASED AGE ✓ BEING FEMALE ✓ CERTAIN AUTOIMMUNE DISORDERS: TYPE 1 DIABETES, RHEUMATOID ARTHRITIS, PSORIASIS AND AUTOIMMUNE THYROID DISORDER ✓ CERTAIN INFECTIONS INCLUDING EPSTEIN-BARR VIRUS AND HUMAN HERPES VIRUS 6 ✓ OBESITY ✓ SMOKING

Overview of Multiple Sclerosis

Although the exact causes of MS are largely unknown, there are some important facts and features about MS that are known. Since MS is an autoimmune disease, it develops as a result of the immune system attacking itself. Specifically, the body attacks myelin, the fatty tissue surrounding and protecting nerve fibers. When this occurs, there is a disturbance in communication between the brain and the rest of the body.

Risk factors for developing multiple sclerosis include having the disorder in the family, having a history of other autoimmune disorders, being diagnosed with certain viral infections, smoking, being female, having chronically low vitamin D levels, and being between the ages of twenty and forty.

As mentioned above, the symptoms of MS can vary, but there are commonly experienced symptoms that most people will have. These symptoms can vary in severity from mild to moderate, severe, and debilitating. One out of three people may lose their ability to walk. Some of the most common symptoms include weakness and fatigue, pain, numbness and tingling sensations, muscle spasms and stiffness, difficulty walking or maintaining balance, dizziness and vertigo, memory and other cognitive issues, and changes in hearing and vision.

Once an individual has had MS for a while, other difficulties can arise, including anxiety and mood changes (including depression), tremor, difficulties with both speech and the ability to swallow, bowel and bladder difficulties, and sexual dysfunction. Individuals diagnosed with MS may experience some of these symptoms and not others. One of the hallmarks of multiple sclerosis is that any of these symptoms are unpredictable, meaning that they will be noticed one day and not the next. In other words, they fluctuate. Since MS is progressive, they will worsen over time. In one form of the disorder, relapsing-remitting MS (RRMS), symptoms will become worse, lessen, and then flare up again.

Diagnosing multiple sclerosis can be challenging, and there is no single or specific test for it. One reason for this is that many of the symptoms appear in other conditions, which means that it takes time for the clinician to rule out other causes and conclude that the condition is indeed MS. Diagnosing begins with a review of the person's medical history and complete physical and neurological examinations. The clinician may also run blood tests and perform a lumbar puncture (spinal tap) and MRI scans. Receiving an early diagnosis is valuable, because it might improve with early treatments and medications that can slow down the progression of the disease.

Traditional Therapies for Multiple Sclerosis

Since there are no known ways to prevent MS or to cure it, treatment focuses on speeding up recovery time from attacks, slowing down the progression, managing symptoms, and improving quality of life. Current methods of treating attacks include corticosteroids to reduce nerve inflammation and plasma exchange if there is poor response to steroids. Some treatments being used to slow the progression of the disease include the use of beta interferons, which can reduce the frequency and severity of relapses and glatiramer acetate, used to stop the body's attack on myelin.

Medications given orally include fingolimod, dimethyl fumarate, teriflunomide, and siponimod. These medications are prescribed to prevent relapse and have several side effects, including infections, headaches, high blood pressure, liver damage, hair loss, heart problems, and blurred vision. Drugs given by infusion include ocrelizumab, natalizumab, alemtuzumab, and mitoxantrone. Side effects may include irritation by the injection site, infections, low blood pressure, fever, nausea, and an increased risk of cancer and autoimmune disorders.

Muscle relaxants may be beneficial for treating muscle spasms and stiffness. Because fatigue is a problem associated with MS, antidepressants might improve energy. Ritalin, OSMOLEX, and Provigil have been used to reduce fatigue. Walking speed slows as MS progresses, and AMPYRA has been shown to increase it in some people, although those with seizure disorders or kidney problems should not take this drug. There are also many drugs that can help with the other symptoms of MS, such as depression, pain, bowel and bladder problems, and sexual dysfunction.

Nonmedication treatments include physical therapy (especially for stretching, mobility, management of leg weakness and strengthening exercises), and lifestyle treatments including rest, relaxation, mindfulness, and stress management. Getting some mild to moderate exercise has shown to be helpful for some people with MS. Nutrition can also help relieve some symptoms of the disorder, and it is well known that vitamin D is especially important to get regularly in one's diet.

Yoga, massage therapy, meditation, and prayer have been found to be effective for some people diagnosed with MS. The American Academy of Neurology recommends the use of medical marijuana to relieve pain and muscle spasticity. Emotional and social support are also important in helping people cope with their disease. Reaching out to friends and family, spiritual leaders within the community, and support groups can be a healthy means to stay active and emotionally healthy. Maintaining daily routines, engaging in meaningful activities and hobbies, and developing a close relationship with a physician, nurse practitioner or counselor can also help manage symptoms and preserve quality of life.

Research Findings on CBD and Multiple Sclerosis
In 2007, a group of researchers from the UK tested the efficacy, safety, and tolerability of an oral spray containing THC and CBD and found that it was

effective in treating painful spasticity.[56] David J. Rog and his team found in their 2007 study that an oral spray containing cannabis and CBD was effective in treating neuropathic pain. Over this two-year study, the only side effects from treatment were mild to moderate dizziness and nausea.[57]

Two studies in 2012 examined the impact of cannabinoids on spasticity associated with multiple sclerosis, since is it greatly associated with pain, disability, and impairment to quality of life. One researcher stated, "Randomized, placebo-controlled trials, as well as longer-term open-label extensions, have shown a clear-cut efficacy to reduce spasticity and their associated symptoms in those patient's refractory to other therapies, with a good tolerability/safety profile. No tolerance, abuse or addictive issues have been found."[58] The other study conducted by researchers in Germany and Austria stress that cannabinoids can be a novel treatment for not only spasticity, but neuropathic pain, tremor, and bladder issues.[59]

One year later, a study from Madrid, Spain, examined the role of CBD for long-lasting protection against inflammation and found that it provided beneficial immunoregulatory effects, improved motor or movement deficits, and had neuroinflammatory effects.[60] A few years later, researchers from the United States found positive results using cannabidiol to treat spasticity, pain, inflammation, fatigue, and depression, and there were no serious interactions when combining CBD with other medications.[61] Another study in 2018 revealed that an oromucosal spray containing THC and CBD was effective in treating MS-related spasticity.[62] A German research team found, after performing a systematic review of observational studies, that the oral spray containing THC and CBD were effective in treating stiffness, pain, spasms, and overall comfort.[63] And finally, a group of researchers from the United States and Spain reviewed the effectiveness of cannabis-based therapy on multiple sclerosis. They found consistency, safety, and efficacy in cannabis-based treatment for spasticity and pain associated with MS. They also cite that this type of therapy reduces inflammation and has neuroprotective qualities.[64]

Summary

Multiple sclerosis is a chronic and progressive disease of the central nervous system that causes a myriad of negative symptoms that can decrease an individual's quality of life. Symptoms may vary between people, but pain and depression are among the most commonly experienced. While there are various medications available, they all come with negative side effects. Alternative and home-based remedies may help manage symptoms of the disease and improve quality of life. It has been shown in research that both a combination of THC and CBD, and CBD alone, have produced good results and without the risk of dependency.

Conclusion

I included this chapter and covered each neurodegenerative disorder for personal as well as academic reasons. As you know by now, my mother lost her life after struggling for years with Alzheimer's disease. Decades earlier, her father, John, was also diagnosed with some form of dementia, lived in a nursing home for a couple of years, and died. My interest in the aging process and associated diseases and disorders began in that sterile nursing home "ward" where my grandfather roomed with two other men who had severe dementia. I've always had a soft spot in my heart for those living with or caring for people with Alzheimer's, Parkinson's, Huntington's, MS, and ALS. While there are many methods for managing symptoms and improving quality of life, I hope that CBD and other cannabinoids receive more research and one day help millions of people diagnosed with neurodegenerative conditions.

11

CBD and End-of-Life Care

Death ends a life, not a relationship.

—Mitch Albom

Introduction

Mitch Albom, the acclaimed author of *Tuesdays with Morrie*, *The Five People You Meet in Heaven*, and many other best sellers, is absolutely correct. When someone close to you passes away, their body may be gone, but you never stop loving or thinking about them. This holds especially true for me, as I reflect on the death of my father many years ago, the more recent passing of my mother, and my experiences working in hospice for the past few years.

My father, Jim Collins, was a WWII vet, an electrical engineer for two large car manufacturers, and a man who reminded me of John Wayne. He was over six feet tall and had pure silver hair from the time it prematurely changed in his twenties. He also had crystal blue eyes. There has been a running joke in my family because my mother, Mary, was much shorter and had brown eyes: "Am I truly my father's son?" Turns out I am. My father also ate and drank like a typical man from his generation—a shot and a beer after work, two packs of cigarettes a day, and meat and potatoes for dinner. After many years maintaining this unhealthy lifestyle, he developed cardiac problems. During one weekend at home, he had multiple mini-heart-attacks. This brought him to a local hospital, where he then had a massive heart attack, underwent surgery, lost

60% of his heart muscle, and lay in a coma attached to various life-support machines and tubes.

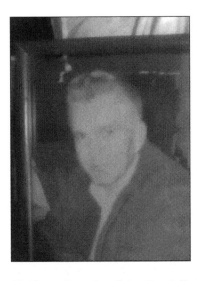

An old, blurry photo of my father, Jim Collins Sr.

After waiting for some time, the surgeon came out to talk with our family and let us know that Dad would never be the same. He may remain in a coma for the rest of his life. If he came out of it, he would be incapable of caring for himself and would require twenty-four-hour nursing care. His chances of survival were extremely low. What should we do? Did I want to see John Wayne exist on machines with no quality of life? My family was torn, but I stepped up to make the decision that the machines should be turned off, and Dad should die like he lived—a man. Once I voiced this to the surgeon, he agreed. We all went in to see Dad, alive, so to speak, one last time. As the medical team turned his life support off, I kissed his cheek, held his hand, and told him to not worry about Mom. "I'll take care of her for the rest of her life," I told him, and with that, he died moments later.

That was a long time ago, back in 1993. Most recently, my mother, Mary Collins, lived twenty-two years after the death of my dad and made it to ninety-two years of age. She had a great life: casinos; concerts (Rod Stewart concerts ten times and Andrea Bocelli four times); breakfast, lunch, and dinner out; and shopping anytime she wanted. She also worked as a nursing assistant in a skilled nursing facility until she was eighty. There were times family members mistook her as a resident! Still, she loved her residents and her role as a professional caregiver. She also died in the same facility where she had worked for thirty years.

Mom lived with me, my wife, and my daughter for almost sixteen years. When she started leaving the stove on, and burning pots and pans and then hiding them in the trash can, we knew we had to do something to help her. She had fallen several times, but since she was a bit bottom heavy, she always landed on her butt. She was the luckiest faller I've ever seen! Then, one day, she fell and hit her head, and there was blood. Lots of it. After some time in the ER, we discussed the possible necessity of an assisted living. Of course, she was not happy with this, so we dropped the subject for a few weeks. But the fires and falls continued, and now it was officially time to stop procrastinating, so we looked into local assisted-living communities.

We are all Catholic in my family, and since my mother worked for a Catholic skilled nursing facility, we chose the assisted-living community on the same campus. It was beautiful. She had her own private "apartment," as she called it, the activities were plentiful and fun, and the food was good. There were lots of white-haired Italian ladies living there, so she blended in nicely and made friends. After a couple of years, her cognitive function began to decline. She became more confused and disoriented, and after being prescribed a particular drug for Alzheimer's disease, she started hallucinating. Her behavior started to deteriorate once again, and she became more aggressive and agitated. Her time in assisted living had come to an end, and it was time for skilled nursing.

Mom moved into the skilled nursing facility up the hill from the assisted-living community. She wasn't happy, but my family, the director and I felt it was best. After a week or so, she settled in and began to enjoy life, even more than in the assisted-living community. There seemed to be more activity and life at the skilled facility. At first, she lived in the main part of the building, but after a couple of years and more cognitive and physical decline, she had to move into the memory care unit, where residents with more severe dementia lived together. After another year or so, she had a massive stroke on a Sunday morning. I was called by the staff, whom I had developed wonderful, trusting relationships with. They really took great care of Mom.

The stroke was severe and left her in a sleeplike state for nine days before she died, surrounded by her family, friends, and the staff she had worked with for thirty years. The office staff, director of nursing, nursing assistants, director of housekeeping, and more—they were all there to kiss her, hold her hand, and say goodbye. She had a beautiful death. The care she gave to her residents for so many years came right back to her. What goes around, comes around.

During the final few weeks of her life, I was invited to take a leadership position in a hospice company in Ohio. I was completely new to hospice but learned as quickly as I could. I had the privilege of working with outstanding directors, nurses, nursing assistants, social workers, and chaplains. I got to train them in areas I've come to know well, like neurodegenerative disorders, mental and emotional issues, behavior management, the aging process, and more. I was lucky to hear the stories about the peaceful passing of so many seniors and how we provided the most tender and loving care during their final hours. My appreciation for life, the dying process, and death has never been more profound as it is now.

Overview of End-of-Life Care

This chapter is about end-of-life care and how CBD may help with certain aspects of the dying process. A good place to start this section is to explain the differences between palliative care and hospice, because both are involved prior to and during the dying process.

The primary goal of palliative care is to provide comfort through medical care and other services to individuals who are either terminally ill or who do not expect to improve. For instance, all care in skilled nursing (besides those receiving short-term rehab and returning home) is considered palliative care. Residents diagnosed with Alzheimer's disease are not expected to be cured; therefore, they receive this type of care and service. Palliative care can begin anytime throughout one's illness, but it's best to start as soon as the diagnosis is made. Conditions like cancer, Parkinson's, Huntington's, and ALS would be appropriate for palliative care.

A team of health care professionals works closely with the resident, family, physicians, and others to ensure choice and options in one's care. It should be delivered with a person-centered approach, with a focus on quality of life and management of symptoms. There is a point at which palliative care becomes end-of-life care, and this is when hospice is called in to help. If the physician believes the individual may only have six months or less to live, a hospice consult is performed, and the individual begins receiving services from a multidisciplinary team. At this time, it is clear that the individual's condition cannot be cured and that aggressive treatment will be futile.

Hospice provides care and support to everyone involved with the individual, including a strong focus on educating the family concerning what to expect and how to cope during the dying process and eventual death of their lived one. Hospice provides person-centered care and services, and the focus is on quality of life, death, and pain management. This kind of care can be delivered anywhere, including the person's home, an assisted-living community, a skilled-nursing home, a hospital, or an inpatient hospice facility.

Research Findings on CBD and End-of-Life Care

The leading question that drives research in this area is this: "Can cannabis-based treatments including CBD be effective at managing pain and other symptoms (e.g., anxiety, depression, sleeplessness, nausea) and improve quality of life and death?" Researchers in 2009 reported that cannabinoids not only have diverse pharmacological activities, but they also may have potential applications as antitumor drugs in cancer treatment.[1] A research team reported in the *Journal of Clinical Nursing* that cannabis-based treatments can improve the individual's quality of life. They examined the pharmaceutical qualities and use of cannabis in people receiving palliative care for conditions including multiple sclerosis (MS), motor neuron disease (MND), and amyotrophic lateral sclerosis (ALS).[2]

The following year, Canadian researchers asked a question in the title of their article: "Is there a legitimate role for the therapeutic use of cannabinoids for symptom management in chronic kidney disease?" They stress that many symptoms, some being severe, are associated with this illness, including chronic pain and emotional disturbance. The use of opioids can exacerbate these symptoms and cause nausea, insomnia, and anorexia, all of which negatively influence quality of life. They believe that cannabis-based medicine may be effective in treating severe pain, nausea, insomnia, and overall well-being.[3]

TIMELINE OF CANNABIDIOL-BASED MEDICATIONS

MARINOL (DRONABINOL)
- SYNTHETIC THC
- PILLS OR CAPSULES USED TO TREAT ANOREXIA, WEIGHT LOSS DUE TO AIDS, AND CHEMO-INDUCED NAUSEA AND VOMITING
- 1985 FDA APPROVED FOR NAUSEA
- 1992 FDA APPROVED AS AN APPETITE STIMULANT
- 1999 FDA APPROVED AS A SCHEDULE III DRUG (LIKE TYLENOL)

SATIVEX (NABIXIMOL)
- COMBINATION OF SYNTHETIC CBD AND THC
- OROMUCOSAL SPRAY USED TO TREAT SPASTICITY AND NERVE PAIN ASSOCIATED WITH MULTIPLE SCLEROSIS
- MAY BE APPROVED SOON FOR CANCER-RELATED PROBLEMS
- 1985 FDA APPROVED

CESAMET (NABILONE)
- SYNTHETIC CANNABINOID SIMILAR TO THC
- USED TO TREAT CHEMO-INDUCED NAUSEA AND VOMITING (ANTIEMETIC)
- 1985 FDA APPROVED TO TREAT NAUSEA AND VOMITING

EPIDIOLEX (CANNABIDIOL)
- PHARMACEUTICAL-GRADE CANNABIDIOL (CBD)
- LIQUID SOLUTION
- USED TO TREAT TWO RARE AND SEVERE FORMS OF EPILEPSY: LENNOX-GASTAUT SYNDROME AND DRAVET SYNDROME
- PRESCRIBED TO CHILDREN AS YOUNG AS ONE YEAR
- 2018 FDA APPROVED

Dr. S. K. Aggarwal, from Adult Palliative Medical Services, MultiCare Auburn Medical Center and MultiCare Institute for Research and Innovation in Auburn, Washington, states, "Globally, about 60% of all people who die would benefit from palliative care before death." He believes that cannabinoids have a significant role in oncological palliative care now, and that greater acceptance using cannabinoids as medicine will follow with more knowledge and research findings. He calls the use of cannabinoids in medicine, or "cannabinoid integrative medicine," because it better identifies cannabinoid use within medical trends occurring today. Integrative medicine combines traditional medicine with complementary and alternative therapies, such as including botanicals and cannabinoids in the treatment of many medical conditions.[4]

Dr. Thomas Strouse, from the UCLA Department of Psychiatry, and Resnick Neuropsychiatric Hospital in Los Angeles, California, states that there is reasonable evidence that cannabinoids can be beneficial in treating various types of pain, including chronic pain, chemotherapy-induced nausea, and multiple-sclerosis-related spasticity. He writes:

> It is worthwhile for palliative care clinicians who may be endorsing cannabinoid use by their patients to familiarize themselves with the clinical picture of intoxication, abuse, dependence, and withdrawal states, and to encourage their patients to allow themselves to be clinically monitored as we might do for any other new course of treatment.[5]

In 2019, a scientist from Poland wrote that there has been an increased interest in using cannabinoids for patients in palliative care situations. Since they tend to work in many ways, they are attractive in treating multiple symptoms. He provides evidence that cannabis-based medicine has been shown to be effective in treating pain, spasticity, nausea and vomiting, seizures, sleep disorders, HIV, digestive disorders, epilepsy, and Tourette's syndrome. There is also research evidence that cannabinoids can help with neuropathic pain management. He concludes that cannabinoids possess a relatively favorable effect profile without depressive effects on the respiratory system.[6]

Summary

End-of-life care is something that most of us will encounter with our families and friends as well as experience for ourselves. If we live long enough, many of us may need or desire palliative care to manage symptoms and improve our quality of living. When we enter the final few months of life, some may choose hospice services to benefit from additional pain management, social and spiritual services, and more frequent visits from nursing staff. Although there are traditional medications and treatments to help ease pain and suffering, will cannabis-based medicine and CBD become mainstream, and can they improve both quality of life as well as quality of death?

12

CBD for Your Pets

If there are no dogs in Heaven, then when I die, I want to go where they went.

—Gilda Radner

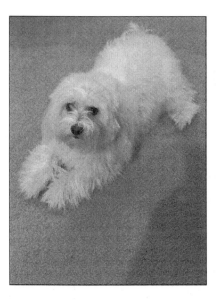
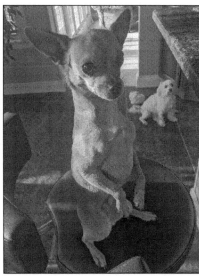

Meet Our Dogs, Buddy and Kitty!

We have always loved animals, especially dogs. Pictured above is Buddy on the left, a Havamalt, and Kitty on the right, a Chiweenie, always begging for food. Chiweenies are a mixed breed dog crossing a Chihuahua with a dachshund. Kitty was a rescue dog, had an injured back leg and separation anxiety, and didn't discriminate where she relieved herself. Buddy, on the other hand, was chosen for our daughter Karina by our neighbors who felt that she needed a little buddy. He came from a local pet store. We brought him home when he was eight weeks old, and as he began to grow a little older, we noticed that his hind legs shook. We brought him to a veterinarian, who diagnosed him with "white dog shaking disorder." That was a new one on me; I had never heard of such a thing.

Our family began giving CBD dog chews to each dog on a daily basis. Each chew contained 2 mg of CBD, which is appropriate for dogs under nine pounds. Larger dogs require higher doses. Within a week to ten days, we all noticed that Kitty had significantly lower anxiety-related behaviors and wasn't peeing on the newly installed hardwood floor, and Buddy's shaking diminished almost completely. We were impressed and continue to give them CBD treats every day.

Every time we go away for a short or extended trip, we have a family member watch the house and care for Buddy and Kitty. Buddy has no anxiety issues and will bond with whomever is there, but Kitty now exhibits almost no separation anxiety after being on CBD treats for several months. She made fewer messes around the house as well and appeared to be rather calm while we were away. Anecdotally speaking, it seems that 2 mg of CBD in a dog treat every day made some impressive improvements in our dogs' quality of physical and emotional health.

What Experts Report about CBD and Dogs

I'm not the only one who believes that CBD is effective in treating various conditions in dogs. Dr. Caroline Coile, the best-selling author of *Barron's Encyclopedia of Dog Breeds*, inductee into the Dog Writer's Association of America Hall of Fame, and winner of eight Maxwell Medallion Awards, thinks so too. She writes in her book *Cannabis and CBD Science for Dogs: Natural Supplements to Support Healthy Living and Graceful Aging* that dogs have an endocannabinoid system, including CB1 and CB2 receptors throughout their body and brain, and that CBD can be beneficial for dogs, much like it is for humans.[1]

Dr. Coile shares some stories from dog owners she knows. One such dog, Georgia, suffered from a painful and progressive neurological disorder called syringomyelia (fluid-filled cysts in the spinal cord) and after trying several traditional medications, found no relief. Georgia's owner was then encouraged by her veterinarian to try CBD, and she was so glad she did. She reported that after some time on CBD, Georgia became a completely different dog. It decreased her anxiety and pain, and she started playing with her dog toys more often.

Another dog, Charlie, was in bad shape and had congestive heart failure. He wasn't expected to live long. He had developed seizures, and things looked grim. Seizure medications worked at first but then lost their effectiveness. Charlie was then given CBD for a few days, and he started to perk up and play, and even though he still had seizures, they reduced from four to one per day. His life drastically improved thanks to CBD.

Many other success stories reveal that pet owners are confident about using CBD for their dogs' ailments, including joint pain and arthritis, degenerative myelopathy (the equivalent of amyotrophic lateral sclerosis, or ALS, in humans), anxiety, and seizure disorder. They also believe that CBD has improved their dogs' quality of life significantly and has helped manage these symptoms.

In her book, Coile provides results of a Department of Clinical Sciences at the Colorado State University College of Veterinary Medicine pet owners' survey of 475 dog owners. The results, although not scientifically supported, are impressive. The majority of those surveyed reported that CBD provided pain relief, relieved seizures or convulsions, reduced muscle spasms, aided in digestive issues, helped with skin problems, reduced inflammation, improved sleep, reduced nausea and vomiting, and helped reduce anxiety.

Dr. Jerry Klein, American Kennel Club's chief veterinarian officer, also believes there is anecdotal evidence from dog owners who indicate that CBD helps their dog's condition. He points out that CBD has shown to be an effective anti-inflammatory, anti-anxiety, and antinausea agent. It also stimulates appetite and has cardiac benefits and possible anticancer properties. When we give CBD to our dogs, he reminds us to start with a low dose or small amounts and closely monitor the effects. It's important to talk to your veterinarian as well. An interesting fact is that dogs possess an unusually high number of CB1 receptors in their cerebellums. In both cats and dogs, he states that CBD can be effective in treating anxiety and phobias, arthritic pain, and inflammation and may be especially beneficial for geriatric pets.[2]

In 2018, a large team of researchers from New York and Colorado examined the pharmacokinetics (the branch of pharmacology concerned with the movement of drugs within the body), safety, and clinical efficacy of CBD in a group of osteoarthritic dogs. They found that 2 mg of CBD taken twice per day significantly helped to decrease pain and increased activity in dogs with osteoarthritis. In terms of pharmacokinetics and efficacy, no side effects were reported by the pet owners.[3]

Dr. Jeffrey Powers, vice chairman of the American Veterinary Medical Association's Council on Biologic and Therapeutic Agents, credits CBD for helping his ten-year-old Saint Bernard, Ella, with her anxiety caused by loud noises. When fireworks went off, Ella would start panting and pacing around the house. She'd also run somewhere to hide. After giving her CBD, her distress started to diminish.[4]

Another large team of researchers from Florida, New York, and Colorado in 2019 examined over a twelve-week period whether CBD was safe for dogs and cats with disorders including anxiety, seizures, cancer, and pain. They found that cats had lower absorption and elimination of CBD compared to dogs, so dosing should be taken into consideration for both animals. They also found that CBD was safe over the twelve-week period. More research is needed in cats to fully understand utility and absorption.[5]

A study in 2019 was conducted to determine how much information and knowledge veterinarians had concerning the use of CBD in dogs. A total of 2,130 participants completed an anonymous survey online. Most veterinarians were comfortable talking about CBD and knew the differences between it and THC. Overall, the participants shared that CBD was mostly discussed with their clients concerning canine health issues including pain, anxiety, and seizures. Those in states where medical marijuana has been legalized were comfortable suggesting CBD for dog owners to use. The most commonly used forms of CBD are oils and edibles. In the end, most of the participants agreed that CBD should be available for dog owners to use for their pets' physical and emotional health.[6]

A research team from Spain examined the effects of Sativex, including movement of the drug through the body, in adult beagles. Sativex, which is currently used in some countries and is being tested by the FDA in the United States, is used to treat multiple-sclerosis-related spasticity and pain in humans. The team believes that it may be effective in treating dogs with a variety of pathologies, including humanlike pathological conditions that produce muscle spasms and pain. The dogs were treated with three consecutive sprays of Sativex. The team found that the drug acted in dogs much like it does in humans and that after multiple doses, it accumulated in in the dogs' systems, supporting the use of Sativex for animals experiencing muscular problems and painful conditions.[7]

Another human condition, epilepsy, is also experienced in dogs and is in fact the most common neurological condition in dogs. It has been shown in several studies that CBD is effective at producing anticonvulsant effects in humans who are diagnosed with the disorder, and a research team wanted to find out whether it could be as effective in dogs. The study is ongoing, and there are currently no results to share. It is hoped that the team will find that CBD can produce anticonvulsant effects in canines to improve their quality and length of life.[8]

Researchers from the Yamazaki University of Animal Health Technology in Japan examined the effects of CBD on three dogs experiencing epileptic seizures. They point out that the most common treatment for epileptic dogs is the use of antiepileptic drugs but that they have undesirable side effects. The researchers administered CBD twice a day for eight weeks, monitoring the dogs closely. They found a decrease in the amount of seizure activity in two dogs, while the other dog showed no reduction in seizures. Interestingly, that dog's owners reported that their dog got no worse, and symptoms remained unchanged. All of the dog owners had positive impressions about the use of CBD for their dogs' seizure disorders.[9]

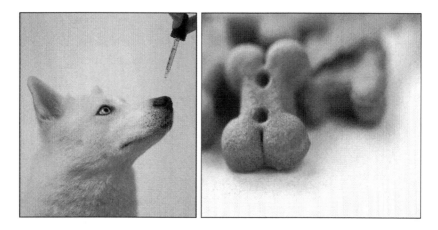

Pets have their choice of CBD liquid, as shown on the left, or edibles, which are usually biscuits or chews. Both are flavorful.

Conclusion

According to the American Veterinary Medical Association (AMVA), pet owners have over seventy-six million dogs and over fifty-eight million cats in their households.[10] It is clear that a large portion of the country loves their pets. There are many reasons why. Studies have shown that having a pet reduces loneliness, blood pressure, depression, stress, and anxiety. Some pet owners find purpose and meaning in caring for their furry little friends.

Since dogs and cats, as well as every animal on the planet (except for insects) possess endocannabinoid systems, it makes intuitive sense that CBD and other cannabinoids may hold physical, emotional, and neurological health benefits for them. Throughout this book, we have seen medical and academic studies that support CBD's use for a number of health conditions, many of which also affect dogs and cats. After all, animals experience pain and inflammation, vomiting and nausea, skin disorders, tumor growth and cancers, seizures and convulsions, digestive problems, nervous system disorders, and anxiety.

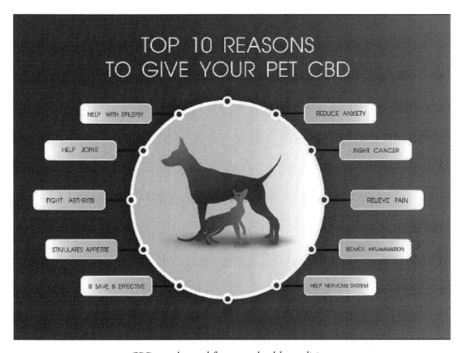

CBD can be used for many health conditions.

We need more robust studies examining how CBD works in the bodies and brains of dogs and cats. We need answers to questions like these:

"How long does it take to start working?"
"Does it accumulate in the animal's system? And for how long?"
"Is it safe to use CBD for long periods of time—perhaps the animal's entire life span?"

Only more time and research will tell. But as of right now, it looks like CBD is here to stay for dogs, cats, and many other animals. You can find CBD pet products at most CBD stores and online.

13

How to Buy and Use CBD

The bitterness of poor quality remains long after the sweetness of low price is forgotten.

—Benjamin Franklin

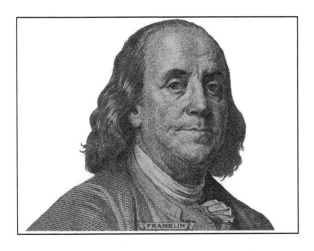

Introduction
What Benjamin Franklin said so very long ago is still true today, especially when it comes to selecting and purchasing CBD products. The market is absolutely flooded with CBD companies located all around the world, competing for sales. It is critical to note that CBD products are not all equal in quality.

The world of CBD can be very confusing, and there are many things to consider when choosing a product that's right for you. My goal in this chapter is to take much of the mystery out of buying and using CBD.

CBD PURCHASING CHECK LIST
☐ THINK ABOUT WHY YOU ARE GOING TO USE CBD (ACHES, PAIN, STRESS, SLEEP)
☐ LOOK FOR THE PERCENTAGE OF CBD IN THE PRODUCT (MORE IS BETTER)
☐ IDENTIFY HOW MUCH THC IS IN THE PRODUCT (LEGAL LIMIT IS 0.3%)
☐ LOOK FOR A "CERTIFICATE OF ANALYSIS" AT THE COMPANY'S WEBSITE
☐ FIND OUT WHERE THE HEMP WAS GROWN (COUNTRY AND STATE)
☐ FIND OUT ABOUT THE COMPANY'S EXTRACTION PROCESS
☐ FIND OUT IF THE PRODUCT IS FULL SPECTRUM, BROAD SPECTRUM, OR AN ISOLATE
☐ REVIEW THE PACKAGING (BOX, BOTTLE, ETC.)
☐ GO TO THE COMPANY'S WEBSITE AND LOOK FOR CUSTOMER SERVICE CONTACT INFORMATION
☐ CONSIDER THE PRICE OF THE PRODUCT (IS IT WORTH IT?)
☐ CHECK TO SEE IF THERE IS A 100% MONEY-BACK GUARANTEE

Buying CBD

In terms of choosing a CBD brand, it's good to take some time and do some research about the company. Most companies have websites, so visit and read about the company's history, founders, location, and extraction process and whether they add any unnatural ingredients to their CBD formulas. Is the company selling hemp oil or CBD oil? It's important to know the differences between the two because some hemp oil products are made solely from hemp seeds, which can contain very little CBD. And if you're looking for an all-natural, organic, or organically grown hemp-based product, the addition of artificial flavors can defeat the purpose of taking something with all-natural ingredients. These are just some things to think about and look for, and there are many others.

How Much THC and CBD Are in the Product?

It's important to find out how much THC is in the product. As you know, THC is the molecule in the plant that produces the feeling of being "high" or euphoric. Most people don't want that sensation. They prefer the benefits without the high. The product should identify whether it has 0.3% or zero THC. It's equally—or perhaps even more—important to find out how much CBD is in the product. Look for brands that clearly indicate how much CBD or cannabidiol is in the product. Some will list only the total amount of "cannabinoids," but this can include compounds other than CBD. It's also good to know how many milligrams of CBD are in the product. The higher the milligram, the more CBD you are getting for your money.

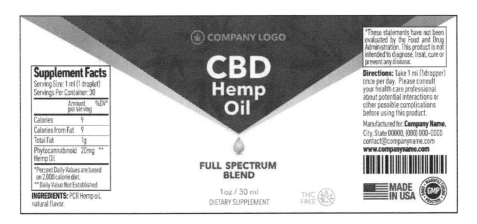

Generic CBD label

This is a generic and typical label you'd find on a bottle (tincture) of CBD oil. There's a lot of information to look for on the label. This product is "full spectrum," meaning that it contains CBD, other cannabinoids, and trace elements, or 0.3%, of THC. This is important to know if you can be drug tested at your workplace. The label also indicates there is a full 1 oz or 30 ml of the oil in the bottle. There are some directions as to how to use the oil and the FDA statement. The oil appears to have been made in the United States and has a "Good Manufacturing Practice" stamp, meaning this is an ethical company. Finally, supplemental facts are provided on the label.

How to Measure Doses

Say you want to use 30 mg of CBD daily, and you want your bottle of oil to last for a month. Here is an easy formula to use. A 500 mg bottle will last 30 days if you take a full dropper, or 16.66 mg daily (500 divided by 30 days). A 1,000 mg bottle will last 30 days if you take 33.33 mg daily—a little bit over your 30 mg per day goal. And a 1,500 mg bottle will last all month if you take 50 mg daily (1,500 divided by 30). By dividing the milligram size by 30, you can find how much CBD oil to take daily and make it last for a month. An easier solution is to take softgels, which are already measured out at 10 mg or 25 mg per gel.

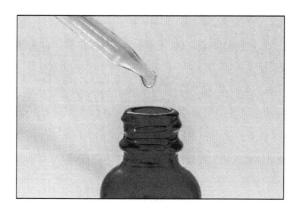

Dosing generally refers to how much CBD oil by milligram is in the actual dropper, as shown here. Depending upon the total CBD milligram portion in the bottle (e.g., 1,000 mg), the amount of CBD in a full dropper will vary.

Look for a Certificate of Analysis…and Read It!
When you're checking out the company's website, look for third-party lab reports. Some CBD companies go a step further than obtaining a certificate of analysis (COA) from their product source and hire a third-party lab to run another analysis. They do this to ensure high-quality products that give customers peace of mind. You definitely want to know that the product you are using is clean, free of contaminants (e.g., insecticides, heavy metals, fungus), is natural, and is organically grown.

Find Out Where the Hemp Was Grown
You should also find out where the hemp was grown. The United States has nutrient-rich soil and superior cultivation standards and is considered to be the best geographical location to grow hemp. Colorado, in particular, stands out as a superior state for growing hemp. Hemp is also a heavily regulated commodity in the United States, making it likely that hemp-based products are Farm Bill compliant.

Find Out How the Hemp Was Extracted
Not only is it important to find out where the hemp was grown, but it's equally important to find out how the oil was extracted from the plants. How the oil is extracted from the plant affects the genetic makeup of the final product. Extraction involves applying pressure to the plant, which then excretes oils. While some companies use steam or solvents like hydrocarbons and butane, the best practice is to extract the oils by using CO_2. This ensures all cannabinoids and terpenes remain intact. CO_2 extraction is more efficient, yields the highest concentration of CBD when compared to the other methods, and produces no toxic residues or chlorophyll. The other methods tend to be less efficient, yield inconsistent amounts of CBD, and may produce some toxic residues and a chlorophyll taste in the final product. The photo identifies equipment used in the extraction process.

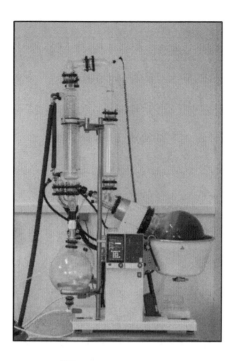

CO_2 extraction equipment

Is the Product Full Spectrum, Broad Spectrum, or Isolate?

In my experience, these terms are confusing to some people, but they don't have to be. The differences between them are quite simple. "Full spectrum" refers to a CBD product that contains CBD, many other cannabinoids, terpenes, and trace amounts of THC (0.3%), which is not enough to produce euphoria. Think of full spectrum as being "full" of everything from the plant. It is also sometimes called "whole-plant" hemp. Broad spectrum, contains everything that full spectrum has except for the THC. And in terms of isolate, think of the term "isolated," because that's exactly what it means. CBD is extracted and isolated from all other cannabinoids, terpenes, and THC and is left all on its own. An important point to remember is that CBD needs the other parts of the plant to produce the "entourage effect," so most people prefer either full spectrum or broad spectrum, depending on whether they can be drug tested at work or not. If you can be drug tested, broad spectrum is the way to go.

Look for Brands with Adequate Packaging
CBD, when exposed to heat or light for prolonged periods of time, can lose some of its potency and quality. Look for brands that contain CBD oil in amber, blue, or dark-colored glass. Darker glass bottles protect the integrity of the product for longer periods of time, and if they come in a box, that's even better.

Check into the Brand's Customer Service Support
Brands that stand behind their products should offer excellent customer service and support. In choosing a CBD brand, this may help you make your decision. Customer support should be able to answer your questions and explain the benefits of taking their products. Ask questions, and see if they know their stuff!

Look for Fairly Priced Brands
In the CBD market, there are wide variations in price, with some brands being priced low and others high. There are also brands in the middle. Do some research to compare products. Generally speaking, higher-priced brands may offer higher quality and better health benefits. CBD is one of those products that fall into the "You get what you pay for" category.

Look for Brands That Have a 100% Money-Back Guarantee
A company that stands behind their product should offer their customers a 100% money-back guarantee. Look to see if they offer a refund if you are not satisfied with their product.

Avoid Brands Making Dramatic Health Claims
This may be one of the most important things to look for. CBD products are not FDA approved for drug-type benefit claims, so no company should be making health claims like "cures headaches, heart disease, or cancer." The more dramatic the claim, the more skeptical the consumer should be. There are some CBD companies making these wild claims, and the FDA is clamping down on them.

Using CBD: What Symptoms Are You Targeting?

When people ask me about trying CBD for the first time, my first question is, "What health condition are you trying to improve?" This is important, because after using CBD for a week or so, there should be some effect or improvement in symptoms. The rule of thumb is to choose a symptom that you'd like to improve, like sleeplessness. You may want to start with 25 mg in either an oil or softgel. Monitor your sleep for a week or so. Is it better? Are you falling asleep quicker and staying asleep longer? If you find good improvement with your quality of sleep, remain on the 25 mg dose. On the other hand, if you feel you can do a little better, most experts say to double the dose. Now take 50 mg daily for a week, and see what happens. This is exactly what my wife, Anabel, did for her sleep problems. But, after doubling her dose from 25 mg to 50 mg, she had to take it one step further and doubled her dose to 100 mg. She had to titrate the milligram size up until her endocannabinoid system found the right amount of CBD for her to take daily. Her sleep was greatly improved.

If there are no symptoms or issues to work on, I let people who are interested in CBD know that it is also a wonderful preventive supplement, which can be taken daily just like a vitamin. Prevent what? CBD is an anti-inflammatory, and as we age, we inflame. CBD has also been shown to possess neuroprotective qualities, meaning that it may help ward off, delay, or reduce risk of developing neurodegenerative conditions like Alzheimer's, Parkinson's, Huntington's, multiple sclerosis, and others. While there are impressive research findings, more research is needed to determine just how effective CBD and other cannabinoids can be concerning these disorders.

Conclusion

The world of CBD is big, and it's predicted to grow even more dramatically in the coming years. It can be very confusing to someone new to CBD who is looking for prevention or help managing certain physical or emotional issues. Always remember to target exactly what you're trying to achieve by using CBD. Is it to reduce stress or anxiety, to improve sleep, or to reduce pain, or used as a preventive supplement? Monitor your symptoms, take notes or start a journal, and measure the benefits of taking CBD.

Since there are so many companies out there, it also important to do your homework and look into these companies. Find out what they're all about.

- Who started the company?
- Where are they located?
- Where do they get their hemp?
- How is it extracted?
- How much CBD and THC are in their products?
- Do they have third-party certificates of analysis on their website?
- Is it hemp oil or CBD oil?
- Are their products full or broad spectrum, or CBD isolates?
- What kinds of containers or bottles do their products come in?
- Do they look high quality or like a bargain brand?
- Are they all natural, organic, and organically grown, or do they contain unnatural added ingredients?
- Do they offer good customer service and support?
- Do they sound like they know what they're talking about?
- Are they fairly priced?
- Do they have a 100% money-back guarantee?
- Do they make wild, dramatic health claims?

After doing your own research into different companies and brands, you should feel more confident about trying CBD products for your health and wellness. It's smart to know what you're taking and why you're taking it. When it comes to CBD, investing in the best, highest-quality product for your health is what matters most. After all, according to lots of research, you might live longer and stronger with CBD!

14

The Future of CBD and Other Cannabinoids

The future belongs to those who can hear it coming.

—David Bowie

The 2018 Farm Bill and the FDA

While it's impossible to accurately predict the future of these products, we may have clues based on what's trending today. The 2018 Farm Bill officially removed hemp from the Controlled Substances Act and opened the floodgates to production, research, and sales of hemp-based products. The bill allows hemp-derived products, including CBD, to be transferred across state lines for commercial and other purposes. There are also no restrictions on the sale, transport, or possession of hemp-derived products. New markets are opening around the country as well as the rest of the world, and people can freely purchase CBD for health and wellness with no fear of breaking the law. Sales are phenomenal now, at around $646 million annually, and it is projected that by the year 2021, they will surpass $2 billion. This is a booming market that is only poised to continue to grow. That growth should stimulate more research, more products, and greater interest.

While CBD is not currently regulated by the US Food and Drug Administration (FDA), it is most likely to happen soon. The only drug that contains CBD approved by the FDA is EPIDIOLEX, which is used for two rare forms of epilepsy, Lennox-Gastaut syndrome, and Dravet syndrome. On the other hand, Sativex (Nabiximols), which is a cannabis-based oral spray and used for muscle stiffness and spasms due to multiple sclerosis, is not yet approved by the FDA. It is possible to buy Sativex in states that have legalized marijuana.

As I write this book, it is illegal to market CBD that is added to foods or beverages or to label it as a dietary supplement. Some companies make unproven medical claims, and this, too, is forbidden by the FDA. The FDA has stated that it's committed to the development of new drugs, including those containing cannabis and CBD, and there is a great need for more research about the uses and safety of these compounds. The question is: For which physical and emotional health conditions will the FDA approve the use of CBD? When they begin to regulate the market, how many companies will go out of business for unethical or illegal practices? Will only the most honest and transparent CBD companies be left standing? Time will tell. And to make matters a little more complicated, the US Department of Agriculture (USDA) is making moves to regulate hemp as well as the CBD industry.

Nutraceuticals and CBD

An incredibly interesting area in which CBD may grow in the future is the nutraceutical market, which includes functional foods, fortified foods, fiber, plant extracts, amino acids, vitamins, and minerals. What are nutraceuticals, and what do they have to do with living longer and stronger? According to Esther Bull and her colleagues, *nutraceuticals* is a broad term describing medicinally or nutritionally functional foods. They also go by other names such as medical foods, designer foods, phytochemicals, functional foods, and nutritional supplements. Examples include bioyogurts, fortified breakfast cereals, herbal remedies, vitamins, and genetically modified foods and supplements.[1]

A recent article in *Cannabis and Cannabinoid Research* supports the idea of hemp being regarded as both a food and nutritional supplement. The researchers point out that hemp is a "valuable source of essential amino acids and fatty acids, minerals, vitamins, and fibers."[2] They also report that the cannabis plant is the most studied plant in human history, and because of all the research surrounding it, hundreds of different compounds with potential health benefits have been identified. This plant contains more than 120 terpenoids; over 100 cannabinoids; 50 hydrocarbons; 34 glycosidic compounds; 27 nitrogenous compounds; 25 noncannabinoid phenols; 22 fatty acids; 21 simple acids; 18 amino acids; 13 simple ketones; 13 simple esters and lactones; 12 simple aldehydes; 11 proteins, glycoproteins, and enzymes; 11 steroids; 9 trace elements; 7 simple alcohols; 2 pigments; and vitamin K. And that's not all! It has also been found that the plant contains 189 lipids, including 52 phospholipids and 80 sulfolipids; and 147 compounds belonging to the classes of flavonoids, proanthocyanidins, and phenolic acids. And besides containing a large amount of CBD, the cannabis plant also has cannabichromene (CBC), cannabigerol (CBG), cannabinol, cannabicyclol, cannabielsoin, and many others. Added up, all of these have shown to have possible health benefits.

Researchers in Spain and Italy have examined the potential for hemp to be used as a nutraceutical or functional food ingredient specifically for the treatment or prevention of gastrointestinal disorders. They report:

> Available experimental data show that the ECS [endocannabinoid system] is implicated in the control of motility, secretion, epithelial barrier function and viscerosensitivity, being a key component in the maintenance of GI homeostasis and a significant player in several pathophysiological states implicating a neuro-immuno-endocrine dysregulation of the GI tract.[3]

CBD may be beneficial in treating such disorders as irritable bowel syndrome, inflammatory bowel syndrome, gastrointestinal cancer, gastroesophageal reflux disease, nausea, and pain. They close by stating, "The eventual introduction and wide use of hemp-derived non-psychoactive phytocannabinoids as food ingredients will require clearer (and more flexible) regulations, based on clear, evidence-based, scientifically demonstrated, knowledge of their effects and mechanisms of action, which are urgently needed."

In a recent editorial piece, the authors indicate that countries like Denmark, Ireland, and Germany already consider CBD to be a food product, which is regulated by various food laws. They also stress that any CBD food-related product must be safe to consume and be clearly labeled.[4]

A fascinating use of CBD as a "dietary modification" or "nutraceutical prescription" is proposed in the journal *Brain, Behavior and Immunity*. The authors discuss the role inflammation has in psychiatric disorders like depression, bipolar disorder, schizophrenia, alcohol-induced dementia, and anorexia nervosa and state that CBD as a dietary supplement may be effective due to its anti-inflammatory effects.[5] While there are numerous pharmacological treatments for these disorders, some are ineffective, and others produce many unwanted side effects. There is still an urgent need for better medicine with fewer negative outcomes. Will CBD as a nutritional prescription be used by psychologists and psychiatrists to treat a number of emotional and mental disorders?

CBD Cosmetics and Cosmeceuticals

Another interesting trend that is expected to continue into the future is the use of CBD in beauty and therapeutic products. In their article "Cannabidiol (CBD)—An Update," the authors point out CBD's ability to help manage flare-ups in certain skin conditions, provide moisture to the skin, and soothe inflammation.[6] Currently CBD is allowed to be added to topical products like skin lotions, creams, salves, and balms. The researchers believe that CBD, although very popular in the United States and around the world, is expected to grow dramatically in its use as a food, medicine, and cosmetic.

Recall the section of this book summarizing studies of CBD for skin conditions like acne, dermatitis and eczema, and psoriasis. While more research needs to be conducted, right now numerous scientists and companies are working on skin care, anti-aging and beauty products, and formulas containing CBD and other cannabinoids. Will dermatologists begin using CBD as medicine for various skin conditions? Will CBD be proven to be an effective anti-aging cosmeceutical? Because of its antioxidant and anti-inflammatory properties, I am predicting this space will only grow as people search for ways to manage skin issues and slow down the aging of their skin.

Expect More CBD and Cannabinoid Research

The future is most likely going to see more research on the physical, mental, emotional, and neurological benefits of CBD and many other cannabinoids. While there are plenty of medications on the market for just about every ailment, they all come with unwanted side effects. Some people stop taking their prescription medications because of the negative side effects. Some medications work for a while, and then their therapeutic effects wear off. And for some people, there are no effective medications for their conditions, and they continue to suffer.

This book is about living longer and stronger with CBD and has provided an overview of the many conditions that may improve by using CBD. More research will focus on physical health issues, including arthritis, cancer, heart disease, diabetes, endocrine disorders, fibromyalgia, gastrointestinal disorders, headaches and migraines, lupus, menopause, pain, respiratory disorders, seizures and epilepsy, and skin disorders.

AREAS OF FUTURE CBD RESEARCH
ARTHRITIS
CANCER
HEART DISEASE
DIABETES
ENDOCRINE DISORDERS
FIBROMYALGIA
GASTROINTESTINAL DISORDERS
HEADACHES AND MIGRAINES
LUPUS
MENOPAUSE
PAIN
RESPIRATORY DISORDERS
SEIZURES AND EPILEPSY
SKIN DISORDERS

As we age, we want to extend the periods of time in our lives where we continue to do what we want. We all want to remain active and as healthy as possible. Most of us will develop arthritis, as it is the most chronic health condition among humans. It also affects a large majority of our pets as well, so expect more research examining the effects of CBD on arthritis for people and pets. Heart disease and cancer affect far too many people. Diabetes is on the rise; lots of people deal with gastrointestinal and breathing problems. Children diagnosed with certain seizure disorders face an uphill battle in finding a treatment that will work for them. Regardless of the physical health problem, isn't it good to know that natural, CBD-based medicine and other cannabinoids might help to manage or improve symptoms, relieve suffering, and increase quality of life?

Based on the success found in numerous studies, future research findings should continue looking into the many emotional and mental disorders that can be helped through the use of CBD and other cannabinoids. In this book, we examined a handful of the most common ailments, including the following:

- Addiction
- Anxiety
- Depression
- Eating disorders
- Obsessive-compulsive disorder (OCD)
- Post-traumatic stress disorder (PTSD)
- Schizophrenia and late-life schizophrenia
- Sleep disorders

More high-quality, controlled studies are needed to determine just how effective CBD can be in treating these disorders and others.

And as the population in the United States ages, more research should focus on the diseases that develop later in life, like these:

- Alzheimer's disease
- Amyotrophic lateral sclerosis
- Parkinson's disease

- Huntington's disease
- Multiple sclerosis

Increased Variety of CBD Products

VARIETY OF CBD PRODUCTS
- Tinctures (drops, oils) - Water-soluble drops - Patches - Suppositories - Capsules and softgels - Chocolates, candy, and gum - Gummies - Honey - Cereal - Massage oils - Bath bombs - Face masks - Vapes - Water - Coffee and tea - Energy drinks - Pet oils, treats, and topicals

As the FDA begins regulation of CBD products, it can be expected that some items will no longer be legal, while others will be developed and flood the market even more than today. Supplements, edibles, drinks, beauty products, and CBD for pets are all available now, and the list keeps growing.

It is expected that this list will quadruple and then some within the next few years. Again, the growth of this industry does depend on the FDA to a large degree. New and improved CBD pain-relief products are sure to be developed soon. Patches will become more effective and popular. CBD sprays for anxiety and pain and CBD-infused activewear will come on the market, and the list of foods and beverages will grow. Beer, wine, and champagne companies will race to the market with the latest and greatest adult "healthy" beverages. The beauty and cosmetic industry will generate billions of dollars and continue to grow. Mainstream drugstores will carry full lines of CBD products.

The health and wellness industry will promote and use more CBD and cannabinoid products, including those specializing in weight loss, exercise, bodybuilding, and yoga. The market for CBD products for pets should continue to grow, as Americans love their pets and spare no expense lavishing them with the best products on the market.

From Seed to Sale

Most people are savvy shoppers and want to know where their products come from. Many want those made in the United States. In the future, it will become increasing important for companies to showcase the farms where the hemp was grown. They will need to tell consumers that the hemp was grown organically, that it's all natural and contains no genetically modified organisms (GMOs), and that they work closely with the local community. Tomorrow's consumer will want to know that the CBD they are ingesting and rubbing on their skin is safe, of the highest quality, and worth the price tag on the container. Consumers will want to know each step of the CBD-producing process, from the seed that goes into the soil to how the oils are extracted, packaged, and delivered to the store.

More Older Adults and Seniors Will Purchase CBD

As a gerontologist, I am particularly interested in this future trend. I must say that I was quite surprised when, after asking dozens and dozens of older adults if they would try CBD for their aches and pains, mood, GI problems, and other issues, the vast majority of them immediately indicated they would indeed try it and that they were neither put off nor afraid to use it. Some didn't even care if THC was in their CBD! Thank you, 1960s!

Regardless of my observations, many experts in the CBD market expect older adults and seniors to lead the charge and purchase CBD much more than they do today. Why? One reason is that older adults and seniors take more prescription medications than any other age group, and they might be looking for something that is natural and doesn't have the side effects of most prescribed medications. Another reason they may jump on the CBD bandwagon is that their older adult children use CBD with good results.

More Physicians, Chiropractors, and Pain Specialists Will Recommend CBD

The Arthritis Foundation may have opened the floodgates by becoming the first large professional organization to issue guidelines using CBD. It is expected that more health agencies and medical organizations will follow. And within these organizations are doctors, nurses, physical and occupational therapists, and others who will recommend CBD for a variety of health problems. Chiropractors and pain specialists are expected to endorse and promote CBD as well. Researchers in 2019 reported on the success of CBD used by individuals suffering from chronic pain after being in car accidents. Even though they reviewed only two case studies, both men reported that the cannabinoids they used during the study provided more relief from pain than the analgesic medications they had used before the study.[7] Most medical schools, while currently not teaching medical students about the endocannabinoid system, will eventually catch up and make it part of their standard curriculum.

Science Will Catch Up with the Market

Even though there are numerous studies on the health benefits of CBD, science has been lagging in terms of the massive number of CBD products available on the market. It seems like more products enter the market without enough science reporting the benefits. Science is already beginning to catch up slowly, with the extensive use of various types of CBD products. A team of researchers points out that while there are some preclinical studies using animals (primarily mice), more human studies are needed to see whether CBD is effective for specific disorders, such as PTSD.[8]

CBD Will Be Used More In Addiction and Recovery

According to an article published by the Mayo Foundation for Medical Education and Research in 2019, "There is a growing body of preclinical and clinical evidence to support use of CBD oils for many conditions, suggesting its potential role as another option for treating opioid addiction."[9] CBD can also be effective for co-occurring conditions associated with addiction and recovery, like anxiety, depression, pain, and sleep difficulties. CBD is particularly attractive because it is safe, is nonaddictive, and has very few to no side effects.

Veterinarians Will Use and Recommend CBD

Although veterinarians are currently not allowed to administer, dispense, prescribe, or recommend CBD or any cannabinoids for animals, perhaps the American Veterinary Medical Association will change their minds in the not-too-distant future. More research on the use of CBD for animal health will be needed before this happens. Regardless, there are veterinarians who believe in the benefits of CBD, and one of them is Dr. Caroline Coile, mentioned earlier. She is a best-selling author of *Barron's Encyclopedia of Dog Breeds*, an inductee into the Dog Writer's Association of America Hall of Fame, and the winner of eight Maxwell Medallion Awards.

Conclusion

While it is difficult to predict the future of CBD, there are a number of trends today that may provide a glimpse of what CBD's future might look like. Thanks to the Farm Bill of 2018, hemp is legal and can be grown around the country, and more research can be performed both now and in the future.

With the success of the CBD/THC drugs EPIDIOLEX for seizure disorders, and Sativex for multiple sclerosis-related spasms, more cannabis-derived medications may be in the works. Research examining the use of CBD for physical, emotional, mental, and neurodegenerative disorders will provide the evidence-based results medical professionals need before recommending it to their patients. Markets in nutraceuticals, functional foods, cosmetics, and cosmeceuticals are expected to grow, and the markets will also see an increase in these types of CBD products, including supplements, edibles and drinks, body care, and pet care.

It is also anticipated that older adults and seniors will become more curious about the benefits of CBD and will begin purchasing it on a regular basis. And as they inquire about it with their doctors, health care and medical professionals will learn more about CBD and other cannabinoids and will recommend it along with traditional treatments and therapies. Chiropractors, pain specialists, and others will have CBD in their offices and will also recommend it for the many physical, emotional, and neurological issues that accompany aging. And as this is all taking place, science will have more answers regarding the effects of CBD in human studies. Addiction and recovery services will implement the use of CBD to wean patients off opioids, heroin, and alcohol. Veterinarians will also catch up and carry CBD products in their offices and recommend it for aches and pains, inflammation, anxiety, and other commonly diagnosed disorders among cats, dogs, and other animals.

Acknowledgments

This book was written as part of a wider mission to spread education and information to as many people as possible. Sharing information about the physical and mental health benefits of CBD or cannabidiol can be life changing for some. As a gerontologist, I have spent almost thirty years teaching health care professionals how to better care for older adults in senior care. I'm aware of the diseases and disorders that affect the aging body and mind. I've lectured to roomfuls of older adults and delivered presentations on aging well and how to effectively deal with depression, anxiety, Alzheimer's, and other age-related disorders. Recently, I have become extremely interested in CBD and have read countless articles and books on the topic. This book is only the beginning. I intend to continue learning and sharing information with as many people as I possibly can for as long as I can.

    I am incredibly grateful to so many wonderful people in my life who have supported and encouraged my work in senior care. My wife and the love of my life, Anabel Esparra-Collins, is a licensed social worker with decades of experience working in senior care communities. She has gained much insight and wisdom about aging and quality of life and shares her knowledge with me each day. We worked together on a very difficult case in a skilled-nursing facility for over a year and slowly fell in love. You never know where love will find you. For us, it was in a skilled-nursing center! How romantic! Thank you for making me a better husband and human being.

    The gratitude I have for my daughter, Karina Bella Collins, cannot be put into words. It's impossible to properly describe the life-changing effects she has had on me. She is a smart, artistic, talented, kind, loving, and very generous soul, and I could not image life without her. Plus, she takes after me quite a bit; she plays guitar and spins vinyl classics. Thank you for making me a better and more patient person and father.

And speaking of living life without someone, I give special thanks to my mother, Mary Collins, who passed away several years ago. Mom was a dedicated and compassionate nursing assistant who worked in the same nursing home for almost three decades. She never complained about her work and loved her elderly residents and the health care professionals she worked with all those years. I am a gerontologist because of my mother, and what she instilled in me is priceless. Thank you for making me a better professional and son.

I also thank Brian Colleran, a fearless pioneer in senior living, who has taught me many lessons about senior care, business, finance, and economics, and the art of living and working with a great sense of urgency. "Later is now" is one of my favorite "Brianisms," but he does have plenty more ("Chop, chop," "Put the fork down," and maybe my favorite: "This drink isn't going to pour itself!"), and it seems like each one is about moving faster and getting somewhere quicker. There are friends, and then there are those who bring such adventure and challenge into your life that you feel like you can never repay them. Thank you for making me feel that sense of urgency to get things done and to live a fuller life, and for making me a better friend.

To the countless health care professionals whom I have been surrounded by for decades, I thank you for your friendship, mentoring, and fellowship. Your energy has sustained and motivated me to be a better and more caring gerontologist. I thank the nurses and nursing assistants who put in the physically and emotionally challenging work of providing care to seniors. Nursing assistants have always held a special place in my heart, as my mother was a nursing assistant for the better part of thirty years. My gratitude is deep for the executive directors, clinical directors, social workers, activity professionals, HR directors, and regional directors whom I have worked with for many years. I have also worked with case managers; psychologists and psychiatrists; physicians and medical directors; and physical, occupational, and speech therapists and learned a lot from them. Activity professionals who provide the fun factor in senior living—you are a special breed, and your work is greatly needed and appreciated. These are not the only people I thank. Countless maintenance, laundry, housekeeping, and dietary professionals have shed light on forgotten areas of senior care.

About the Author

Jim Collins, PhD, is a gerontologist from Ohio who has worked in senior care for almost thirty years. He is an educator, speaker, and author. His areas of expertise include geropsychiatry and mental health issues in later life and trains health care professionals to effectively work with seniors who have depression, anxiety, or Alzheimer's disease. He has studied the aging process and provides education concerning neurodegenerative disorders and other age-related physiological illnesses. Dr. Collins has published numerous articles and written a book entitled *The Person-Centered Way: Revolutionizing Quality of Life in Long Term Care*. He assists senior care communities in implementing person-centered care models with the goal of deinstitutionalizing life and creating places to call home.

Early in his career, he formed a management company with a friend for geropsychiatrists who practiced in northeastern Ohio. For seven years, he traveled with the doctors, assisting with psychiatric evaluations and medication reviews for elderly adults living in senior care centers. One psychiatrist in particular was a phenomenal role model and mentor: Dr. Roy Fischer, who went to medical school in Vienna with Sigmund Freud's daughter Anna. The education, training, and lessons Jim learned during these years are irreplaceable.

Jim develops continuing education courses for licensed health care professionals that are delivered both live and online. He owns and operates Collins Learning, an online learning management system that provides compliance training requirements to employees in senior care, and CEU Academy, which provides continuing education courses to licensed health care professionals. Jim also has experience in hospice care and has focused on training and education concerning end-of-life care.

He has been the keynote speaker at large health care and assisted-living conferences and presents often at the Ohio Health Care Association and the Ohio Assisted Living Association. He has recently presented at the Georgia Senior Living Association and the District of Columbia Health Care Association annual conferences. Jim holds seminars and workshops virtually and in person.

For the past six years, he has intensely studied the use of medical marijuana and phytocannabinoids (CBD) for the treatment of physical, emotional, mental, and neurodegenerative disorders. He provides presentations on the use of cannabis and CBD to medical and health care professionals, and much to his surprise, this topic is very well received by the medical community. This book was written in part to fill the void in science-based education on the many health benefits of CBD. He continues to investigate medical cannabis and CBD in medicine and psychiatry as new information regularly emerges.

Jim also spent twelve years in college and university classrooms in Ohio and Pennsylvania as an instructor in gerontology, psychology, sociology, and anthropology. In his spare time, he enjoys playing guitar, reading, eating, studying, and drinking wines from around the world. Jim became a level 1 sommelier with a good friend, J. T., from the Court of Master Sommeliers. Cheers! He also spent six months earning a master certificate from the Cannabis Training University Program.

His passions include spending time with his family and dogs, promoting his daughter's art, reading, being obsessed with David Bowie, picking up one of many guitars in his collection and playing, practicing the laws of attraction and mindfulness, and traveling. He always looks for ways to reinvent himself.

References

Chapter 1 Cannabidiol (CBD)—An Introduction

1. Smith, Gregory, L. Cannabidiol (CBD). What you need to know. 2017.
2. Corroon, Jamie, and Joy A. Phillips. A cross-sectional study of cannabidiol users. *Cannabis and Cannabinoid Research*. 3.1: 152–161, 2018.
3. Moskowitz, Michael, H. *Medical Cannabis: A Guide for Patients, Practitioners and Caregivers.* Koehlerbooks: VA.
4. The World Health Organization (WHO). Critical Review Report. Expert Committee on Drug Dependence Fortieth Meeting. Geneva, 4–7 June 2018.

Chapter 2 The Very Long and Fascinating History of Cannabis as Medicine

1. Pen Ts'ao Ching. *The Classic of Herbal Medicine.* AD 1.
2. Sun Simiao. *Prescriptions Worth a Thousand Gold.* AD 652.
3. *The Vedas.* 1500–1000 B.C.
4. *Homeopathic Pharmacopoeia of India.* 1971.
5. *The Ebers Papyrus (Papyrus Ebers).* 1550 BC.
6. Pedanius Dioscorides. *De Materia Medica.* AD 40–90.

Chapter 3 The Endocannabinoid System and Phytocannabinoids Explained

1. Pacher, P., and George Kunos. Modulating the endocannabinoid system in human health and disease: successes and failures. *FEBS Journal.* 280(9): 1918–1943. 2013.

Chapter 4 The Connection Between CBD and the Aging Process

1. World Health Organization. Mental Health of Older Adults. 2018.
2. Guarldo, L. Inappropriate medication use among the elderly: a systematic review of administrative databases. *BMC Geriatrics*. 11:79. 2011.
3. Fillit, Howard, M., Kenneth Rockwood, and John Young. Introduction: Aging, Frailty, and Geriatric Medicine. In Brocklehurst's *Textbook of Geriatric Medicine and Gerontology, Eighth Edition*. Philadelphia: Elsevier. 2017.
4. Price, Emily. *Forbes*. February 2019.

Chapter 5 CBD and Arthritis, Cancer, Cardiovascular Disease, Diabetes, Endocrine Disorders, Fibromyalgia, and Gastrointestinal Disorders

1. Wolf, S. M., et al. *Worts Pills, Best Pills—A Consumer's Guide to Avoiding Drug-Induced Death or Illness*. NY: Pocket Books. 1999.
2. Malfait, A. M., et al. The nonpsychoactive cannabis constituent cannabidiol is an oral anti-arthritic therapeutic in murine collagen-induced arthritis. *Proceedings of the National Academy of Sciences of the United States of America*. 97(17): 9561–9566. 2000.
3. Sumariwalla, P. F. et al. A novel synthetic, nonpsychoactive cannabinoid acid (HU-320) with anti-inflammatory properties in murine collagen-induced arthritis. *Arthritis and Rheumatism*. 50(3): 985–998. 2004.
4. Woodhams, S. G., et al. The role of the endocannabinoid system in pain. *Handbook of Experimental Pharmacology*. 227: 119–143. 2015.
5. Schuelert, N., and J. J. McDougall. Canabinoid-mediated antinociception is enhanced in rat osteoarthritic knees. *Arthritis and Rheumatism*. 58(1): 145–153. 2008.
6. Blake, D. R., et al. Preliminary assessment of the efficacy, tolerability and safety of a cannabinoid-based medicine (Sativex) in the treatment of pain caused by rheumatoid arthritis. *Rheumatology*. 45(1): 50–52. 2006.
7. La Porta, C., et al. Involvement of the endocannabinoid system in osteoarthritis pain. *The European Journal of Neuroscience*. 39(3): 485–500. 2014.
8. Katz-Talmor, D., et al. Cannabinoids for the treatment of rheumatic diseases—where do we stand? *National Review of Rheumatology*. 14: 488–498. 2018.

9. National Academies of Sciences, Engineering, and Medicine. *The Health Effects of Cannabis and Cannabinoids: The Current State of Evidence and Recommendations for Research.* Washington, DC: National Academies Press. 2017.
10. Torsten, Lowin, M. Schneider, and G. Pongratz. Joints for joints: Cannabinoids in the treatment of rheumatoid arthritis. *Current Opinion in Rheumatology.* 31(3): 271–278. 2019.
11. Holly, T. P., M. O'Brien, and Jason J. McDougall. Attenuation of early phase inflammation by cannabidiol prevents pain and nerve damage in rat osteoarthritis. *Pain.* 158: 2442–2451. 2017.
12. Munson, A. E., et al. Antineoplastic activity of cannabinoids. *Journal of the National Cancer Institute.* 55: 597–602. 1975.
13. Blesching, Uwe. *The Cannabis Health Index.* Berkeley: North Atlantic Books. 2015.
14. Shrivastava, A., et al. Cannabidiol induces programmed cell death in breast cancer cells by coordinating the cross-talk between apoptosis and autophagy. *Molecular Cancer Therapy.* 10(7): 1161–1172. 2011.
15. Aviello, G., B. Romano, and F. Borrelli, et al. Chemoprotective effect of the non-psychotropic phytocannabinoid cannabidiol on experimental colon cancer. *Journal of Molecular Medicine of Berlin Germany.* 90(8): 925–34. 2012.
16. Izzo, A. A., et al. Increased endocannabinoid levels reduce development of precancerous lesion in the mouse colon. *Journal of Molecular Medicine of Berlin Germany.* 86: 89–98. 2008.
17. Orellana-Serradell, O. et al. Proapoptotic effect of endocannabinoids in prostate cancer cells. *Oncology Reports.* 33: 1599–1608. 2015.
18. Massi, P., et al. Cannabidiol as a potential anticancer drug. *British Journal of Clinical Pharmacology.* 75(2): 303–312. 2013.
19. Satoshi, Yamaori, et al. Structural requirements for potent direct inhibition of human cytochrome P450 1A1 by Cannabidiol: Role of Pentylresorcinol Moeity. *Biological and Pharmacological Bulletin.* 36(7): 1197–1120. 2013.
20. Armstrong, J. L., et al. Exploiting endocannabinoid-induced cytotoxic autophagy to drive melanoma cell death. *Journal of Investigative Dermatology.* 135: 1629–1637. 2015.

21. Salazar, M. A., et al. cannabinoid action induces autophagy-mediated cell death through stimulation of ER stress in human glioma cells. *Journal of Clinical Investigation.* 119: 1359–1372. 2009.
22. Vara, D. M. et al. Anti-tumoral action of cannabinoids on hepatocellular carcinoma: role of AMPK-dependent activation of autophagy. *Cell Death and Differentiation.* 18: 1099–1111. 2011.
23. Sayeda, Y. K., et al. Enhancing the treatment efficacy of cancer treatment with cannabinoids. *Frontiers in Oncology.* 8(114): 1–8. 2018.
24. Scott, K. A., A. G. Dalgleish, and William Liu. The combination of cannabidiol and delta9-tetrahydrocannabidiol enhances the anticancer effects of radiation on an orthotopic murine glioma model. *Molecular Cancer Therapy.* 13(12): 2955–2967. 2014.
25. Leinow, Leonard, and Juliana Birnbaum. *CBD: A Patient's Guide to Medical Cannabis.* Berkeley: North Atlantic Books. 2017.
26. National Comprehensive Cancer Network. *NCCN Clinical Guidelines in Oncology: Antiemesis.* V. 2. Fort Washington, PA. 2017.
27. Hesketh, P. J., M. G. Kris, E. Basch, et al. Antiemetics: American Society of Clinical Oncology Clinical Practice Guideline Update. *Journal of Clinical Oncology.* 35(28): 3240–3261. 2017.
28. Alfulaij, Naghum, et al. Cannabinoids, the Heart of the Matter. *Journal of the American Heart Association.* 7: 1–10. 2018.
29. He, J., and P. K. Whelton. Epidemiology and prevention of hypertension. *Medical Clinics of North America.* 81(5): 565–568. 1997.
30. Kazuhide, H., K. Mishihiro, and M. Fujiwara. *Pharmaceuticals.* 3: 2197–2212. 2010.
31. Ronen, D., et al. Cannabidiol, a nonpsychoactive Cannabis constituent, protects against myocardial ischemic reperfusion injury. *American Journal of Physiological-Heart and Circulatory Physiology.* 293: 3602–3607. 2007.
32. Khalid, A. J., Garry D. Tan, and S. E. O'Sullivan. A single dose of cannabidiol reduces blood pressure in healthy volunteers in a randomized crossover study. *Journal of Clinical Investigation Insight.* 2(12): 1–11. 2017.
33. Lamontagne, D., et al. The endogenous cardiac cannabinoid system: A new protective mechanism against myocardial ischemia. *Archives des Maladies du Cœur et des Vaisseaux.* 99(3): 242–246. 2006.

34. Ashton, L. C., and P. F. Smith. Cannabinoids and cardiovascular disease: The outlook for clinical treatments. *Current Vascular Pharmacology.* 5(3) 175–185. 2007.
35. Resstel, L. B., et al. 5-HT receptors and involved in the cannabidiol-induced attenuation of behavioural and cardiovascular responses to acute restraint stress in rats. *British Journal of Pharmacology.* 156(1): 181–188. 2009.
36. Montecucco, F., et al. CB2 cannabinoids receptor activation is cardioprotective in a mouse model of ischemic/reperfusion. *Journal of Molecular and Cellular Cardiology.* 46(5): 612–620. 2009.
37. The United States of America as represented by the Department of Health and Human Services. Cannabinoids as antioxidants and neuroprotectants. 2003.
38. Hayakawa, K., et al. Delayed treatment with cannabidiol has a cerebroprotective action via a cannabinoid receptor-independent myeloperoxidase-inhibiting mechanism.
39. Blesching, Uwe. *The Cannabis Health Index.* Berkeley: North Atlantic Books. 2015.
40. CDC National Diabetes Statistics Report. 2017.
41. Sobenin, I. A., et al. Metabolic effects of time-released garlic powder tablets in type 2 diabetes mellitus: The results of double-blinded placebo-controlled study. *Acta Diabetologica.* 45(1): 1–6. 2008.
42. Al-Amin, Z. M., et al. Anti-diabetic and hypolipidaemic properties of ginger (Zingiber officinale) in Streptozotocin-induced diabetic rats. *British Journal of Nutrition.* 96(4): 660–666.
43. Horvath, Bela, et al. The endocannabinoid system and plant-derived cannabinoids in diabetes and diabetic complications. *The American Journal of Pathology.* 180(2): 432–441. 2012.
44. Bujalska, M. Effects of cannabinoid receptor agonists on streptozotocin-induced hyperalgesia in diabetic neuropathy. *Pharmacology.* 82(3): 193–200. 2008.
45. Zhang, F., S. C. Challapalli, and P. J. Smith. Cannabinoid CB(1) receptor activation stimulates neurite outgrowth and inhibits capsaicin-induced Ca(2+) influx in an in vitro model of diabetic neuropathy. *Neuropharmacology.* 57(2): 88–96. 2009.

46. Weiss, L., et al. Cannabidiol arrests onset of autoimmune diabetes in NOD mice. *Neuropharmacology.* 54(1): 244–249.
47. American Thyroid Association. https://www.thyroid.org/media-main/press-room/. Accessed on June 9, 2019.
48. American Psychiatric Association. *DSM-5 Diagnostic and Statistical Manual of Mental Disorders, Fifth Edition.* American Psychiatric Publishing, Washington, DC. 2013.
49. Pagotto, Uberto, et al. The emerging role of the endocannabinoid system in endocrine regulation and energy balance. *Endocrine Reviews.* 27(1): 73–100. 2006.
50. Bifulco, M., et al. Endocannabinoids in endocrine and related tumors. *Endocrine Related Cancer.* 15(2): 391–408. 2008.
51. Li, C., et al. Role of the endocannabinoid system in food intake, energy homeostasis and regulation of the endocannabinoid pancreas. *Pharmacology and Therapeutics.* 129(3): 307–320. 2011.
52. Bermudez-Silva, F. J., et al. The role of the endocannabinoid system in the neuroendocrine regulation of energy balance. *Journal of Psychopharmacology.* 26(1): 114–124. 2012.
53. Borowska, M., et al. The effects of cannabinoids on the endocrine system. *Endokrynologia Polska.* 69(6): 705–719. 2018.
54. Chakrabarty, S., et al. Fibromyalgia. *American Family Physician.* 76(2): 247–254. 2007.
55. Walitt, B., et al. *Cannabinoids for Myalgia (Review).* Cochrane Library. 2016.
56. Habib, George, and Irit Avisar. The consumption of cannabis by fibromyalgia patients in Israel. *Pain Research and Treatment:* 1–5. 2018.
57. Fiz, J., et al. Cannabis use in patients with fibromyalgia: Effect on symptom relief and health-related quality of life. *Plos One.* 6(4): 18,440–18,445. 2011.
58. Skrabek, R. Q., et al. Nabilone for the treatment of pain in fibromyalgia. *Journal of Pain.* 9(2): 164–173. 2008.
59. Ware, M. A., et al. The effects of Nabilone on sleep in fibromyalgia: results of a randomized controlled trial. *Anesthesia and Analgesia.* 110(2): 604–610. 2010.

60. Burnstein, S. H. et al. Cannabinoids, endocannabinoids, and related analogs in inflammation. *AAPS Journal.* 11(1): 109–119. 2009.
61. American Nutrition Association web page. Accessed June 1, 2019.
62. Saltzman, John R. Burden and costs of gastrointestinal disease in the U.S. *Gastroenterology: NEJM Journal Watch.* October 2018.
63. Russo, Ethan B. Clinical endocannabinoid deficiency reconsidered: current research supports the theory in migraine, fibromyalgia, irritable bowel, and other treatment-resistant syndromes. *Cannabinoid and Cannabinoid Research.* 1(1): 154–165. 2016.
64. Pagano, E., et al. An orally active cannabis extract with high content in cannabidiol attenuates chemically-induced intestinal inflammation and hypermotility in the mouse. *Frontiers in Pharmacology.* 7(341): 1–12. 2016.
65. Borrelli, F., et al. Cannabidiol, a safe and non-psychotropic ingredient of the marijuana plant cannabis sativa, is a protective in a murine model of colitis. *Journal of Molecular Medicine Berlin.* 87(11): 1111–1121. 2009.
66. De Filippis, D. Cannabidiol reduces intestinal inflammation through the control of neuroimmune axis. *Plos One.* 6(12): 1–8. 2011.
67. Izzo, A. A., and K. A. Sharkey. Cannabinoids and the gut: new developments and emerging concepts. *Pharmacology and Therapeutics.* 126(1): 21–38. 2010.
68. Esposito, G., et al. Cannabidiol in inflammatory bowel diseases: a brief overview. *Phytotherapy Research.* 27(5): 633–636. 2012.
69. Schicho, R., and Martin Storr. Cannabis finds its way into treatment of Crohn's disease. *Pharmacology.* 93(0): 1–3. 2014
70. Ahmed, Waseem, and Seymour Katz. Therapeutic use of cannabis in inflammatory bowel disease. *Gastroenterology and Hepatology.* 12(11): 668–679. 2016.
71. Aviello, G., B. Romano, and A. A. Izzo. Cannabinoids and gastrointestinal motility: animal and human studies. *European Review for Medical and Pharmacological Sciences.* 1: 81–93. 2008.
72. Borrelli, F., et al. Cannabidiol, a safe and non-psychotropic ingredient of the marijuana plant cannabis sativa, is a protective in a murine model of colitis. *Journal of Molecular Medicine Berlin.* 87(11): 1111–1121. 2009.
73. Smith, Gregory, L. Cannabidiol (CBD). What you need to know. 2017.

Chapter 6 CBD and Headaches and Migraines, Lupus, Menopause, Pain, Respiratory Disorders, Seizures and Epilepsy, and Skin Conditions

1. Akermnan, S., et al. Endocannabinoids in the brainstem modulate dural trigeminovascular nociceptive traffic via CB1 and "triptan" receptors: implications in migraine. *Journal of Neuroscience.* 33(37): 14,869–14,877. 2013.
2. Baron, E. P. Comprehensive review of medicinal cannabis, cannabinoids, and therapeutic implications in medicine and headache: what a long strange trip it's been. *Headache.* 55(6): 885–916. 2015.
3. Greco, R., et al. Activation of CB2 receptors as a potential therapeutic target for migraine" evaluation in an animal model. *The Journal of Headache and Pain.* 15: 14. 2011.
4. Rhyne, D. N., et al. Effects of cannabinoids on migraine headache frequency in an adult population. *Pharmacotherapy.* 36(5): 505–510. 2012.
5. Boychuk, D. G. The effectiveness of cannabinoids in the management of chronic nonmalignant neuropathic pain: a systematic review. *Journal of Oral and Facial Pain and Headache.* 29(1): 7–14. 2015.
6. Greco, R., et al. Effects of anandamide in migraine data from an animal model. *The Journal of Headache and Pain.* 12(2): 177–183. 2011.
7. Russo, Ethan B. Hemp for headache: an in-depth historical and scientific review of cannabis in migraine treatment. *Journal of Cannabis Therapeutics.* 1(2). 2001.
8. Russo, Ethan B. Clinical endocannabinoid deficiency (CECD): can this concept explain therapeutic benefits of cannabis on migraine, fibromyalgia, irritable bowel syndrome and other treatment-resistant conditions? *Neuroendocrinology Letters.* 25(1/2). 2004.
9. https://www.lupus.org/understanding-lupus. Last accessed on December 10, 2020.
10. https://www.cdc.gov/lupus/basics/index.html. Last accessed on December 10, 2020.
11. https://www.corbuspharma.com/our-science/lenabasum. Last accessed on December 10, 2020.
12. Russo, Ethan, et al. Cannabis, pain, and sleep: lessons from therapeutic

clinical trials of Sativex, a cannabis-based medicine. *Chemistry and Biodiversity.* 4(8): 1729–1743. 2007.
13. How Cannabis Helps Menopause. *Impact Network.* www.impactcannabis.org/medical-marijuana-menopause. 2017.
14. Reynolds, J. Russell. On the therapeutic uses of Indian hemp. *Archives of Medicine.* 2: 154.
15. Manzanares, J. Role of the cannabinoid system in pain control and therapeutic implications for the management of acute and chronic pain episodes. *Current Neuropharmacology.* 4: 239–257. 2006.
16. Richardson, Denise, et al. Characterization of the cannabinoid receptor system in synovial tissue and fluid in patients with osteoarthritis and rheumatoid arthritis. *Arthritis Research and Therapy.* 10(R43): 1–14. 2007.
17. Russo, Ethan, B. Cannabinoids in the management of difficult to treat pain. *Therapeutics and Clinical Risk Management.* 4(1), 245–259. 2008.
18. Elikotti, J., et al. The analgesic potential of cannabinoids. *Journal of Opioid Management.* 5(6): 341–357. 2009.
19. Hammell, D. C., et al. Transdermal cannabidiol reduces inflammation and pain-related behaviors in a rat model of arthritis. *European Journal of Pain.* 2015.
20. O'Brien, Melissa. Cannabis and joints: scientific evidence for the alleviation of osteoarthritis pain by cannabinoids. *Current Opinion in Pharmacology.* 40: 104–109. 2018.
21. Hauser, W., et al. European Pain Federation (EFIC) position paper on appropriate use of cannabis-based medicines and medical cannabis for chronic pain management. *European Journal of Pain.* 22: 1547–1564. 2018.
22. CDC. Asthma. CDC.gov. 2019. Accessed on May 30, 2019.
23. American Lung Association. https://www.lung.org/lung-health-and-diseases/lung-disease-lookup/copd/learn-about-copd/how-serious-is-copd.html. Accessed on May 30, 2019.
24. Burnstein, S. H., and R. B. Zurier. Cannabinoids, endocannabinoids, and related analogs in inflammation. *The AAPS Journal.* 11(1): 109. 2009.
25. Staino, R. I., et al. Human lung-resident macrophages express CB1 and CB2 receptors whose activation inhibits the release of angiogenic and lymphangiogenic factors. *Journal of Leukocyte Biology.* 99(4): 531–540. 2016.

26. Yoshihara, S., et al. The cannabinoid receptor agonist WIN 55212-2 inhibits neurogenic inflammations in airway tissues. *Journal of Pharmacological Sciences.* 98(1): 77–82. 2005.
27. Tashkin, D. P., et al. Acute effects of smoked cannabis and oral delta9-tetrahydrocannabidiol on specific airway conductance in asthmatic subjects. *The American Review of Respiratory Disease.* 109(4): 420–428. 1974.
28. Grassin-Delyle, S. Cannabinoids inhibit cholinergic contraction in human airways through prejunctional CB1 receptors. *British Journal of Pharmacology.* 171(11): 2,767–2,777. 2014.
29. Ribeiro, A., et al. Cannabinoid improves lung function and inflammation in mice submitted to LPS-induced acute lung injury. *Immunopharmacology and Immunotoxicology.* 37(1): 1–7. 2014.
30. Pini, A., et al. The role of cannabinoids in inflammation modulation of allergic respiratory disorders, inflammatory pain and ischemic stroke. *Current Drug Targets.* 13(7): 984–993. 2012.
31. Makwana, Raj, et al. The effect of phytocannabinoids on airway hyper-responsiveness, airway inflammation and cough. *The Journal of Pharmacology and Experimental Therapeutics.* 353: 169–180. 2015.
32. Vuolo, F., et al. Evaluation of serum cytokines levels and the role of cannabinoid treatment in animal model of asthma. *Mediators of Inflammation.* 2015.
33. Centers for Disease Control and Prevention. https://www.cdc.gov/epilepsy/data/index.html. Accessed on June 3, 2019.
34. Smith, Gregory, L. Cannabidiol (CBD). What you need to know. 2017.
35. Epilepsy Foundation. https://www.epilepsy.com/learn/types-seizures. Accessed on June 3, 2019.
36. Leinow, Leonard, and Juliana Birnbaum. *CBD: A Patient's Guide to Medical Cannabis.* Berkeley: North Atlantic Books. 2017.
37. Smith, Gregory, L. Cannabidiol (CBD). What you need to know. 2017.
38. Cilio, Maria R. The case for assessing cannabidiol in epilepsy. *Epilespia.* 55(6): 787–790. 2014.
39. Leo, Antonio, et al. Cannabidiol and epilepsy: rationale and therapeutic potential. *Pharmacological Research.* 107: 85–92. 2016.
40. Pamplona, F. A., et al. Potential clinical benefits of CBD-rich cannabis

extracts over purified CBD in treatment-resistant epilepsy: observational data meta-analysis. *Frontiers in Neurology.* 9(759): 1–9. 2018.
41. Zaheer, Sidra, et al. Epilepsy and cannabis: A literature review. *Cureus.* 10(9) 3,278–3,285. 2018.
42. Perucca, Emilio. Cannabinoids in the treatment of epilepsy? Hard evidence at last? *Journal of Epilepsy Research.* 7(2): 61–76. 2017.
43. Biro, T., et al. The endocannabinoid system of the skin in health and disease: novel perspectives and therapeutic opportunities. *Trends in Pharmacological Sciences.* 30(8): 411–420. 2009.
44. Li, Shan-Shan, et al. Cannabinoid CB2 receptors are involved in the regulation of fibrogenesis during skin wound repair in mice. *Molecular Medicine Reports.* 13: 3,441–3,450. 2016.
45. Derakhshan, N., and M. Kazemi. Cannabis for refractory psoriasis—high hopes for a novel treatment and a literature review. *Current Clinical Pharmacology.* 11(2): 146–147. 2016.
46. Olah, Attila. Cannabidiol exerts sebostatic and anti-inflammatory effects on human sebocytes. *The Journal of Clinical Investigation.* 124(9): 3,713–3,774. 2014.
47. University of Colorado Anschultz Medical Campus. Cannabinoids may soothe certain skin diseases, say researchers. *Science Daily.* 2017. Accessed on June 9, 2019.
48. Eagleston, L. R. M., et al. Cannabinoids in dermatology: a scoping review. *Dermatology Online Journal.* 24(6). 2018.
49. Stander, S. Topical cannabinoid agonists. An effective new possibility for treating chronic pruritus. *Hautarzt.* 57(9): 801–807. 2006.
50. Karsak, M., et al. Attenuation of allergic contact dermatitis through the endocannabinoid system. *Science.* 316: 1494–1497. 2007.
51. Wilkinson, J. D., and E.M. Williamson. Cannabinoids inhibit human keratinocyte proliferation through a non-CB1/CB2 mechanism and have a potential therapeutic value in the treatment of psoriasis. *Journal of Dermatological Science.* 45: 92. 2007.
52. Telek, A., et al. inhibition of human hair follicle growth by endo- and exocannabinoids. *FASEB Journal.* 21(13): 3,534–3,541. 2007.

Chapter 7 CBD and Addiction, Anxiety, Depression, and Eating Disorders

1. Substance Abuse and Mental Health Services Administration. Key substance use and mental health indicators in the United States: results from the 2017 National Survey on Drug Use and Health. 2018.
2. National Institute on Drug Abuse. https://www.drugabuse.gov/related-topics/trends-statistics. Accessed on June 17, 2019.
3. Substance Abuse and Mental Health Services Administration. Results from the 2017 National Survey on Drug Use and Health: Detailed Tables. 2017.
4. American Psychiatric Association. *DSM-5 Diagnostic and Statistical Manual of Mental Disorders, Fifth Edition.* American Psychiatric Publishing, Washington, DC. 2013.
5. National Institute on Drug Abuse. https://www.drugabuse.gov/publications/drugfacts/treatment-approaches-drug-addiction. Accessed on June 17, 2019.
6. Ren, Yanhua, et al. Cannabidiol, a non-psychotropic component of cannabis, inhibits cue-induced heroin-seeking and normalizes discrete mesolimbic neuronal disturbances. *Journal of Neuroscience.* 29(47): 14,764–14,769. 2009.
7. Alvaro-Bartolome, M., and J. A. Garcia-Sevilla. Dysregulation of cannabinoid CB1 receptor and associated signaling networks in brains of cocaine addicts and cocaine-treated rodents. *Neuroscience.* 247: 294–308. 2013.
8. Crippa, J. A. S., et al. Cannabidiol for the treatment of cannabis withdrawal syndrome: a case report. *Journal of Clinical Pharmacy and Therapeutics.* 38(2): 162–164. 2012.
9. Katsidoni, V., et al. Cannabidiol inhibits the reward-facilitating effect of morphine: involvement of 5-HT1A receptors in the dorsal raphe nucleus. *Addiction Biology.* 18(2): 286–296. 2013.
10. Marcus, A., et al. Medical Cannabis Laws and Opioid Analgesic Overdose Mortality in the United States. *JAMA International Medicine.* 174(10). 2014.
11. Leinow, Leonard, and Juliana Birnbaum. *CBD: A Patient's Guide to Medical Cannabis.* Berkeley: North Atlantic Books. 2017.
12. Prud'homme, Melissa, et al. Cannabidiol as an intervention for addictive

behaviors: a systematic review of the evidence. *Substance Abuse Research and Treatment.* 9: 33–38. 2015.
13. Fabricio, M. A., et al. Endocannabinoids and striatal function: implications for addiction-related behaviors. *Behavioral Pharmacology.* 26(1 and 2), Special Issue: 59–72. 2015.
14. Hurd, Yasmin L., et al. Early phase in the development of cannabidiol as a treatment for addiction: opioid relapse takes initial center stage. *Neurotherapeutics.* 12: 807–815. 2015.
15. Smith, Gregory, L. Cannabidiol (CBD). What you need to know. 2017.
16. Hayase, T. Epigenetic mechanisms associated with addiction-related behavioral effects of nicotine and/or cocaine: implication of the endocannabinoid system. *Behavioral Pharmacology.* 28(7): 493–511. 2017.
17. Lee, Jonathan L. C., et al. Cannabidiol regulation of emotion and emotional memory processing: relevance for treating anxiety-related and substance abuse disorders. *British Journal of Pharmacology.* 174: 3,242–3,256. 2017.
18. Weiss, Friedbert. Cannabidiol: lasting attenuation of ethanol seeking. National Institutes of Health. Scripps Research Institute, California. 2018.
19. Gonzalez-Cuevas, Gustavo, et al. Unique treatment potential of cannabidiol for prevention of relapse to drug use: preclinical proof of principle. *Neuropsychopharmacology.* 43: 2,036–2,045. 2018.
20. Hurd, Yasmin L., et al. Cannabidiol for the reduction of cue-induced craving and anxiety in drug-abstinent individuals with heroin use disorder: a double-blind randomized placebo-controlled trial. *The American Journal of Psychiatry.* Published online, May 21, 2019.
21. Anxiety and Depression Association of America. https://adaa.org/about-adaa/press-room/facts-statistics. Accessed on June 10, 2019.
22. Crippa, J. A. S, et al. Neural basis of anxiolytic effects of cannabidiol (CBD) in generalized anxiety disorder: a preliminary report. *Journal of Psychopharmacology*, 25(1). 2010.
23. Kessler, RC. The global burden of anxiety and mood disorders: putting the European Study of the Epidemiology of Mental Disorders (ESEMeD) findings into perspective. *Journal of Clinical Psychiatry.* 68(2): 10–19. 2007.

24. Blanco, C., et al. Pharmacology of social anxiety disorder. *Biological Psychiatry*. 51: 109–120. 2002.
25. Campos, A. C., et al. Multiple mechanisms involved in the large-spectrum therapeutic potential of cannabidiol in psychiatric disorders. *Philosophical Transactions of the Royal Society B*. 367: 3364–3378. 2012.
26. Campos, A. C., and F. S. Guimaraes. Activation of 5HT1A receptors medicates the anxiolytic effects of cannabidiol in a PTSD model. *Behavioral Pharmacology*. 20, S54. 2009.
27. Casarotto, P. C., et al. Cannabidiol inhibitory effect on marble-burying behavior: involvement of CB1 receptors. *Behavioral Pharmacology*, 21: 353–358. 2010.
28. Yehuda, R., et al. The memory paradox. *Nature Reviews Neuroscience*. 11: 837–839. 2010.
29. De Mello Sheir, A.R., et al. Cannabidiol: a cannabis sativa constituent, as an anxiolytic drug. *Revista Brasileira de Psiquitria*. 34(1): 104–117. 2012.
30. Zuardi, A. W., et al. Action of cannabidiol on the anxiety and other effects produced by delta 9-THC in normal subjects. *Psychopharmacology Berlin*. 76: 245–250. 1982.
31. Blessing, Esther M., et al. Cannabidiol as a potential treatment for anxiety disorders. *Neurotherapeutics*. 12: 825–836. 2015.
32. Jurkus, R., et al. Cannabidiol regulation of learned fear: implications for treating anxiety-related disorders. *Frontiers in Pharmacology*. 7(454): 1–8. 2016.
33. Shannon, Scott, et al. Cannabidiol in anxiety and sleep: a large case series. *The Permanente Journal*. 23: 18–41. 2019.
34. American Psychiatric Association. *DSM-5 Diagnostic and Statistical Manual of Mental Disorders, Fifth Edition*. American Psychiatric Publishing, Washington, DC. 2013.
35. National Institute of Mental Health. https://www.nimh.nih.gov/health/topics/depression/index.shtml. Last accessed on June 15, 2019.
36. Dhingra, D., and A. Sharma. Anti-depressant-like activity of n-hexane extract of nutmeg (Myristica fragrans) seeds in mice. *Journal of Medicinal Food*. 9(1): 84–89. 2006.

37. Young, Simon N. How to Increase Serotonin in the Human Brain without Drugs. *Journal of Psychiatry and Neuroscience.* 32(6): 394–399. 2007.
38. Carlsson, et al. Seasonal and circadian monoamine variations in human brains examined post mortem. *Acta Psychiatrica Scandinavica.* 280: 75–85. 1980.
39. Beal, J. E., et al. Dronabinol as a treatment for anorexia associated with weight loss in patients with AIDS. *Journal of Pain and Symptom Management.* 10(2): 89–97. 1995.
40. Neff, G. W. Preliminary observation with dronabinol in patients with intractable pruritus secondary to cholestatic liver disease. *The American Journal of Gastroenterology.* 97(8): 2,117–2,119. 2002.
41. Hill, M. N., et al. The therapeutic potential of the endocannabinoid system for the development of a novel class of antidepressants. *Trends in Pharmacological Sciences.* 30(9): 484–493. 2009.
42. Linge, R., et al. Cannabidiol induces rapid-acting antidepressant-like effects and enhances cortical 5-HT/glutamate neurotransmission: role of 5-HT^{1A} receptors. *Neuropharmacology.* 103. 2016.
43. De Mello Schier, A. R., et al. Antidepressant-like and anxiolytic-like effects of cannabidiol: a chemical compound of Cannabis sativa. *CNS and Neurological Disorders Drug Targets.* 13(6): 953–960. 2014.
44. McLaughlin, R. J., et al. Local enhancement of cannabinoid CB1 signaling in the dorsal hippocampus elicits an antidepressant-like effect. *Behavioral Pharmacology.* 18(5–6): 431–438. 2007.
45. Bambico, F. R., et al. Cannabinoids elicit antidepressant-like behavior and activate serotonergic neurons through the medial prefrontal cortex. *Journal of Neuroscience.* 27(43): 11,700–11,711. 2007.
46. Leinow, Leonard, and Juliana Birnbaum. *CBD: A Patient's Guide to Medical Cannabis.* Berkeley: North Atlantic Books. 2017.
47. Huang, Wen-Juan, et al. Endocannabinoid system: role in depression, reward and pain control (review). *Molecular Medicine Reports.* 14: 2,899–2,903. 2016.
48. Haj-Dahmane, S., and Roh-Yu Shen. Endocannabinoid signaling and the regulation of the serotonin system. In *Endocannabinoid Regulation of*

Monoamines in Psychiatric and Neurological Disorders. Van Brockstaele, E. J. (ed). New York: Springer. 239–254. 2013.

49. Hill, M. N., et al. The therapeutic potential of the endocannabinoid system for the development of a novel class of antidepressants. *Trends in Pharmacological Sciences.* 30(9): 484–493. 2009.

50. Hilliard, Cecilia J., and Qing-song Liu. Endocannabinoid signaling in the etiology and treatment of major depressive illness. *Current Pharmaceutical Design.* 20(3): 3,795–3,811. 2014.

51. Sales, Amanda J. et al. *Progress in Neuro-Psychopharmacology and Biological Psychiatry.* 86(30): 255–261. 2018.

52. Zanelati, T. V., et al. Antidepressant-like effects of cannabidiol in mice: possible involvement of 5-HT$_{1A}$ receptors. *British Journal of Pharmacology.* 159: 122–128. 2010.

53. Wade, T. D., et al. *Epidemiology of Eating Disorders, in Textbook of Psychiatric Epidemiology.* (3rd Ed.; Eds Tsuang, M., et al.) John Wiley and Sons, Ltd. Chichester, UK. 2011.

54. Hudson, J. I., et al. The prevalence and correlates of eating disorders in the National Comorbidity Survey Replication. *Biological Psychiatry.* 61(3): 348–358. 2007.

55. Kalisvaart, J. L., and Hergenroeder, A. C. Hospitalization of patients with eating disorders on adolescent medical units is threatened by current reimbursement systems. *International Journal of Adolescent Medicine and Health.* 19(2): 155–165. 2007.

56. American Psychiatric Association. *DSM-5 Diagnostic and Statistical Manual of Mental Disorders, Fifth Edition.* American Psychiatric Publishing, Washington, DC. 2013.

57. Lapid, Maria I., et al. Eating disorders in the elderly. *International Psychogeriatrics.* 22: 523–536. 2010.

58. Robertston, Russell G., and Marcos Montagnini. Geriatric failure to thrive. *American Family Physician.* 15(7): 343–350. 2004.

59. Minaglia, Cecilia. Cachexia and advanced dementia. *Journal of Cachexia, Sarcopenia and Muscle.* 10: 263–277. 2019.

60. Zayed, M., and Joseph P. Garry. Geriatric anorexia nervosa. *Journal of the American Board of Family Medicine.* 30(5): 666–669. 2017.

61. Tetsuka, S., et al. Anorexia due to depression in the elderly from the viewpoint of primary care. *Journal of Medical Cases.* 8(4): 119–123. 2017.
62. Landi, Francesco, et al. Anorexia of aging: risk factors, consequences, and potential treatments. *Nutrients.* 8(69): 1–10. 2016.
63. Plasse, T. F., et al. Recent clinical experience with Dronabinol. *Pharmacology Biochemistry Behavior.* 40(3): 695–700. 1991.
64. Beal, J. E., et al. Dronabinol as a treatment for anorexia associated with weight loss in patients with AIDS. *Journal of Pain and Symptom Management.* 10(2): 89–97. 1995.
65. Gomez, R. et al. A peripheral mechanism for CB1 cannabinoid receptor-dependent modulation of feeding. *Journal of Neuroscience.* 22(21): 9,612–9,617. 2002.
66. Kirkam, T. C. Endocannabinoids in the regulation of appetite and body weight. *Behavioral Pharmacology.* 16(5–6): 297–313. 2005.
67. Maida, V. The synthetic cannabinoid Nabilone improved pain and symptom management in cancer patients. Paper presented at the San Antonio Breast Cancer Symposium, December, 2006.
68. Dejesus, E., et al. Use of Dronabinol improves appetite and reverses weight loss in HIV/AIDS-infected patients. *Journal of the International Association of Providers of AIDS Care.* 6(2): 95–100. 2007.
69. Wilson, M. M., et al. Anorexia of aging in long-term care: Is Dronabinol an effective appetite stimulant? A pilot study. *Journal of Nutrition, Health and Aging.* 11(2): 195–198. 2007.
70. Costiniuk, C. T., et al. Evaluation of oral cannabinoid-containing medications for the management of interferon and ribavirin-induced anorexia, nausea and weight loss in patients with AIDS. *Canadian Journal of Gastroenterology.* 22(4): 376–380. 2008.
71. Stoving, R. K. et al. Leptin, ghrelin, and endocannabinoids: potential therapeutic targets in anorexia nervosa. *Journal of Psychiatric Research.* 43(7): 671–679. 2009.
72. Marco, Eva M., et al. Endocannabinoid system and psychiatry: in search of a neurobiological basis for detrimental and potential therapeutic effects. *Frontiers in Behavioral Neuroscience.* 5(63): 1–23. 2011.
73. Viveros, M. P., et al. The endocannabinoid system as pharmacological

target derived from its CNS role in energy homeostasis and reward. Applications in eating disorders and addiction. *Pharmaceuticals.* 4: 1,101–1,136. 2011.
74. Marco, E. M., et al. The role of the endocannabinoid system in eating disorders: pharmacological implications. *Behavioral Pharmacology.* 23(5–6): 526–536. 2012.
75. Scherma, Maria, et al. The role of the endocannabinoid system in eating disorders: neurochemical and behavioral preclinical evidence. *Current Pharmaceutical Design.* 29(13): 2089–2099. 2014
76. Andries, A., et al. Dronabinol in severe, enduring anorexia nervosa: a randomized controlled trial. *International Journal of Eating Disorders.* 47: 18–23. 2014.
77. Mickle, Kelly. Can marijuana really help treat anorexia? *Cosmopolitan.* June 23, 2015.
78. Monteleone, A. M., et al. Deranged endocannabinoid responses to hedonic eating in underweight and recently weight-restored patients with anorexia nervosa. *The American Journal of Clinical Nutrition.* 101: 262–269. 2015.
79. Devon, Natashia. Obesity is an eating disorder just like anorexia and it's time we started treating it that way. *The Independent.* February 23, 2016.
80. Parray, H. J., and J. W. Yun. Cannabidiol promotes browning in 3T3-L1 adipocytes. *Molecular and Cellular Biochemistry.* 416: 131. 2016.
81. Landi, Francesco, et al. Anorexia of aging: risk factors, consequences, and potential treatments. *Nutrients.* 8(69): 1–10. 2016.
82. Milano, Walter, et al. The role of endocannabinoids in the control of eating disorders. *Diseases and Disorders.* 1(1): 1–6. 2017.

Chapter 8 CBD and Obsessive-Compulsive Disorder, Post-Traumatic Stress Disorder, Schizophrenia, and Late-Onset Schizophrenia

1. Anxiety and Depression Association of America. https://adaa.org/about-adaa/press-room/facts-statistics. Accessed on June 10, 2019.
2. International OCD Foundation. www.iocdf.org. Last accessed on June 24, 2019.

3. American Psychiatric Association. *DSM-5 Diagnostic and Statistical Manual of Mental Disorders, Fifth Edition.* American Psychiatric Publishing, Washington, DC. 2013.
4. Crippa, J. A., et al. Effects of cannabidiol (CBD) on regional cerebral blood flow. *Neuropsychopharmacology.* 29: 417–426. 2004.
5. Plinio, Casarotto C., et al. Cannabidiol inhibitory effect on marble-burying behavior: involvement of CB1 receptors. 21(4): 353–358. 2010.
6. Deiana, Serena. Plasma and brain pharmacokinetic profile of cannabidiol (CBD), cannabidivarine (CBDV), Delta-9 tetrahydrocannabivarian (THCV) and cannabigerol (CBG) in rats and mice following oral and intraperitoneal administration and CBD action on obsessive-compulsive behavior. *Psychopharmacology.* 219(3): 859–873. 2012.
7. De Mello Sheir, A. R., et al. Cannabidiol: a cannabis sativa constituent, as an anxiolytic drug. *Revista Brasileira de Psiquitria.* 34(1): 104–117. 2012.
8. Nardo, Mirella, et al. Cannabidiol reverses the mCPP-induced increase in marble-burying behavior. *Fundamental and Clinical Pharmacology.* 28: 544–550. 2014.
9. Casarotto, Linio C., et al. Cannabinoids and obsessive-compulsive disorder. In *Cannabinoids in Neurologic and Mental Disorders.* Fattore, L. (ed.). Elsevier: Brazil. 2015.
10. U.S. Department of Veterans Affairs. https://www.ptsd.va.gov/understand/common/common_adults.asp and https://www.ptsd.va.gov/understand/common/common_veterans.asp. Last accessed on June 26, 2019.
11. Abbot, C., et al. What's killing our medics? Ambulance Service Manager Program. Conifer, CO. www.revivingresponders.com/originalpaper. Accessed on June 26, 2019.
12. Stanley, I. H., et al. A systematic review of suicidal thoughts and behaviors among police officers, firefighters, EMTs, and paramedics. *Clinical Psychology Review.* 44: 25–44. 2016.
13. Badge of Life. A study of police suicide 2008–2016. www.policesuicidalitystudy.com. Last retrieved on June 26, 2019.
14. Hartley, Tara A., et al. PTSD symptoms among police officers: associations with frequency, recency, and types of traumatic events. *International Journal of Emergency Mental Health.* 15(4): 241–253. 2013.

15. American Psychiatric Association. *DSM-5 Diagnostic and Statistical Manual of Mental Disorders, Fifth Edition.* American Psychiatric Publishing, Washington, DC. 2013.
16. Shin, L. M., et al. Amygdala, medial prefrontal cortex, and hippocampal function in PTSD. *Annals of the New York Academy of Sciences.* 1,071: 67–79. 2006.
17. Harloe, J. P., et al. Differential endocannabinoid regulation of extinction in appetitive and aversive Barnes maze tasks. *Learning and Memory.* 15(11): 806–809. 2008.
18. Fraser, G. A. The use of a synthetic cannabinoid in the management of treatment-resistant nightmares in posttraumatic stress disorder (PTSD). *CNS Neuroscience and Therapeutics.* 15(1): 84–88. 2009.
19. Ganon-Elazar, E., and I. Akirav. Cannabinoid receptor activation in the basolateral amygdala blocks the effects of stress on the conditioning and extinction of inhibitory avoidance. *Journal of Neuroscience.* 29(36): 11,078–11,088. 2009.
20. Crippa, Jose A., et al. Translational investigation of the therapeutic potential of cannabidiol (CBD): toward a new age. *Frontiers in Immunology.* 1–16. 2009.
21. Hill, M. N., et al. Reductions in circulating endocannabinoid levels in individuals with post-traumatic stress disorder following exposure to the World Trade Center attacks. *Psychoneuroendocrinology.* 38(12): 2952. 2013.
22. Papini, Santiago, et al. Toward a translational approach to targeting the endocannabinoid system in posttraumatic stress disorder: a critical review of preclinical research. *Biological Psychology.* 104: 8–18. 2015.
23. Mizrachi Zer-Aviv, T., et al. Cannabinoids and post-traumatic stress disorder: clinical and preclinical evidence for treatment and prevention. *Behavioral Pharmacology.* 27(7): 561–569. 2016.
24. Jurkus, R., et al. Cannabidiol regulation of learned fear: implications for treating anxiety-related disorders. *Frontiers in Pharmacology.* 7(454): 1–8. 2016.
25. Loflin, Mallory J. E., et al. Cannabinoids as therapeutic for PTSD. *Current Opinion in Psychology.* 14: 78–83. 2017.

26. Lee, Jonathan L. C., et al. Cannabidiol regulation of emotion and emotional memory processing: relevance for treating anxiety-related and substance abuse disorders. *British Journal of Pharmacology*. 174: 3,242–3,256, 2017.
27. Bitencourt, Rafael M., and R. N. Takahashi. Cannabidiol as a therapeutic alternative for post-traumatic stress disorder: from bench research to confirmation in human trials. *Frontiers in Neuroscience*. 12(502): 1–10. 2018.
28. Elms, Lucas, et al. Cannabidiol in the treatment of post-traumatic stress disorder: a case series. *The Journal of Alternative and Complimentary Medicine*. 25(4): 392–397. 2019.
29. Schizophrenia and Related Disorders Alliance of America. Sardaa.org/resources/about-schizophrenia. Last accessed on June 29, 2019.
30. World Health Organization (WHO). www.who.int/news-room/fact-sheets/detail/schizophrenia. Last accessed on June 29, 2019.
31. American Psychiatric Association. *DSM-5 Diagnostic and Statistical Manual of Mental Disorders, Fifth Edition*. American Psychiatric Publishing, Washington, DC. 2013.
32. Emrich, H. M., et al. Towards a cannabinoid hypothesis of schizophrenia: cognitive impairments due to dysregulation of the endogenous cannabinoid system. *Pharmacology, Biochemistry and Behavior*. 56(4): 803–807. 1997.
33. Giuffrida, A., et al. Cerebrospinal anandamide levels are elevated in acute schizophrenia and are inversely correlated with psychotic symptoms. *Neuropsychopharmacology*. 29(11): 2,108–2,114. 2004.
34. Muller-Vahl, Kirsten. Cannabinoids and schizophrenia: where is the link? *Cannabinoids*. 3(4): 11–15. 2008.
35. Muller-Vahl, Kirsten, and Hindrek M. Emrich. Cannabis and schizophrenia: towards a cannabinoid hypothesis of schizophrenia. *Expert Review of Neurotherapeutics*. 8(7): 1037–1048. 2008.
36. Desfosses, J., et al. Endocannabinoids and schizophrenia. *Pharmaceuticals*. 3: 3,101–3,126. 2010.
37. Parolaro, D., et al. The endocannabinoid system and psychotic disorders. *Experimental Neurology*. 224(1): 3–14. 2010.

38. Coulston, Carissa M., et al. Cannabinoids for the treatment of schizophrenia? A balanced neurochemical framework for both adverse and therapeutic effects of cannabis use. *Schizophrenia Research and Treatment.* 1–9. 2011.
39. Ferretjans, Rodrigo, et al. The endocannabinoid system and its role in schizophrenia: a systematic review of the literature. *Revista Brasileira de Psiquiatria.* 34(Supplement 2): S163–S193. 2012.
40. Zamberletti, E., et al. The endocannabinoid system and schizophrenia: integration of evidence. *Current Pharmacological Design.* 18(32): 4,980–4,990. 2012.
41. Leweke, F. M., et al. Cannabidiol enhances anandamide signaling and alleviates psychotic symptoms of schizophrenia. *Translational Psychiatry.* 2(e94): 1–7. 2012.
42. Zuardi, A. W., et al. A critical review of the antipsychotic effects of cannabidiol: 30 years of a translational investigation. *Current Pharmaceutical Design.* 18: 5,131–5,140. 2012.
43. Kirkpatrick, Brian, and Brian J. Miller. Inflammation and Schizophrenia. *Schizophrenia Bulletin.* 39(6): 1,174–1,179. 2013.
44. Rohleder, Cathrin, and F. Markus Leweke. Cannabinoids and schizophrenia. In *Cannabinoids in Neurologic and Mental Disease.* Lianna Fattore (Ed.). Elsevier, NY: 193–204. 2015.
45. Manseau, Marc W., and Donald C. Goff. Cannabinoids and schizophrenia: risks and therapeutic potential. *Neurotherapeutics.* 12: 816–826. 2015.
46. Muller, Norbert, et al. The role of inflammation in schizophrenia. *Frontiers in Neuroscience.* 9(372): 1–9. 2015.
47. Muller, N., et al. The role of inflammation in schizophrenia. *Frontiers in Neuroscience.* 9: 372. 2015.
48. J. Renard, et al. Cannabidiol counteracts amphetamine-induced neuronal behavioral sensitization of the mesolimbic dopamine pathway through a novel mTOR/p70S6 kinase signaling pathway. *Journal of Neuroscience.* 36(18): 5,160. 2016.
49. Reia, J., and G. Pereira. The role of cannabinoids in schizophrenia: Where have we been and where are we going? *European Psychiatry.* S277. 2017.
50. Ruggiero, Rafael N., et al. Cannabinoids and vanilloids in schizophrenia:

neurophysiological evidence and directions for basic research. *Frontiers in Pharmacology.* 8(399): 1–27. 2017.
51. McGuire, Philip, et al. Cannabidiol (CBD) as an adjunctive therapy in schizophrenia: a multicenter randomized controlled trial. *American Journal of Psychiatry.* 175(3): 225–231. 2018.
52. Pierre, Joseph M. Cannabidiol (CBD) for schizophrenia: promise or pipe dream? *Current Psychiatry.* 18(5): 13–20. 2019.
53. American Psychiatric Association. *DSM-5 Diagnostic and Statistical Manual of Mental Disorders, Fifth Edition.* American Psychiatric Publishing, Washington, DC. 2013.
54. Maglione, Jeanne E., et al. Late-onset schizophrenia: do recent studies report categorizing LOS as a subtype of schizophrenia? *Current Opinion in Psychiatry.* 27(3): 173–178. 2014.
55. Chen, Laura, et al. Risk factors in early and late onset schizophrenia. *Comprehensive Psychiatry.* 80: 155–162. 2018.
56. Assche, Lies Van, et al. The neuropsychology and neurobiology of late-onset schizophrenia and very-late-onset schizophrenia-like psychosis: a critical review. *Neuroscience & Behavioral Reviews.* 83: 604–621. 2017.
57. Lubman, Dan L., and David J. Castle. Late-onset schizophrenia: make the right diagnosis when psychosis merges after age 60. *Current Psychiatry.* 1(12): 35–44. 2002.

Chapter 9 CBD and Sleep Disorders

1. Cleveland Clinic. https://my.clevelandclinic.org/health/drugs/15308-sleeping-pills. Accessed on July 3, 2019.
2. American Sleep Association. https://www.sleepassociation.org/about-sleep/sleep-statistics/. Last accessed on July 2, 2019.
3. American Psychiatric Association. *DSM-5 Diagnostic and Statistical Manual of Mental Disorders, Fifth Edition.* American Psychiatric Publishing, Washington, DC. 2013.
4. Murillo-Rodriguez, E., et al. The nonpsychoactive cannabis constituent cannabidiol is a wake-inducing agent. *Behavioral Neuroscience.* 122(6): 1,378–1,382. 2008.

5. Murillo-Rodriguez, E. The role of the CB1 receptor in the regulation of sleep. *Progress in Neuro-Psychopharmacology & Biological Psychiatry.* 32: 1,420–1,427. 2008.
6. Chagas, M. H., et al. Effects of acute systemic administration of cannabidiol on sleep-wake cycle of rats. *Journal of Psychopharmacology.* 27(3): 312–316. 2013.
7. Prasad, B., et al. Proof of concept trial of dronabinol in obstructive sleep apnea. *Frontiers in Psychiatry.* 4(1): 1–5. 2013.
8. Babson, Kimberly A., James Sottile, and Danielle Morabito. Cannabis, cannabinoids, and sleep: a review of the literature. *Current Psychiatric Reports.* 19(23). 2017.
9. Linares, Ila M. et al. No acute effects of cannabidiol on the sleep-wake cycle of healthy subjects: a randomized, double-blind, placebo-controlled, crossover study. *Frontiers in Pharmacology.* 9(315): 1–8. 2018.
10. Carley, David W., et al. Pharmacotherapy of apnea by cannabimimetic enhancement, the PACE Clinical Trial: effects of dronabinol in obstructive sleep apnea. *Sleep.* 41(1): 1–13. 2018.
11. Murillo-Rodriguez, Eric, et al. Systemic injections of cannabidiol enhance acetylcholine levels from basal forebrain in rats. *Neurochemical Research.* 43(8): 1,511–1,518. 2018.
12. Shannon, Scott, et al. Cannabidiol in anxiety and sleep: a large case series. *The Permanente Journal.* 23: 18–41. 2019.

Chapter 10 CBD and Neurodegenerative Disorders

1. Alzheimer's Association. https://www.alz.org/. Last accessed on July 4, 2019.
2. Fagan, Steven G., and Veronica A. Campbell. Endocannabinoids and Alzheimer's disease. In L. Fattore (Ed): *Cannabinoids in Neurologic and Mental Disease.* Elsevier: NY. 2015.
3. Leinow, Leonard, and Juliana Birnbaum. *CBD: A Patient's Guide to Medical Cannabis.* Berkeley: North Atlantic Books. 2017.
4. Iuvone, T., et al. Neuroprotective effect of cannabidiol, a non-psychoactive component from cannabis sativa, on beta-amyloid-induced

toxicity in PC12 cells. *Journal of Neurochemistry*. 89(1): 131–141. 2004.

5. Bisogno, Tizaiana, and Vincenzo Di Marzo. The role of the endocannabinoid system in Alzheimer's disease: facts and hypotheses. *Current Pharmaceutical Design*. 14(23): 2008.
6. Krishnan, S., R. Cairns, and R. Howard. Cannabinoids for the treatment of dementia. *Cochrane database of Systematic Reviews*. 15(2). 2009.
7. Iuvone, T., et al. Cannabidiol: a promising drug for neurodegenerative disorders? *CNS Neuroscience and Therapeutics*. 15(1): 65–75. 2009.
8. Walther, Sebastian, and Michael Halpern. Cannabinoids and dementia: a review of the clinical and preclinical data. *Pharmaceuticals*. 3: 2,689–2,708. 2010.
9. Esposito, G., et al. Cannabidiol reduces AB-induced neuroinflammation and promotes hippocampal neurogenesis through PPARy involvement. *Plos One*. 6(12): 28,668–28,668. 2011.
10. Howes, M. J., and E. Perry. The role of phytochemicals in the treatment and prevention of dementia. *Drugs & Aging*. 28(6): 439–468. 2011.
11. Karl, T., D. Cheng, B. Garner, and J. C. Arnold. The therapeutic potential of the endocannabinoid system for Alzheimer's disease. *Expert Opinion on Therapeutic Targets*. 16(4): 407–420. 2012.
12. Maroof, N., M. C. Pardon, and D. A. Kendall. Endocannabinoid signaling in Alzheimer's disease. 41(6): 1,583–1,587. 2013.
13. Aso, E., and I. Ferrer. Cannabinoids for treatment of Alzheimer's disease: moving toward the clinic. *Frontiers in Pharmacology*. 5(37). 2014.
14. Bedse, G., et al. The role of the endocannabinoid signaling in the molecular mechanisms of neurodegeneration in Alzheimer's disease. 43(4): 1,115–1,136. 2015.
15. Liu, Celina S., et al. Cannabinoids for the treatment of agitation and aggression in Alzheimer's disease. *CNS Drugs*. 29(8): 615–623, 2015.
16. Libro, Rosaliana, et al. Natural phytochemicals in the treatment and prevention of dementia: an overview. *Molecules*. 21(518): 1–38. 2016.
17. Shelef, Assaf, et al. Safety and efficacy of medical cannabis oil for behavioral and psychological symptoms of dementia: an open label add-on, pilot study. *Journal of Alzheimer's Disease*. 51: 15–19. 2016.

18. Currais, Antonio, et al. Amyloid proteotoxicity initiates an inflammatory response blocked by cannabinoids. *Aging and Mechanisms of Disease.* 2: 1–8. 2016.
19. Mannucci, C., et al. Neurological aspects of medical use of cannabidiol. *CNS Neurological Disorders Drug Targets.* 16(5): 541–553. 2017.
20. Watt, George, and Tim Karl. In vivo evidence for therapeutic properties of cannabidiol (CBD) for Alzheimer's disease. *Frontiers in Pharmacology.* 8(20): 1–7. 2017.
21. Shoemaker, Jennifer L., et al. The CB2 cannabinoid agonist AM-1241 prolongs survival in a transgenic mouse model of amyotrophic lateral sclerosis when initiated at symptom onset. *Journal of Neurochemistry.* 101(1): 2007.
22. Bilsland, Lynsey G., and Linda Greensmith. The endocannabinoid system in amyotrophic lateral sclerosis. *Current Pharmaceutical Design.* 14(23): 2,306–2,316. 2008.
23. Pryce, G., and D. Baker. Endocannabinoids in multiple sclerosis and amyotrophic lateral sclerosis. *Handbook of Experimental Pharmacology.* 231: 213–231. 2015.
24. De Lago, Eva, et al. Endocannabinoids and amyotrophic lateral sclerosis. In. L Fattore (Ed): *Cannabinoids in Neurological and Mental Disease.* 99–123. 2015.
25. Rajan, T. S., et al. Gingival stromal cells as an in vitro model: cannabidiol modulates genes linked with amyotrophic lateral sclerosis. *Journal of Cellular Biochemistry.* 118(4). 2016.
26. Giacoppo, Sabrina, and Emanuela Mazzon. Can cannabinoids be a potential therapeutic tool in amyotrophic lateral sclerosis? *Neural Regeneration Research.* 11(12): 1,896–1,899. 2016.
27. Nahler, Gerhard. Co-medication with cannabidiol may slow down the progression of motor neuron disease: a case report. *Journal of General Practice.* 5(4): 1–3. 2017.
28. Riva, Nilo, et al. Safety and efficacy of nabiximols on spasticity symptoms in patients with motor neuron disease (CANALS): a multicenter, double-blind, randomized, placebo-controlled, phase 2 trial. *The Lancet Neurology.* 18(2): 156–164. 2019.

29. Urbi, B., et al. Effects of cannabinoids in Amyotrophic Lateral Sclerosis (ALS) murine models: a systematic review and meta-analysis. *Journal of Neurochemistry.* 149 (2): 284–297. 2019.
30. Parkinson's New Today. https://parkinsonsnewstoday.com/parkinsons-disease-statistics/. Last accessed on August 9, 2019.
31. Garcia-Arencibia, M., et al. Evaluation of the neuroprotective effect of cannabinoids in a rat model of Parkinson's disease: Importance of antioxidant and cannabinoid receptor-independent properties. *Brain Research.* 1134 (23): 162–170. 2007.
32. Zuardi, A.W., et al. Cannabidiol for the treatment of psychosis in Parkinson's disease. *Journal of Psychopharmacology.* September 18, 2008.
33. Zuardi, Antonio Waldo. Cannabidiol: from an inactive cannabinoid to a drug with a wide spectrum of action. *Bras Psiquiatr.* 30(3): 271–280. 2008.
34. Fagherazzi, Elen V. Memory-rescuing effects of cannabidiol in an animal model of cognitive impairment relevant to neurodegenerative disorders. *Psychopharmacology.* 219(4): 1133–1140. 2012.
35. Gomes, Felope V., et al. Cannabidiol attenuates catalepsy induced by distinct pharmacological mechanisms via 5-HT$_{1A}$ receptor activation in mice. *Progress in Neuro-Pharmacological & Biological Psychiatry.* 46: 43–47. 2013.
36. Chagas, M. H., et al. Effects of cannabidiol in the treatment of patients with Parkinson's disease: an exploratory double-blind trial. *Journal of Psychopharmacology.* 28(11): 1088–1098. 2014.
37. Chagas, M. H., et al. Cannabidiol can improve complex sleep-related behaviors associated with rapid eye movement sleep behavior disorder in Parkinson's disease patients: a case series. *Journal of Clinical Pharmacy and Therapeutics.* 39(5). 2014.
38. Santos, Neife Aparecida Guinaim, et al. The neuroprotection of cannabidiol against MPP$^+$-induced toxicity in PC12 cells involves trkA receptors, upregulation of axonal and synaptic proteins, neuritogenesis, and might be relevant to Parkinson's disease. *Toxicology in Vitro.* 30: 231–240. 2015.
39. Campos, Alline C., et al. Cannabidiol, neuroprotection and neuropsychiatric disorders. *Pharmacological Research.* 112: 119–127. 2016.

40. Bassi, Mario S., et al. Cannabinoids in Parkinson's Disease. *Cannabis and Cannabinoid Research.* 2(1): 21–29. 2017.
41. Mannucci, Carmen, et al. Neurological aspects of medical use of cannabidiol. *CNS & Neurological Disorders—Drug Targets.* 16(5): 541–553. 2017.
42. Milano, Walter, et al. Cannabinoids involvement in Neurodegenerative diseases. *Current Neurobiology.* 8(3): 135–144. 2017.
43. Maroon, Joseph, and Jeff Bost. Review of the neurological benefits of phytocannabinoids. *Surgical Neurology International.* 91(9): 1–26. 2018.
44. Peres, F. F., A. Lima, V. Abilio, et al. Cannabidiol as a Promising Strategy to Treat and Prevent Movement Disorders? *Frontiers in Pharmacology.* 9(482): 1–12. 2018.
45. Bonelli, Paphael M., et al. Pharmacological management of Huntington's disease: An evidence-based review. *Current Pharmaceutical Design.* 12(21): 2,701–2,720. 2006.
46. Sandyk, R., et al. Effects of cannabidiol in Huntington's disease. *Neurology.* 36(Supplemental 1): 342. 1986.
47. Consroe, Paul, et al. Controlled clinical trial of cannabidiol in Huntington's disease. *Pharmacology, Biochemistry and Behavior.* 40(3): 701–708. 1991.
48. Richfield, Eric K., and Miles Herkenham. Selective vulnerability in Huntington's disease: Preferential loss of cannabinoid receptors in lateral globus pallidus. *Annals of Neurology.* 36(4). 1994.
49. Curtis, Adrienne, and Hugh Rickards. Nabilone could treat chorea and irritability in Huntington's disease. *The Journal of Neuropsychiatry and Clinical Neurosciences.* 2006.
50. Micale, Vincenzo, et al. Endocannabinoids and neurodegenerative diseases. *Pharmacological Research.* 56(5): 382–392. 2007.
51. Blazquez, Cristina, et al. Loss of striatal type 1 cannabinoid receptors is a key pathogenic factor in Huntington's disease. *Brain.* 134: 119–136. 2011.
52. Sagredo, O., et al. Neuroprotective effects of phytocannabinoid-based medicines in experimental models of Huntington's disease. *Journal of Neuroscience Research.* 89(9): 1–8. 2011.
53. Fernandez-Ruiz, Javier, et al. Cannabidiol for neurodegeneration disorders: important new clinical applications for this phytocannabinoid? *British Journal of Clinical Pharmacology.* 75(2): 323–333. 2012.

54. Sagredo, O., et al. Cannabinoids: novel medicines for the treatment of Huntington's disease. *Recent Patents on CNS Drug Discovery.* 7(1): 41–48. 2012.
55. Laprairie, Robert B., et al. Biased Type 1 cannabinoid receptor signaling influences neuronal viability in a cell culture model of Huntingtin disease. *Molecular Pharmacology.* 89: 364–375. 2016.
56. Baker, D., S. J. Jackson, and G. Pryce. Cannabinoid control of neuroinflammation related to multiple sclerosis. *British Journal of Pharmacology.* 152: 649–654. 2007.
57. Rog, David J., Turo J. Nurmikko, and C. A. Young. Oromucosal Delta^9—tetrahydrocannabinol/cannabinol for neuropathic pain associated with multiple sclerosis: An uncontrolled, open-label, 2-year extension trial. *Clinical Therapeutics.* 29(9): 2,068–2,079. 2007.
58. Oreja-Guevara. Treatment of spasticity in multiple sclerosis: regarding the use of cannabinoids. *Revista de Neurologia.* 55(7): 421–430. 2012.
59. Leussink, Verena Isabell, et al. Symptomatic therapy in multiple sclerosis: the role of cannabinoids in treating spasticity. *Therapeutic Advances in Neurological Disorders.* 5(5): 255–266. 2012.
60. Mecha, M., et al. Cannabidiol provides long-lasting protection against the deleterious effects of inflammation in a viral model of multiple sclerosis: A role for A^{2A} receptors. *Neurobiology of Disease.* 59: 141–150. 2013.
61. Rudroff, T., and J. Sosnoff. Cannabidiol to improve mobility in people with multiple sclerosis. *Frontiers in Neurology.* 9(183): 1–3. 2018.
62. Manuela, Contin, et al. Tetrahydrocannabinol/Cannabidiol oromucosal spray in patients with multiple sclerosis: A pilot study on the plasma concentration-effect relationship. *Clinical Neuropharmacology.* 41(5): 171–176. 2018.
63. Akgun, K., et al. Daily practice managing resistant multiple sclerosis spasticity with Delta-9-Tetrahydrocannabinol: Cannabidiol oromucosal spray: A Systematic review of observational studies. *Journal of Central Nervous System Disease.* 11: 1–18. 2019.
64. Mecha, M., et al. Perspectives on cannabis-based therapy of multiple sclerosis: a mini-review. *Frontiers in Cellular Neuroscience.* 14(34): 1–7. 2020.

Chapter 11 CBD and End-of-Life Care

1. Pisanti, Simona, et al. Use of cannabinoid receptor agonists in cancer therapy as palliative curative agents. *Best Practice & Research Clinical Endocrinology & Metabolism.* 23(1): 117–131. 2009.
2. Green, A. J., and Kay De-Vries. Cannabis use in palliative care—an examination of the evidence and implications for nurses. *Journal of Clinical Nursing.* 19: 2,454–2,462. 2010.
3. Davison, Sara N., and Joseph S. Davison. Is there a legitimate role for the therapeutic use of cannabinoids for the symptom management in chronic kidney disease? *Journal of Pain and Symptom Management.* 41(4): 768–778. 2011.
4. Aggarwal, S. K. Use of cannabinoids in cancer care: palliative care. *Current Oncology.* 23: 1–8. 2016.
5. Strouse, Thomas B. Cannabinoids in palliative medicine. *Journal of Palliative Medicine.* 20(7): 692–694. 2017.
6. Dzierzanowski, T. Prospects for the Use of Cannabinoids in Oncology and Palliative Practice: A Review of the Evidence. *Cancers.* 11(2): 129. 2019.

Chapter 12 CBD for Your Pets

1. Coile, Caroline, PhD. *Cannabis and CBD Science for Dogs: Natural Supplements to Support Healthy Living and Graceful Aging.* Assisi Bio Press, 2016.
2. Klein, Jerry. CBD oil for dogs: What you need to know. https://www.akc.org/expert-advice/health/cbd-oil-dogs/. Accessed on June 23, 2020.
3. Gamble, Lauir-Jo, et al. Pharmacokinetics, Safety, and Clinical Efficacy of Cannabidiol Treatment in Osteoarthritic Dogs. *Frontiers in Veterinary Science.* 5(165): 1–9. 2018.
4. American Veterinary Medical Association (AMVA). https://www.avma.org/resources-tools/reports-statistics/us-pet-ownership-statistics. Accessed on June 23, 2020.
5. Deabold, Kelly A., Wayne S. Schwark, Lisa Wolf, and Joseph J. Wakshlag. Single-Dose Pharmacokinetics and Preliminary Safety Assessment with

use of CBD-rich hemp nutraceutical in healthy dogs and cats. *Animals.* 9(832): 1–13. 2019.
6. Kogan, Lori, et al. US Veterinarians' knowledge, experience, and perception regarding the use of cannabidiol for canine medical conditions. *Frontiers in Veterinary Science.* 5(338): 1–11. 2019.
7. Fernandez-Trapero, Maria, et al. Pharmacokinetics of Sativex in Dogs: Towards a potential cannabinoid-based therapy for canine disorders. *Biomolecules.* 10(279): 1–8. 2020.
8. Hartsel, J. A., et al. Efficacy of cannabidiol (CBD) for the treatment of canine epilepsy. https://www.pwdfoundation.org/project/efficacy-of-cannabidiol-cbd-for-the-treatment-of-canine-epilepsy/. Accessed on June 23, 2020.
9. Mogi, Chie, and Takaaki Fukuyama. Cannabidiol as a potential anti-epileptic dietary supplement in dogs with suspected epilepsy: three case reports. *Pet Behaviour Science.* 7:11–16. 2019.
10. American Veterinary Medical Association (AMVA). https://www.avma.org/resources-tools/reports-statistics/us-pet-ownership-statistics. Accessed on June 23, 2020.

Chapter 14 The Future of CBD and Other Cannabinoids

1. Bull, Esther, Lisa Rapport, and Brian Lockwood. What is a nutraceutical? *The Pharmaceutical Journal.* July 2000.
2. Cerino, P., et al. A review of hemp as food and nutritional supplement. *Cannabis and Cannabinoid Research.* X(X): 1–9. 2020.
3. Martinez, Vincente, et al. Cabbidiol and other non-psychoactive cannabinoids for prevention and treatment of gastrointestinal disorders: Useful nutraceuticals? *International Journal of Molecular Sciences.* 21(3,067): 1–35. 2020.
4. Lachenmeier, D. W., and Stephen G. Walch. Cannabidiol (CBD): a strong plea for mandatory pre-marketing approval of food supplements. *Journal of Consumer Protection and Food Safety.* April 2020.
5. Need updated reference here.
6. Cernovsky, Zack Z., and Larry Craig Litman. Case studies of analgesic

cannabinoid use by persons with chronic pain from car accidents. *Open Science Journal of Psychology*. 6(1): 1–4. 2019.
7. Sarker, S. D., and Luftin Nahar. Cannabidiol (CBD)—An Update. *Trends in Phytochemical Research (TPR)*. 4(1): 1–2. 2020.
8. Need updated reference here.
9. VanDolah, H. J., B. A. Bauser, and K. F. Mauck. Clinicians' Guide to Cannabidiol and Hemp Oils. *Mayo Clinic Proceedings*. 94(9): 1,840–1,851. 2019.

Living Longer and Stronger with CBD provides the reader with a wealth of information about the miracle molecule known as cannabidiol, or CBD. Whether you are currently using CBD, want to learn more about it, or are a health care provider, this book contains the latest science-based evidence you'll need to understand the potential effectiveness of this plant-derived medicine. Jim Collins, PhD, takes the reader on a long ride from the basics about CBD to its medicinal uses for physical, mental, emotional, and neurological conditions.

Hemp and cannabis plants have been used in virtually every culture on the planet for thousands of years to treat everything from pain and nausea to stress, and even cancer. The resurgence in cannabis-based medicine and CBD is due to its success in hundreds of scientific studies as well as the 2018 Farm Bill, which changed the classification of hemp from a Schedule I substance to a nutritional supplement.

Get ready to learn about how CBD can improve the aging process and help with the following physical health issues:
Arthritis / Cancer / Cardiovascular disease / Diabetes / Endocrine disorders / Fibromyalgia / Gastrointestinal disorders / Headaches and migraines / Pain / Respiratory disorders / Seizures and epilepsy / Skin Conditions

You will also read research results on CBD and its impact on emotional and mental conditions, including the following:
Addiction / Anxiety / Depression / Eating disorders / OCD / PTSD / Schizophrenia / Sleep disorders
Special attention is provided to CBD and how it can help symptoms of the following neurodegenerative diseases:
Alzheimer's / Huntington's / Parkinson's / Multiple sclerosis / ALS

Living Longer and Stronger with CBD also provides the reader with information about end-of-life care and how CBD may be used to better manage difficult symptoms and promote quality of life and death. The book provides practical information on choosing products that are right for you and even your pets. Read about what the future may have in store for CBD in prevention, health and wellness, and medicine. It is a must-read for anyone who uses CBD or wants to learn about its potential to heal the body and mind.

James H. Collins

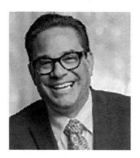

Jim Collins, PhD, is a gerontologist and nationally recognized expert on aging and wellness. He has spent thirty years as an educator, speaker, and author. His first book, *The Person-Centered Way: Revolutionizing Quality of Life in Long-Term Care*, was the first to be published in the United States on this topic. He presents to thousands of health care professionals around the country, both in person and online, from two of his company websites, Collins Learning and CEU Academy. Jim has also provided education to countless older adults and seniors on various topics, including aging successfully, finding the proper diet and nutrition, maximizing physical and emotional health, and improving quality of life. He became interested in the health benefits of CBD several years ago and researched hundreds of scientific studies regarding CBD's impact on physical, emotional, mental, and neurological conditions. So, inspired, Jim founded Sapphire Essentials, which provides high-quality, organically grown THC-free CBD for older adults, seniors, and health care professionals. He lives in Ohio with his wife, Anabel, and daughter, Karina, and their two dogs, Buddy and Kitty. His other interests include music, guitar playing, travel, food, and wine. Jim is also a wine sommelier and is certified in cannabis training.

Made in the USA
Columbia, SC
27 July 2022